Contents

Foreword

A foreword to a book, which is generally written by someone other than the author, is a relatively new practice. Books often begin with a preface written by the authors themselves to explain their purpose in writing the book. The foreword gives an opportunity for someone else to comment on how well the authors have met their objectives. I am very pleased to have been asked to do this for this new edition of *Lecture Notes: Cardiology* (the 5th Edition).

Unusually the book has been written by a whole NHS Cardiology Department, the Wessex Regional Cardiothoracic Unit in Southampton. Drs Gray, Dawkins, Morgan and Simpson are the prime movers. The book is well written, beautifully illustrated and well designed in terms of content and layout. The book is comfortable on the eye and very easy to read.

The book is intended to educate those who are interested in cardiology and it is clear that it has been written with the readers in mind. There is a well balanced combination of fluent text, boxed lists, diagrams, colour photographs and catalogues of further reading for those who would like to take their education further.

The book is comprehensive in its coverage of not only traditional cardiology but also cardiovascular medicine in general. This new edition brings the book fully up-to date in every aspect of diagnosis and treatment. The authors keep the reader in close touch with new developments in cardiology and frequently refer the reader to the recently issued guidelines from national (UK National Institute for Clinical Excellence - NICE) and international sources (the European Society of Cardiology, the American Heart Association, and the American College of Cardiology). *Lecture Notes: Cardiology* manages to stay close to the basics whilst not neglecting important details and new developments.

The book is suitable for any student of modern cardiology/cardiovascular medicine, whether nurse, physiologist or physician. It is ideal for young doctors preparing for the membership, nurses embarking on specialist careers and for general physicians or general practitioners who would like to read about this fast moving subject.

No individual could take such good 'notes' from 'lectures' and this book of pre-written lecture notes will rarely be matched by such fine lecturers in cardiology.

John Camm,
Professor of Clinical Cardiology,
Head of the Divisional Cardiac and
Vascular Sciences,
St. George's University of London

Lecture Notes
Cardiology

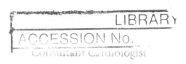

Keith D. Dawkins
BSc MD FRCP FACC FSCAI
Consultant Cardiologist

John M. Morgan
MA MD FRCP FESC
Consultant Cardiologist & Electrophysiologist

Iain A. Simpson
MD FRCP FACC
Consultant Cardiologist

All of
Wessex Regional Cardiothoracic Unit
Southampton University Hospital
Southampton, UK

Fifth Edition

With a foreword by
A. John Camm

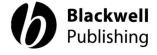

Blackwell
Publishing

Blackwell Publishing, Inc., 350 Main Street, Malden, Massachusetts 02148-5020, USA
Blackwell Publishing Ltd, 9600 Garsington Road, Oxford OX4 2DQ, UK
Blackwell Publishing Asia Pty Ltd, 550 Swanston Street, Carlton, Victoria 3053, Australia

First published 1967
Second edition 1974
Third edition 1991
Fourth edition 2002
Fifth edition 2008

1   2008

Library of Congress Cataloging-in-Publication Data
Lecture notes. Cardiology / Huon H. Gray . . . [et al.]. — 5th ed.
    p. ; cm.
  Rev. ed. of: Lecture notes on cardiology / Huon H. Gray . . . [et al.]. 4th ed. 2002.
  Includes bibliographical references and index.
  ISBN 978-1-4051-5708-7 (alk. paper)
1. Heart–Diseases. I. Gray, Huon H. II. Lecture notes on cardiology.
  [DNLM: 1. Heart Diseases. 2. Heart. 3. Cardiology–methods. WG 200 L4707 2007]

RC681.F54 2007
616.1'2–dc22
                              2007020964

ISBN: 978-1-4051-5708-7

A catalogue record for this title is available from the British Library

Set in 8/12pt Stone Serif by SNP Best-set Typesetter Ltd., Hong Kong
Printed and bound in Singapore by Utopia Press Pte Ltd

Commissioning Editor: Vicki Noyes
Development Editors: Hayley Salter and Laura Murphy
Production Controller: Debbie Wyer

For further information on Blackwell Publishing, visit our website:
http://www.blackwellpublishing.com

Acknowledgements

The authors are grateful to Boston Scientific Corporation for their generous educational grant towards production of the illustrations, to Dr Patrick Gallagher (Reader in Pathology, Southampton) who kindly supplied photographs of pathological specimens, and to the following consultant colleagues within the Wessex Cardiothoracic Unit for their valuable contributions to this edition:

Dr Alison L. Calver MA MD FRCP
Consultant Cardiologist

Dr Peter J. Cowburn MD FRCP
Consultant Cardiologist

Dr Nick Curzen PHD FRCP FESC
Consultant Cardiologist

Dr Charles D. Deakin MA MD FRCP FRCA
Consultant Cardiac Anaesthetist

Dr Tom Pierce MRCP FRCA
Consultant Cardiac Anaesthetist

Dr Paul R. Roberts MD FRCP
Consultant Cardiologist & Electrophysiologist

Dr Anthony P Salmon FRCP FRCPCH
Consultant Paediatric Cardiologist

Abbreviations

AAT aspartate aminotransferase
ACE angiotensin-converting enzyme
ACS acute coronary syndrome
ACT activated clotting time
ACTH adrenocorticotrophic hormone
ADH antidiuretic hormone
ADP adenosine diphosphate
AF atrial fibrillation
AHF acute heart failure
AICD 'automatic' implantable cardiovertor defibrillator
ALS advanced life support
AME authorized medical examiner
ANP atrial natriuretic peptide
APSAC anisoylated plasminogen–streptokinase activator complex
aPTR activated partial thromboplastin time ratio
aPTT activated partial thromboplastin time
AR aortic regurgitation
ARB angiotensin receptor blocker
AS aortic stenosis
ASD atrial septal defect
ASO antistreptolysin-O
ATP adenosine triphosphate
AV atrioventricular
AVN atrioventricular node
AVRT atrioventricular re-entry tachycardia
BHS British Hypertension Society
BLS basic life support
BMI body mass index
BNP brain natriuretic peptide
BP blood pressure
CAA Civil Aviation Authority
CABG coronary artery bypass graft
CAC coronary artery calcification
CAD coronary artery disease
cAMP cyclic adenosine monophosphate
CBP cardiopulmonary bypass
CCS Canadian Cardiovascular Society
CCU Coronary Care Unit

CCMAT counterclockwise macro re-entrant atrial tachycardia
CHB complete heart block
CHD coronary heart disease
CHF chronic heart failure
CNS central nervous system
COPD chronic obstructive pulmonary disease
CPAP continuous positive airway pressure
CPB cardiopulmonary bypass
CPK creatine phosphokinase
CPR cardiopulmonary resuscitation
CRP C-reactive protein
CRT cardiac resynchronization therapy
CT computed tomography
CTR cardiothoracic ratio
Cx circumflex
DA descending aorta
DC direct current
DIC disseminated intravascular coagulation
DNAR do not attempt resuscitation
DVLA Driver and Vehicle Licensing Agency
DVT deep venous thrombosis
EBCT electron beam computed tomography
ECG electrocardiogram
EDRF endothelium-derived relaxing factor
EMF endomyocardial fibrosis
ESR erythrocyte sedimentation rate
ET-1 endothelin-1
FDP fibrin degradation product
GFR glomerular filtration rate
GIK glurose-insulin-potassium
GP glycoprotein
HACEK *Haemophilus, Actinobacillus, Cardiobacterium, Eikenella, Kingella* spp.
HCM hypertrophic cardiomyopathy
HDL high-density lipoprotein
HIT heparin-induced thrombocytopaenia
HIV human immunodeficiency virus
HOCM hypertrophic obstructive cardiomyopathy
HRA high right artium

HRT hormone replacement therapy

5-HT 5-hydroxytryptamine

ICD implantable cardioverter defibrillator

IDC idiopathic dilated cardiomyopathy

INR international normalized ratio

IO interosseal

IP ischaemic pre-conditioning

IPHT idiopathic pulmonary hypertension

IPPV intermittent positive pressure ventilation

iRBBB incomplete right bundle branch block

ISA intrinsic sympathomimetic activity

ISDN isosorbide dinitrate

IVC inferior vena cava

IVS interventricular septum

JVP jugular venous pressure

LA left atrium

LAA left atrial appendage

LAD left anterior descending

LBBB left bundle branch block

LDH lactate dehydrogenase

LDL low-density lipoprotein

LMA laryngeal mask airway

LMWH low molecular weight heparin

LV left ventricle

LVAD left ventricular assist device

LVEDP left ventricular end-diastolic pressure

LVEF left ventricular ejection fraction

LVH left ventricular hypertrophy

LVOTO left ventricular outflow tract obstruction

MI myocardial infarction

MIBI methoxy-isobutyl isonitrile

MIC minimum inhibitory concentration

MPA main pulmonary antery

MRI magnetic resonance imaging

MR mitral regurgitation

MS mitral stenosis

MSA membrane stabilizing activity

MVA mitral valve area

MVO$_2$ myocardial oxygen requirement

NICE National Institute for Health and Clinical Excellence

NIDDM non-insulin-dependent diabetes mellitus

NIH National Institutes of Health

NSAIDs non-steroidal anti-inflammatory drugs

NSTEMI non-ST segment elevation myocardial infarction

NYHA New York Heart Association

OCP oral contraceptive pill

OS opening snap

PA posterior-anterior

PA pulmonary-artery

PAF platelet-activating factor

PCI percutaneous coronary intervention

PDA patent ductus arteriosus

PAP pulmonary artery pressure

PAPVD partial anomalons pulmonary venous drainage

PE pulmonary embolism

PEA pulseless electrical activity

PET positron emission tomography

PFO patent foramen ovale

PHT pulmonary hypertension

PND paroxysmal nocturnal dyspnoea

PPCI primary percutaneous coronary intervention

PR pulmonary regurgitation

PS pulmonary stenosis

PTCA percutaneous transluminal coronary angioplasty

PV pulmonary valve

PVR pulmonary vascular resistance

RA right atrium

RAAS renin-angiotensin-aldosterone system

RBBB right bundle branch block

RCA right coronary artery

rt-PA recombinant tissue-type plasminogen activator

ROSC return of spontaneous circulation

RV right ventricle

RVA right ventricular apex

RVG radionuclide ventriculography

RVOT right ventricular outflow tract

SA sinoatrial

SBP systolic blood pressure

SCD sudden cardiac death

SLE systemic lupus erythematosus

SN sinus node

SNP sodium nitroprusside

SPECT single photon emission computed tomography

SSEP somatosensory evoked potentials

STEMI ST segment elevation myocardial infarction

SVC superior vena cava

SVR surgical ventricular restoration

SVR systemic vascular resistance

SVT supraventricular tachycardIa

TAPVD total amomalous pulmonary venous
  drainage

TEG thromboelastogram

TIA transient ischaemic attack

t-PA tissue plasminogen activator

TOE transoesophageal echocardiography

TR tricuspid regurgitation

TS tricuspid stenosis

TTE transthoracic echocardiography

TV tricuspid valve

UA unstable angina

UA umbilical artery

UFH unfractionated heparin

VA ventriculoatrial

VF ventricular fibrillation

VSD ventricular septal defect

VT ventricular tachycardia

Chapter 1

Taking a cardiovascular history

Introduction

In an era when imaging and other diagnostic techniques have become more numerous and sophisticated, there is a tendency for the clinical assessment of the patient to seem less relevant. This is wrong, for the importance of the clinical examination cannot be overemphasized. However much information is gathered by other means, decisions about the correct management of patients still rely fundamentally on a good overall clinical assessment. It is bad practice to put patients through more than the minimum number of investigations needed to make a diagnosis and allow patient management to be planned, some of which may be uncomfortable and have associated risks. The good clinician selects investigations carefully and sparingly, always balancing the potential value of any information that may be obtained against the risks, cost and discomfort to the patient.

Establishing a good rapport and obtaining the confidence of a patient start at the time of the clinical assessment and are extremely important later, when sometimes distressing information has to be discussed and difficult decisions made about potential treatment. The clinical assessment will often involve obtaining information from relatives or friends of the patient, who may be able to judge more objectively than the patient the extent of their limitations in daily activities.

The clinical assessment consists of obtaining a history to elicit symptoms, and performing a physical examination to observe signs, of cardiovascular disease. In this chapter, broad principles will be covered, but symptoms and signs relating to specific conditions will be detailed in the chapters relating to those conditions.

The art of good history taking involves allowing the patient to tell their story whilst, at the same time, through the questions asked, directing their attention to those aspects of their clinical presentation which are most likely to provide information that is relevant to making a diagnosis and determining treatment. Often a patient will unwittingly give vitally important clinical information almost as an aside remark, information that may never have come to light if the history taking consisted merely of asking numerous predetermined questions or, worse, providing a questionnaire for the patient to complete. Taking time to obtain a clear history, in patients' own words and in their own time, is an important part of clinical training. As the clinician's expertise increases, this process can be achieved in relatively short periods of time. With experience, helpful information can also be gleaned from other sources, such as the patient's attitude, demeanour, emotional state and dress.

Specific symptoms (see Boxes 1.1 and 1.2)

Because cardiac work is so closely related to exercise, many cardiac symptoms are worse during exertion, the effect of which should be enquired about specifically.

Box 1.1 Symptoms of cardiovascular disease

The features most relevant when taking a history are:
- Dyspnoea, cough and haemoptysis
- Chest pain
- Syncope
- Palpitation
- Ankle swelling
- Fatigue
- Cyanosis
- Claudication

Box 1.2 Symptom details

The following information should be obtained about each symptom where relevant:
- Nature and severity
- Chronology
- Onset and duration
- Precipitating, aggravating and alleviating factors
- Associated symptoms
- Site and radiation of any pain

Box 1.3 Causes of dyspnoea

Cardiac causes
Acute
- Myocardial ischaemia or infarction
- Mitral regurgitation due to chordal rupture
- Onset of AF in mitral or aortic valve disease

Chronic
- Left ventricular dysfunction
- Mitral or aortic valve disease
- Atrial myxoma

Non-cardiac
Acute
- Pulmonary embolism
- Pneumothorax
- Asthma
- Hyperventilation syndrome

Chronic
- Obstructive or restrictive lung disease
- Pulmonary hypertension
- Chest wall abnormalities
- Anaemia
- Obesity and lack of fitness

Dyspnoea

Defined as an abnormal and uncomfortable awareness of breathing, dyspnoea is a common symptom of both cardiac and respiratory disease and is most commonly observed on exertion. This is unlike the breathlessness associated with anxiety where a heightened awareness of respiration progresses to hyperventilation, and where the sensation of dyspnoea is often worse at rest or in stressful situations. Hyperventilation also causes other symptoms (many of which are due to the fall in arterial PCO_2 and alkalosis), such as peri-oral and peripheral parasthesiae, clouding of consciousness, stabbing left infra-mammary chest pain and, in extreme cases, tetany. As the underlying cardiac condition progresses, the sensation of dyspnoea becomes present at ever lower levels of exertion, and ultimately occurs at rest (see Box 1.3 for causes of dyspnoea).

Dyspnoea due to cardiac disease arises due to pulmonary venous congestion. Left atrial pressure, and hence pulmonary venous pressure, is normally around 5 mmHg. When it rises, as will occur with mitral and aortic valve disease or left ventricular dysfunction, the pulmonary veins become distended and the bronchial walls congested and oedematous, causing an irritating non-productive cough and wheeze. As pulmonary venous pressure rises further and the plasma oncotic pressure (around 25 mmHg) is exceeded, so the lung tissue becomes stiffer due to interstitial oedema (increasing the muscular work required to inflate the lungs and the sensation of dyspnoea), a transudate collects in the alveoli, and **pulmonary oedema** results. As this worsens, frothy sputum is expectorated, which may be pink due to ruptured small bronchial vessels bleeding into the oedema fluid.

Cardiac dyspnoea is worse when lying flat (**orthopnoea**), may wake the patient from sleep in the early hours of the morning associated with sweating and anxiety (**paroxysmal nocturnal dyspnoea**) and tends to be relieved by sitting upright or standing. Systemic venous return to the right heart is increased in the recumbent position, especially in the early hours of the morning when blood volume is usually at its greatest, resulting in increased pulmonary blood flow and further increase in pulmonary venous pressure. However, if right ventricular contraction is severely impaired, as may occur with the dilated cardiomyopathies or right ventricular infarction, orthopnoea may be lessened because the right heart is unable to increase pulmonary blood flow in response to the increase in venous return.

Although cardiac dyspnoea may occur acutely, for example due to left ventricular failure following acute myocardial infarction, it is more commonly of gradual onset and of a more chronic nature, slowly deteriorating over weeks or months. The sudden onset of dyspnoea should always make one consider alternative causes such as pneumothorax or pulmonary embolism (see Box 1.4 and Box 9.6 for the **New York Heart Association (NYHA) classification**: the most commonly used classification to indicate the degree of disability from dyspnoea due to cardiac disease).

Chest pain

Chest pain or choking discomfort due to myocardial ischaemia (**angina**) typically has certain characteristics: a tight, constricting, band-like, or sometimes burning, retrosternal discomfort, occurring principally on exertion and relieved within minutes by rest or sublingual nitrates. Patients usually describe this as an uncomfortable rather than a truly painful sensation. The discomfort may radiate to either arm (most commonly the left), to the neck and jaw, or through to the back or abdomen.

An attack is normally short lived, lasting up to 20 min. Angina is sometimes atypical, causing neck, throat, jaw, back or abdominal discomfort without chest symptoms.

Angina is due to an imbalance between myocardial oxygen supply (coronary blood flow) and demand (myocardial oxygen consumption). The most common cause of angina is therefore coronary artery disease, but it may occur even with normal coronary arteries in conditions of severe left ventricular hypertrophy or dilatation where myocardial O_2 demand is high (see Chapter 9). Angina that occurs at rest or is rapidly worsening is termed 'unstable angina', and usually indicates critical coronary disease. Anginal pain lasting more than 30 min, and especially if associated with sweating, nausea and vomiting, should make one suspicious of myocardial infarction. Stabbing pain or episodes of pain lasting only seconds suggests a musculoskeletal cause.

Patients may describe exertional breathlessness rather than chest pain but, when pressed to be more precise, it is often the sensation of heaviness of the mid-chest (angina) that gives rise to a feeling of difficulty in expanding the chest. Breathlessness may, however, be due to the associated left ventricular dysfunction that occurs with myocardial ischaemia. Other symptoms that may be associated with myocardial ischaemia include belching, indigestion, nausea and dizziness, although their association with exertion is usually a consistent feature. Symptoms occurring above the mandible and below the umbilicus are very unlikely to be due to myocardial ischaemia. See Box 1.5 for the

---

Box 1.4 New York Heart Association (NYHA) classification of heart failure

Describes the degree of disability from dyspnoea due to cardiac disease:
- Class I: no limitation in physical activity
- Class II: slight limitation of exercise (fatigue, dyspnoea)
- Class III: marked limitation of activity (comfortable at rest but slight exertion causes symptoms)
- Class IV: symptoms even at rest

Box 1.5 Canadian Cardiovascular Society (CCS) classification

Describes the degree of disability caused by angina:
- Class 1 — Angina only on strenuous or prolonged exertion
- Class 2 — Slight limitation due to angina with normal activities
- Class 3 — Marked limitation due to angina with ordinary activity
- Class 4 — Unable to undertake any physical activity. Angina at rest

Canadian Cardiovascular Society (CCS) classification: the most commonly used classification to describe the degree of disability caused by angina.

Almost any structure in the chest may also cause chest pain, but some of the more common are given in Box 1.6. Usually a careful history will allow these causes to be differentiated. Perhaps the most common differentiation lies between cardiac pain and oesophageal spasm or reflux. The character of the pain caused by oesophageal spasm may be indistinguishable from angina and may be relieved by vasodilators, such as the nitrates. Oesophageal causes of pain often last longer than anginal episodes, are rarely related to exertion, and oesophageal reflux tends to be worse on bending or lying down. Functional or psychogenic chest pain (**Da Costa syndrome**) may occur in patients with a fear of heart disease, for instance due to a family history of myocardial infarction. It manifests as a dull, persistent ache in the area of the cardiac apex lasting hours or days, and is often interspersed with more intense stabbing episodes. This pain may be associated with hyperventilation, palpitation and panic attacks. Chest pain is also well described in patients with mitral valve prolapse, although the reason for this is not known.

Syncope

Loss of consciousness may be caused by a number of cardiovascular causes, but their final common pathway is a reduction in cerebral blood flow. A careful history will often suggest the underlying cause, but there are a number of patients who have transient dizzy or syncopal episodes that defy cardiological and neurological diagnosis. See Box 1.7 for cardiovascular causes of syncope and

---

Box 1.6 Non-myocardial causes of chest pain

Acute
- **Oesophageal spasm**: very similar to angina but more prolonged and unrelated to exertion
- **Thoracic aortic dissection**: usually felt interscapularly
- **Pneumonia**: usually pleuritic but may be more diffuse ache
- **Pneumothorax**: localized, intense, pleuritic
- **Pulmonary embolus**: either pleuritic and localized or dull central discomfort
- **Pericarditis**: varies with position and respiration

Chronic
- **Costochondritis (Tietze syndrome)**: localized, tender area of chest wall
- **Peptic ulceration**
- **Gall bladder disease**: usually abdominal symptoms also present
- **Pancreatic disease**
- **Cervical or thoracic spine disease**: related to movement

---

Box 1.7 Cardiovascular causes of syncope and presyncope

- **Aortic stenosis (AS)**: usually exertional, or at rest with the onset of AF (atrial fibrillation) or heart block
- **Left ventricular outflow tract obstruction (LVOTO)**: as occurs with hypertrophic obstructive cardiomyopathy (HOCM). Syncope may be due to associated arrhythmias as well as LVOTO
- **Tachyarrhythmias**: may be associated with awareness of palpitation
- **Heart block**: patient may be aware of bradycardia or pauses
- **Hypotensive drugs**: symptoms often postural
- **Vasovagal syndrome**: often occurs in painful situations, after standing up or prolonged standing, with emotional stress. Attacks often occur over many years
- **Carotid sinus syndrome**: sensitivity of carotid sinus to neck movement or palpation results in vagal stimulation, causing bradycardia and hypotension
- **Myocardial ischaemia**: rarely causes syncope in the absence of other cardiac disease (e.g. aortic stenosis) except if left main stem coronary artery is stenosed
- **Severe pulmonary hypertension**: usually exertional. Mechanism comparable with hypertension or AS. Fixed obstruction to circulatory blood flow
- **Acute pulmonary embolism**: only when massive embolism produces circulatory obstruction
- **Subclavian steal syndrome**: due to severe subclavian artery stenosis or occlusion causing 'steal' of blood by retrograde flow down the vertebral artery. Occurs with ipsilateral arm movement
- **Cerebrovascular disease**: often causes dizzy spells (transient ischaemic episodes), and mainly in the elderly
- **Atrial myxoma**: rare. Symptoms may be posturally related. Produces intermittent mitral valve obstruction

---

presyncope. Cardiac syncope is usually of rapid onset, without an aura, and is usually not associated with convulsions or incontinence. Recovery is typically rapid (unlike the slower recovery of neurological causes which may cause postsyncopal confusion), and may be associated with profound vasodilatation as blood supply is restored to arterioles that have become vasodilated by the accumulation of local metabolites. A gradual reduction of consciousness is more suggestive of vasodepressor syncope or postural hypotension.

Palpitation (see also Chapter 13)

This is a common symptom and is defined as an unpleasant awareness of the heart beating. At the outset it is important to determine exactly what sensation the patient is describing. It may be an awareness of the heart beating more forcefully than usual, more rapidly, more slowly, erratically, or a combination of these.
- An awareness of a forceful beat may suggest an increased stroke volume (e.g. aortic or mitral regurgitation) or may just represent an individual's heightened awareness of their heart.
- Rapid palpitation suggests a tachycardia.
- An erratic palpitation may be fast, as in atrial fibrillation, or slower, as in an awareness of ectopic beats.
- With ectopics the patient may be aware of the prematurely occurring 'extra beat' (ectopic), the compensatory pause after the ectopic which may give the sensation of a 'missed beat', or of the post-ectopic beat which is accentuated and felt as a 'more forceful' beat because, occurring later, it has a larger stroke volume than the preceding sinus or ectopic beats.

Palpitation associated with a slow rate may be due to atrioventricular block or sinus node disease. Rapid palpitations usually start and stop suddenly, and imply an atrial, atrioventricular nodal or ventricular tachycardia. A gradual termination of the palpitation is more in keeping with a sinus tachycardia.

Oedema

An elevation in right heart pressure increases systemic venous pressure in the inferior and superior venae cavae, and this will be greatest in the most dependent parts of the body, most usually the feet and ankles, but will be the sacral region in those confined to bed. Oedema occurs when plasma oncotic pressure is exceeded by the raised intravascular pressure, a situation which is exacerbated in hypoalbuminaemic states.
- Elevation of right heart pressure may be secondary to left heart disease (left ventricular failure, mitral or aortic valve disease) or may be due to right heart failure as a consequence of pulmonary hypertension, right ventricular or constrictive pericardial disease.
- Oedema due to superior vena cava obstruction (usually caused by malignancy) is obviously confined to the head, neck and arms.
- A history of periorbital oedema is characteristic of renal disease (nephrotic and nephritic syndromes).
- Unilateral oedema of a limb implies local vascular or lymphatic obstruction, as occurs following deep venous thrombosis or chronic venous insufficiency due to varicose veins.
- Other causes of oedema include the cyclical oedema that may occur perimenstrually and angioneurotic oedema that occurs as an allergic reaction to various stimuli, including seafood.

Fatigue

This is a non-specific but common symptom in cardiac disease. It may arise due to a low cardiac output or an inability to raise cardiac output sufficiently on exercise. Drug therapy may cause fatigue, either directly as in the case of β-blockers, or indirectly such as that due to hypokalaemia caused by diuretic therapy.

Cyanosis

As well as being a sign which should be sought on examination, patients may complain of a bluish discoloration of the skin and mucous membranes, and thus cyanosis may also be a presenting symptom. The blue discoloration arises as a result of the presence of increased amounts of deoxygenated haemoglobin in the blood perfusing the tissues. Cyanosis can be divided into 'peripheral' and 'central', terms which indicate the cause of the cyanosis rather than where it is observed.

• **Peripheral cyanosis** is usually due to cutaneous vasoconstriction, because of either exposure to cold or Raynaud's phenomenon. Cyanosis is most readily seen when cardiac output is reduced for any reason. Whereas cyanosis of central origin usually worsens on exercise, peripheral cyanosis is usually unchanged if cardiac output is poor, or may improve with reflex vasodilatation if the principal abnormality is vasoconstriction.

• **Central cyanosis** is characterized by decreased arterial oxygen saturation, due to central venous–arterial admixture of blood in conditions causing right-to-left shunting, or due to pulmonary disease causing impaired arterial oxygen uptake. Right-to-left shunting may be intra-cardiac in origin (**cyanotic congenital heart disease involving absence of or defects in ventricular or atrial septa**) or may be extra-cardiac (**pulmonary arteriovenous malformations**). Central cyanosis is best observed by examining the oral mucous membranes and is clinically apparent when >40 g/L of deoxygenated (reduced) haemoglobin is present. Cyanosis of central origin is usually not improved by giving higher concentrations of inspired O_2, whereas peripheral cyanosis may be. In darker skinned individuals, cyanosis may not be observed until greater levels of reduced haemoglobin are present. More rarely cyanosis may be due to the presence of abnormal haemoglobin pigments, such as methaemoglobin. When there is a central cause for the cyanosis, peripheral cyanosis must also be present, whereas cyanosis due to a peripheral cause will not result in cyanosis of the mucous membranes.

Claudication

This aching discomfort in the legs, usually the calves, occurs after varying amounts of exercise, and is due to skeletal muscle ischaemia as a consequence of peripheral vascular disease. Since this is almost always atheromatous, the presence of claudication should alert one to the probability that the patient also has underlying coronary artery disease.

Additional history

A full medical history should be obtained from the patient. Box 1.8 details what this should include.

Box 1.8 Patient history

A full medical history for the patient should include:
• **Systems review**: for urinary, menstrual and gastrointestinal symptoms
• **Drug history**: specific cardiovascular drugs, contraceptive pill, other medication (e.g. treatment for indigestion)
• **Past medical history**: for tuberculosis, rheumatic fever, diabetes mellitus, hypertension, stroke, venereal or tropical diseases, thyroid disease, asthma, previous operations
• **Social history**: exercise, occupation, smoking, alcohol consumption, family/partner
• **Family history**: for any cardiovascular or other possibly genetically linked disease

---

Chapter 2

Examination of the cardiovascular system

Introduction

The examination of a patient should be thorough but, when applied in routine and busy clinical practice, must also be undertaken quickly. The goal of the examination is to obtain clinical information that advances diagnosis and is not merely an exercise in repeating a set series of tasks. The examiner should have a clear understanding of why a particular part of the examination may be relevant to that patient and how to interpret the physical signs when present. There are various ways by which the cardiovascular system can be examined, the pattern of which is less important than consistency and thoroughness. Table 2.1 gives details of a suggested approach to eliciting cardiovascular signs and the observations that should be made.

General approach
(see Tables 2.1 and 2.2)

On approaching the patient, the examiner should make an appropriate introduction and attempt to put the patient at ease. The patient should be asked to lie semi-recumbent (30–40°) and the examiner should ensure that it is possible to examine the patient's chest, abdomen and legs without the interference of clothing, whilst maintaining the patient's dignity using bedclothes and removable garments. The examiner should already be making general observations about things such as the patient's demeanour, any obvious confusion and degree of co-operation. Once the patient is comfortably positioned, specific observations should be made such as the pattern of respiration, the presence of any distress and the patient's general appearance and body habitus. For example, it may be obvious that the patient has features of **Marfan syndrome** (tall with arm-span greater than height, arachnodactyly, and skeletal deformities such as pectus carinatum and kyphoscoliosis), or may look thyrotoxic or dysmorphic (e.g. **Down syndrome**). The patient may be morbidly obese or cachectic, may have malar flushing (**mitral valve disease, systemic lupus erythematosus**) or look generally unwell.

Examination of the head and neck
(see Tables 2.1 and 2.2)

Hands and arms

The patient should be asked to raise their arms, outstretched with palms downwards, and the fingers should be examined for nail clubbing, splinter haemorrhages, Janeway lesions, peripheral cyanosis (see Chapter 1) or xanthomata (**hypercholesterolaemia**) over extensor tendons. Observe any tar staining suggesting past cigarette consumption and therefore the possibility of coronary and peripheral vascular disease. Palpate both radial pulses to confirm their presence, and use one to

Table 2.1 Summary of the examination process.

1 General approach	
Introduce yourself	
Position the patient	
Ensure patient's comfort	
Make general observations — dyspnoea, distress, build, body habitus	
2 Examination of arms, head and neck	
Hands	Clubbing, splinter haemorrhages, cyanosis, tar staining
Arms	Radial and brachial pulses, scars, blood pressure, xanthomata
Face	Malar flush
Eyes	Anaemia, jaundice, corneal arcus, fundoscopy, xanthelasmata
Mouth	Palate, dentition, cyanosis
Neck	Thyroid, carotid pulse, jugular venous pulse
3 Cardiac examination	
Inspect anterior chest wall	General appearance, scars
Palpate precordium	Cardiac impulses, thrills, apex beat
Auscultate	Heart sounds (S1, S2, added sounds)
	Systole (murmurs)
	Diastole (murmurs)
4 Examination of the chest	
Inspect posterior chest wall	General appearance, scars
Palpate	Lung expansion
Percuss	Pleural effusion
Auscultate	Bronchial breathing, crepitations
5 Examination of the abdomen	
Palpate	Liver, spleen, kidneys, aorta
Percuss	Ascites
Auscultate	Bowel sounds, bruits
6 Examination of the legs	
Pulses	Presence, femoro-radial synchrony, bruits
Oedema	
Toes	Splinter haemorrhages, clubbing

assess the heart rate and rhythm (**regularity**). Palpate the elbows for xanthomatous eruptions (**hypercholesterolaemia**), inspect the antecubital fossa for evidence of scars (**previous cardiac catheterization**) and palpate the brachial pulse for its **presence and character**.

Taking the blood pressure is a vital part of the cardiovascular examination, and care should be taken to ensure that the sphygmomanometer cuff is inflated to well above systolic blood pressure before slowly deflating (see Chapter 5). A discrepancy of >10 mmHg between the two arms should raise the possibility of obstruction (**intimal dissection, stenoses**) in the aorta, innominate, subclavian or brachial arteries. If aortic coarctation is suspected, measure the blood pressure in the leg for comparison.

Head

Make general observations (**malar flush, dysmorphic features, cushingoid or acromegalic, exophthalmic**) and then examine the eyes. Observe the skin bordering the medial aspect of the eyes for xanthelasmata (**hypercholesterolaemia**), inspect the conjunctivae (**anaemia, jaundice**) and anterior eyes (**corneal arcus, cataracts, lens dislocation and rarities such as blue sclera, Kayser–Fleischer**

Table 2.2 Non-cardiac physical signs in cardiovascular disease.

Sign	Causes	Comments
Finger clubbing	Infective endocarditis Cyanotic heart disease Suppurative lung disease Bronchial carcinoma Gastrointestinal disease Idiopathic	Usually seen as finger clubbing but may occur in the toes
Splinter haemorrhages (subungual)	Infective endocarditis Local trauma	Less likely to be traumatic if seen near nail bed rather than nail tips
Janeway lesions	Infective endocarditis	Slightly raised, non-tender haemorrhagic lesions on the palms of hands and soles of feet
Peripheral cyanosis	Vasoconstriction Low cardiac output	Vasoconstriction due to cold or Raynaud's phenomenon
Central cyanosis	Venous–arterial admixture of blood	Intracardiac and extracardiac shunts
Malar flush	Mitral stenosis SLE	Mechanism uncertain. SLE can be associated with valve disease and sterile endocarditis
Facial dysmorphism	Down syndrome Turner syndrome Noonan syndrome	Associated with various congenital cardiac abnormalities
Cushingoid fascies	Hyperadrenalism	Hypertension, oedema
Paget's skull or long bones	Paget's disease	High cardiac output heart failure
Myopathic fascies	Myopathies and muscular dystrophies	Various types (dystrophia myotonica, Friedreich's ataxia, Duchenne, Becker, facio-scapulohumeral) associated with cardiomyopathies
Acromegalic fascies	Acromegaly	Associated with cardiomyopathies
Thyrotoxic appearance	Hyperthyroidism	Sinus tachycardia, palpitations, atrial fibrillation, high cardiac output cardiomyopathy if severe
Hypothyroid appearance	Hypothyroidism	Sinus bradycardia, dilated cardiomyopathy Coronary disease due to associated hypercholesterolaemia
Corneal arcus	Hyperlipidaemia Ageing	Significant if present in those <60 years
Cataracts	Age Congenital rubella	Rubella associated with patent ductus, ASD or pulmonary stenosis
Lens dislocation	Marfan syndrome	Associated with aortopathy and mitral valve prolapse
Kayser–Fleischer ring	Wilson disease	Copper overload and rare cause of cardiomyopathy
Argyll Robertson pupil	Syphilis	May have associated aortopathy
Roth spots	Infective endocarditis	Retinal haemorrhages near the discs and with white spots in centre
Angioid streaks and blue sclerae	Pseudoxanthoma elasticum	Pink retinal streaks and/or blue scleral discoloration Associated with aortopathy and/or coronary lesions

ASD, atrial septal defect; SLE, systemic lupus erythematosus.

ring and Argyll Robertson pupils) and then use an ophthalmoscope to examine the fundi (**diabetic or hypertensive retinopathy, Roth spots, angioid streaks**). Examine the mouth for the presence of mucosal cyanosis (**central cyanosis**), state of the dentition (**poor dentition predisposes towards bacterial endocarditis**) and presence of a high-arched palate (**Marfan syndrome**). Facial oedema and engorgement of the neck veins may be present in cases of obstruction to the superior vena cava (SVC).

Neck

Palpate the thyroid and, if a goitre is suspected, auscultate the thyroid for bruits, then examine the carotid pulse and jugular venous waveform.

Carotid pulse (see Figs 2.1 and 2.2)

Using the thumb, palpate the carotid arteries separately on both sides to confirm their presence and also to assess the character of the pulse. The normal waveform consists of an upstroke, a peak and a decline, which is less steep than the upstroke and is interrupted soon after the peak by the incisura (dicrotic notch) which coincides with closure of the aortic valve. Various abnormalities may be detected.

The pulse may be **slow rising** due to aortic stenosis or subaortic obstruction (subaortic membrane or hypertrophic obstructive cardiomyopathy), with a peak which occurs later and is more sustained than usual, and is often associated with a **thrill** (palpable bruit). A notch may occur on the upstroke (**anacrotic notch**) and may be so prominent as to produce two distinct peaks (**anacrotic pulse**). In elderly patients, the carotid artery wall may be so inelastic that the upstroke may be normal even in the presence of significant aortic stenosis.

The pulse may be **low volume** due to a low cardiac output, for whatever reason, or **high volume** (hyperdynamic) due to any high cardiac output state (fever, pregnancy, anaemia, hyperthyroidism).

A **collapsing** (**water hammer or Corrigan's**) **pulse** has a rapid upstroke and then abrupt col-

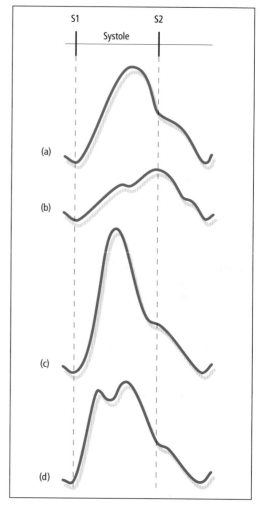

Fig. 2.1 The arterial pulse waves. (a) Normal. (b) Slow rising. (c) Sharp ('water hammer'). (d) Bisferiens. S1, first heart sound; S2, second heart sound.

lapse, and is typically due to aortic regurgitation. When severe, this may be associated with a number of eponymous clinical signs, such as pistol shot femoral pulses (**Traube's sign**), an audible diastolic murmur over the femoral artery when it is compressed (**Duroziez' sign**), and visible pulsation of the nail capillaries (**Quincke's sign**), retinal vessels (**Becker's sign**) and uvula (**Mueller's sign**).

A **bisferiens** pulse has two systolic peaks (percussion and tidal waves) separated by a mid-systolic dip. This occurs in conditions where a large stroke

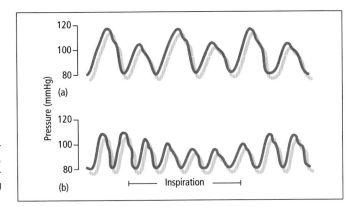

Fig. 2.2 (a) Pulsus alternans — alternate large and small amplitude pulses. (b) Pulsus paradoxus — marked diminution of pulse amplitude during inspiration.

volume is ejected rapidly from the left ventricle (**aortic regurgitation or combined aortic stenosis and regurgitation**), and disappears as heart failure develops. Contrary to general teaching, it is not usually clinically detectable in hypertrophic cardiomyopathy except by using the Valsalva manoeuvre, though it may be seen on intra-arterial pressure recordings, where it is due to early left ventricular ejection being halted as the left ventricular outflow tract obstruction (**septal hypertrophy**) occurs, and is followed by a reflected (**tidal**) wave.

A **dicrotic** pulse occurs when the dicrotic notch is exaggerated, as may occur when a low stroke volume is ejected into an elastic aorta under lower than usual pressure, in conditions such as cardiac tamponade, severe heart failure and hypovolaemic shock. It is rarely seen if the systolic pressure exceeds 120 mmHg. The normal carotid systolic wave is reduced but the dicrotic notch is preserved, giving a double peak to the palpated pulse, one systolic and one early diastolic. This should not be confused with a bisferiens pulse where both peaks are systolic.

Pulsus alternans consists of alternating strong and weak pulse waves on consecutive beats and is a sign of severe left ventricular dysfunction. The alternating intensity can also be heard on sphygmomanometry. It is clinically detectable if systolic pressures differ by >20 mmHg between beats, and is best assessed in held mid-respiration, to avoid the effects of the respiratory cycle on stroke volume.

Pulsus bigeminus is due to an ectopic beat, usually ventricular, occurring after each sinus beat. The ectopic beat is weaker than the preceding sinus beat and occurs prematurely (in contradistinction to pulsus alternans where the weaker beat occurs when the beat would normally be expected). The sinus beat following the ectopic may be stronger than usual due to **post-ectopic accentuation**.

Pulsus paradoxus is an exaggeration of a normal phenomenon. Systolic pressure normally falls slightly on inspiration due to the effects of negative intrathoracic pressure on the aorta and on left ventricular stroke volume, but if this fall is >10 mmHg during quiet respiration then it is considered abnormal, and when >25 mmHg is often detectable even by palpation. It is characteristic of pericardial tamponade, is seen in approximately 50% of patients with pericardial constriction, and may also be seen in conditions with wide swings in intrathoracic pressure (**asthma, emphysema**), or less commonly in hypovolaemic shock, pulmonary embolism, pregnancy and severe obesity. A reverse paradox, a rise in systolic pressure with inspiration, may occur in hypertrophic obstructive cardiomyopathy.

Having palpated the carotids, they should next be **auscultated**. When an artery becomes >50% stenosed, the sound of blood passing through the stenotic segment in systole may be heard (**bruit**). When aortic valve disease is present, it is usually impossible to distinguish between a radiated systolic murmur and intrinsic arterial stenosis, and carotid ultrasound scanning may be required.

Jugular venous pulse

Both internal jugular veins lie deep to the sterno-cleidomastoid muscles. The right internal jugular drains directly into the SVC whereas the left drains first into the innominate vein and thereafter into the SVC, with the SVC draining directly into the right atrium. The jugular venous column of blood therefore allows a clinical assessment of right atrial pressure to be made at the bedside. Careful observation of the jugular venous pulse should be made, but clinically it can often be difficult to see visually what is classically described below, and students should not be disheartened if the more subtle observations remain obscure. However, understanding the jugular venous pressure (JVP) and waveform assists greatly in an understanding of cardiac physiology.

JVP

The normal JVP is <4 cm H_2O above the manubri-osternal joint (sternal angle) when the patient is lying semi-recumbent (30–40°), and so the upper end of the column of systemic venous blood will either be below or only just be visible above the level of the sternal notch. The top of the venous column may be seen more easily if the patient reclines closer to the horizontal, and some recommend using hepatojugular reflux. This is a potentially uncomfortable manoeuvre whereby firm pressure is exerted by the examiner's hand in the patient's right hypochondrium for 10–30 s. This manoeuvre will tend to raise the JVP transiently by up to 3 cm H_2O, sometimes making it visible when at normal or low pressure. More simply, confirmation that the JVP is low may be undertaken by exerting moderate pressure on the base of the patient's neck using the ulnar edge of the examiner's hand. By doing this, venous drainage from the jugular vein is obstructed and the vein above the level of compression will be seen to fill from above and become engorged. By releasing compression, the examiner should be able to see clearly that the venous column disappears rapidly by normal drainage into the SVC, thus confirming a normal pressure.

The JVP is elevated in conditions causing a rise in right atrial pressure (**right heart failure, reduced right ventricular diastolic compliance, pericardial disease, hypervolaemia, pulmonary hypertension**), or if the SVC is compressed (**usually due to mediastinal tumour involvement**). When the JVP is very high it may be difficult to see the top of the column of venous blood but this may be easier if the patient is asked to sit vertically. Pulsation may be seen near the angle of the jaw, or the ear lobes may be seen to pulsate. When the patient is obese, or in those with short, thick necks, it may be difficult to see the engorged jugular vein even when it is dilated. The JVP normally falls with inspiration as a result of an increase in negative intra-thoracic pressure, augmenting venous return. Paradoxically, an abnormal rise in JVP on inspiration (**Kussmaul's sign**) occurs when the right heart cannot accommodate the additional venous return. Classically, this occurs n pericardial constriction, but may also occur in pericardial tamponade.

Jugular venous waveform (Fig. 2.3)

In normal sinus rhythm the waveform consists of two main parts, the 'a' and 'v' waves.

The '**a' wave** coincides with right atrial contraction and consists of a rise to a peak followed by a decline ('**x' descent**), occurring just before the first heart sound (S1) (**closure of the tricuspid and mitral valves**). A small '**c' wave** occurs on the 'x' descent and coincides with carotid pulsation, but is of little importance and is usually undetectable at the bedside. The SVC opens directly into the right atrium without any intervening valve, and so contraction of the right atrium causes a transient increase in SVC and jugular venous pressure.

The 'a' wave is prominent when there is resistance to right atrial emptying (right ventricular hypertrophy, right ventricular restriction, pulmonary hypertension, tricuspid stenosis (TS)).

It is described as a '**cannon wave**' when the right atrium contracts against a closed tricuspid valve, as occurs intermittently in atrioventricular dissociation (complete heart block).

The 'a' wave is absent in atrial fibrillation since co-ordinated atrial contraction does not occur.

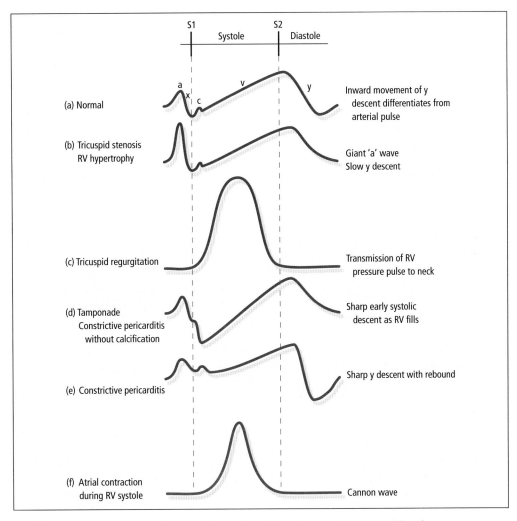

Fig. 2.3 Jugular venous pulse waveforms in relation to S1 and S2, and ventricular systole and diastole.

The 'x' descent occurs as a result of the right atrium relaxing (atrial diastole) at the end of its contraction together with the effects of right ventricular contraction (RV systole), which tends to pull the right atrioventricular ring and closed tricuspid valve downwards. The 'x' descent will therefore be rapid in conditions where the 'a' wave is increased in association with an enlarged right ventricle due to volume overload, as typically occurs with an atrial septal defect and significant left-to-right shunting.

The **'v' wave** upstroke coincides with the later half of atrial diastole, as the right atrium becomes more distended with venous blood. It is followed by the **'y' descent**, which coincides with opening of the tricuspid valve and consequent passive emptying of the right atrium into the right ventricle at the start of atrial systole. It occurs after the second heart sound (S2). Later in diastole, atrial contraction occurs again ('a' wave) and the cycle is repeated.

In mild to moderate tricuspid incompetence, blood regurgitates into the right atrium in ventricular systole (atrial diastole) and results in accentuation of the 'v' wave. In severe tricuspid incompetence, this accentuation occurs early in atrial diastole causing the normally invisible 'c' wave to become prominent, the 'x' descent to be abolished and resulting in the so-called giant 'cv' wave.

The 'y' descent is typically rapid in pericardial constriction but also occurs in tricuspid regurgitation and any condition associated with right ventricular dilatation and dysfunction. The descent is typically slow in tricuspid stenosis.

The jugular venous pulse can usually be differentiated from carotid pulsation because of its double waveform (if in sinus rhythm), the ability of the examiner to abolish venous pulsation with light-to-moderate external compression and the fact that venous pressure alters visibly with phases of the respiratory cycle and position of the patient.

Cardiac examination

Inspection (see Table 2.3)

Assess the respiratory rate and observe any thoracic deformities, such as pectus excavatum (**depressed sternum**), which may displace the cardiac apex to the left and give the false impression of cardiomegaly, or cause 'innocent' ejection flow murmurs due to mild compression of the right ventricular outflow tract. Pectus carinatum (**prominent sternum**) and kyphoscoliosis may be associated with Marfan syndrome. The presence of a median sternotomy scar suggests previous surgery on the heart (**valvular or coronary bypass grafting**) or ascending aorta (**aneurysms, aortic dissection**). Large ventricular or aortic **aneurysms** may produce visible pulsations, and either superior or inferior **vena cava obstruction** may produce prominent venous collateral channels of the chest wall.

Palpation (see Table 2.3)

The widespread use of chest radiographs and more specialized cardiac investigations has meant that percussion of the precordium is now rarely undertaken. Firstly, determine the **position** of the apex beat using the tips of the fingers, and then palpate it using the palm of the hand to assess its **character**. The apex beat usually consists of the left

Table 2.3 Findings on precordial inspection and auscultation.

Action	Observation	Association
Inspection	Kyphoscoliosis or pectus carinatum	Marfan syndrome
	Ankylosing spondylitis (kyphosis)	Aortic regurgitation
	Wide-spaced nipples	Turner syndrome
		Noonan syndrome
	Median sternotomy scar	Approach for most modern cardiac operations
	Lateral thoracotomy scar	Old mitral valvotomy or present approach for coarctation, patent ductus or descending thoracic aortic aneurysm surgery
	Respiratory rate	Normal 16–20 per min at rest
Palpation	Apex beat displaced	Left ventricular dilatation or aneurysm
	Apical heave (lift)	Left ventricular hypertrophy or dilatation
	Tapping apex	Mitral stenosis
	Double apical impulse	Hypertrophic obstructive cardiomyopathy
	Left parasternal heave	Right ventricular dilatation
	Hyperdynamic precordium	Severe mitral or aortic regurgitation, large left-to-right shunts, fever, hyperthyroidism
	Pulsation right second ICS	Dilated aorta
	Pulsation left third ICS	Dilated main pulmonary artery
	Knocking sensation	Mechanical prosthetic heart valve

ICS, intercostal space.

ventricular impulse, and normally lies slightly me-dial and superior to the fifth intercostal space in the mid-clavicular line. It is often impalpable in the supine position, especially in older individuals, but may more easily be felt if the patient is turned towards the left side. The apex beat consists of a brief outward motion, followed by a more sus-tained inward one. With moderate or severe left ventricular hypertrophy, the outward thrust per-sists throughout ejection (**left ventricular heave or lift**), although this is even more obviously detected when the left ventricle (LV) is dilated or aneurysmal, where the lift is over a larger area and is displaced laterally. The apical impulse reduces as stroke volume declines. In significant mitral steno-sis (MS), the apex beat is described as 'tapping' in nature (the tapping being due to accentuated mi-tral valve closure), or may have a double impulse in hypertrophic obstructive cardiomyopathy. Palpa-tion of the rest of the precordium using the palm or ulnar border of the hand is intended to detect such things as a left parasternal heave, generally hyper-dynamic precordium or abnormal pulsations in specific areas. Mechanical prosthetic cardiac valves create sounds which can often also be felt on pal-pation of the chest wall.

Auscultation

Auscultation of the heart is the skill which students find the most difficult to acquire, and there is no substitute for experience. The more times and the greater the variety of cardiac conditions in which auscultation is undertaken, the more comfortable and accurate the examiner becomes. Theory is important, but without the ability to put it into clinical practice it is of little value. Before describing the signs that occur in cardiac disease, it is helpful to describe the normal cardiac cycle and the events that occur.

Cardiac cycle (see Fig. 2.4)

Atrial emptying of blood into the ventricles starts when the atrioventricular (**mitral and tricuspid**) valves open, and for most of this period blood flows passively from the atria across the valves. A later phase of active atrial contraction (**atrial sys-tole**) occurs, during which approximately the last

Fig. 2.4 The heart sounds and their relation to the LV and aortic pressure pulses (RV pulse occurs 10–20 ms later). Left-sided events precede right except for RA contraction (sinus node in RA). Events within the pink-shaded area are inaudible when normal but may become audible when pathologi-cal. S4 and A, atrial sounds (right and left); S1, first sound — mitral (M) and tricuspid (T) components; Ej, ejection sounds (pulmonary and aortic); S2, second sound — aortic (A) and pulmo-nary (P) components; OS, opening snaps of mitral and tricuspid valves; S3, third sounds (left and right). Only those sounds spreading beyond the shaded area are audible in a normal subject.

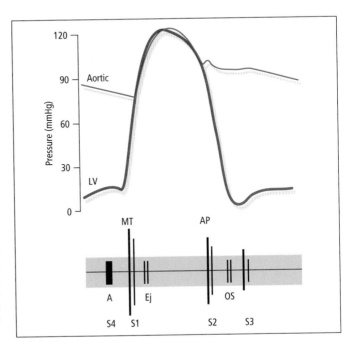

20% of atrial emptying and ventricular filling takes place. The opening of normal atrioventricular valves is clinically inaudible. At the end of atrial contraction the atria start to relax (atrial diastole), intra-atrial pressure starts to fall and ventricular diastolic pressure then exceeds atrial pressure. Because of this reversal in pressure gradient, the atrioventricular (AV) valves close. Closure of the AV valves generate S1, which is made up of mitral (M1) and tricuspid (T1) components, and mitral closure occurs fractionally before tricuspid. Almost immediately, ventricular contraction (**ventricular systole**) starts.

Just before the onset of left ventricular systole, pressure in the LV is low (5–10 mmHg) but very rapidly increases in early systole until it exceeds aortic diastolic pressure (approximately 80 mmHg) and, once it does so, the aortic valve opens. This short phase in early systole, when left ventricular pressure is rising but the aortic valve is still closed, is termed '**isovolumic contraction**' because the volume of blood in the LV is not changing. Opening of a bicuspid, as opposed to the more usual tricuspid, aortic valve may result in an audible ejection click even in the absence of any stenosis. Once the aortic valve is open, left ventricular stroke volume (approximately 45 mL/m^2) is quickly ejected and aortic pressure rises to a peak (equal to systolic blood pressure, around 110–140 mmHg).

When the LV starts to relax, ventricular and aortic pressures fall and the aortic valve closes, creating the aortic component (A2) of the second sound (S2). This precedes the pulmonary component (P2) by a short period. Ventricular diastole starts at S2 and, for a short period of time, diastolic ventricular pressure, whilst falling, is still higher than atrial pressure. This short period of time, when both atrioventricular (**mitral, tricuspid**) and ventriculoarterial (**aortic, pulmonary**) valves are closed, is termed **isovolumic relaxation** because ventricular volumes remain constant.

These principles also apply to right ventricular function, except that right ventricular pressure is considerably lower, at around 20% of left ventricular, and events in the cardiac cycle usually occur a short time after corresponding events in the left heart.

Principles of auscultation

The stethoscope has two components, the bell and the diaphragm. Low frequency sounds are best heard with the bell and high frequencies with the diaphragm. When using the bell, just enough pressure should be applied to form skin contact around its circumference. Greater pressure stretches the underlying skin and makes it more like a diaphragm.

Respiration

Inspiration increases the amount of lung tissue around the heart and, as such, if unopposed by other factors, would tend to muffle all cardiac sounds and murmurs. However, inspiration also augments negative intrathoracic pressure and increases systemic venous return. For a few cardiac cycles this results in increased right heart volumes and pressure and delays pulmonary valve closure (P2), which causes increased splitting of S2. Right heart murmurs (**tricuspid stenosis and regurgitation, pulmonary stenosis and regurgitation**) and added sounds tend to be accentuated by the inspiratory effect on venous return, but offset by the 'muffling' effect of an increase in lung volume. Overall, **right-sided** murmurs and added sounds are either **accentuated or not diminished** on inspiration. On the other hand, for the first few cardiac cycles after inspiration, left heart volumes are unchanged and **left-sided** murmurs and added sounds will be **diminished** because of the muffling effect of increased lung volume. On full expiration this muffling effect is reduced, and left heart murmurs and added sounds become accentuated.

Valsalva manoeuvre

This is forced expiration against a closed glottis followed by a release from straining, and can be employed to affect the intensity and timing of some murmurs and added sounds. It consists of four sequential phases:
- **phase 1** is associated with an increase in blood pressure;
- **phase 2** with a fall in systemic venous return and blood pressure, and a reflex tachycardia;

- **phase** 3 starts as the straining phase ends and expiration is allowed to occur, and is associated with a further small fall in systemic venous return and blood pressure;
- **phase** 4 follows, during which there is a considerable increase in blood pressure (overshoot) and a reflex bradycardia.

Effects of posture and exercise

Sudden lying down from a standing position or leg raising will increase systemic venous return. Initially this augments right ventricular stroke volume, and a few cardiac cycles later also results in an increase in left ventricular stroke volume. Sudden changes from a standing to a squatting position initially increase systemic venous return and systemic vascular resistance simultaneously, increasing both stroke volume and blood pressure. Handgrip exercise (**isometric exertion**) increases systemic vascular resistance, heart rate and cardiac output. Treadmill or bicycle exercise normally results in a gradual increase in heart rate and blood pressure.

General comments

Areas of the precordium are often described as 'mitral', 'tricuspid', 'aortic' and 'pulmonary'. This tends to imply that murmurs originating from these valves are always best heard in these defined areas. This is often not the case and it is probably a better discipline to describe the anatomical position on the chest wall where a particular murmur is best heard, such as lower left sternal edge, upper right sternal edge or cardiac apex. Such an ap-

proach encourages the examiner to decide the origin of the murmur by its characteristics and not by imprecise surface landmarks. Placing the patient in different positions (supine, semi-recumbent, leaning forward or lateral decubitus) is designed to maximize the chances of gaining as much auscultatory information as possible and, after an initial learning phase, the examiner should be flexible in approach, selecting a position and determining the radiation of any murmur so as best to identify its origin. Such an approach can only come with practice.

Starting auscultation (see Table 2.4)

Try to ensure surrounding quiet when auscultating, and initially listen briefly over the precordium with the diaphragm and bell and the patient in the semi-recumbent (40°) position; this allows an initial impression to be gained. To accentuate sounds and murmurs originating from the aortic and pulmonary (and possibly the tricuspid) valves, the patient should lean forward, and for the mitral valve should be asked to turn on their left side. In each position, the appropriate phase of respiration (inspiration or expiration) should be used to maximize the information gained. Once a murmur has been identified, its **radiation** should be determined. Mitral regurgitation may radiate posteriorly towards the axilla or anteriorly towards the sternum depending on the principal valve leaflet affected, and aortic stenosis generally radiates towards the upper right sternal edge and carotids. Timing of events in relation to the cardiac cycle can be helped by knowing that S1 approximately coincides with the carotid pulse.

Table 2.4 Auscultation of cardiac murmurs.

Murmur	Patient position	Phase of respiration	Bell or diaphragm
Aortic	Sitting forward	Expiration	Diaphragm
Mitral	Lying on left side	Expiration	MS = Bell, MR = Diaphragm
Pulmonary	Sitting forward	Inspiration	PS = Diaphragm, PR = Bell or Diaphragm depending on PA pressure
Tricuspid	Sitting forward	Inspiration	TS = Bell, TR = Diaphragm

MR, mitral regurgitation; MS, mitral stenosis; PA, pulmonary artery; PR, pulmonary regurgitation; PS, pulmonary stenosis; TR, tricuspid regurgitation; TS, tricuspid stenosis.

Table 2.5 Heart sounds.

Heart sound	Increased	Decreased
S1	MS or TS	Severe MS or TS when valve immobile
Ejection clicks	Bicuspid aortic valve or PS	Severe AS or PS when valve immobile
	Mechanical aortic prosthetic valves	
Mid- and late systolic sounds	Mitral valve prolapse	
S2		
Intensity	Systemic hypertension (A2)	Severe aortic or pulmonary stenosis with immobile valve
	Pulmonary hypertension (P2)	Decreased in expiration, pulmonary hypertension
Splitting	Increased in inspiration, and in right bundle branch block	Reversed split in left bundle branch block, right ventricular pacing
	Fixed split in atrial septal defect	
Early diastolic sounds		
Opening snap	Mitral or tricuspid stenosis	Severe MS or TS with immobile valve
Other	Mechanical aortic valves	
	Pericardial constriction	
	Atrial myxoma	
Mid- and late diastolic sounds		
S3	Youth	
	Ventricular dysfunction	
S4	Elderly	
	LV fibrosis or hypertrophy	

AS, aortic stenosis; LV, left ventricle; MS, mitral stenosis; PS, pulmonary stenosis; TS, tricuspid stenosis.

Heart sounds (see Table 2.5 and Fig. 2.5)

These are vibrations of varying intensity (**loudness**), frequency (**pitch**) and quality (**timbre**). S1 marks the start of ventricular systole and S2 the start of ventricular diastole.

S1

This high-pitched sound consists of mitral (M1) and tricuspid (T1) components and is due to abrupt restraint of the papillary muscles of the respective valve. It is best heard at the lower left sternal edge. M1 is dominant and occurs just before T1, which is often inaudible. M1 is accentuated in MS when the valve still retains some mobility. TS is rare but similarily will accentuate T1.

Early systolic sounds

Aortic and pulmonary **ejection clicks** are high frequency and are usually due to congenital abnormalities, such as a bicuspid aortic valve or pulmonary stenosis. They coincide with the fully opened position of the valve, and the valve must retain some mobility for the sound to be heard. Timing of these clicks is simulated by mechanical aortic prosthetic valves (ball and cage or tilting disc varieties) which make audible opening sounds.

Mid- to late systolic sounds

The most commonly heard of these is the **mitral click** of mitral valve prolapse, caused by the sudden cessation of movement of the prolapsing component of the mitral valve.

S2 (Fig. 2.6)

This high-pitched sound consists of aortic and pulmonary components, with the aortic component (A2) being louder and occurring earlier than the pulmonary component (P2). A2 is heard widely

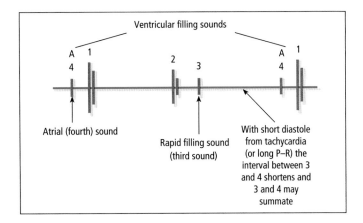

Fig. 2.5 Ventricular filling sounds.

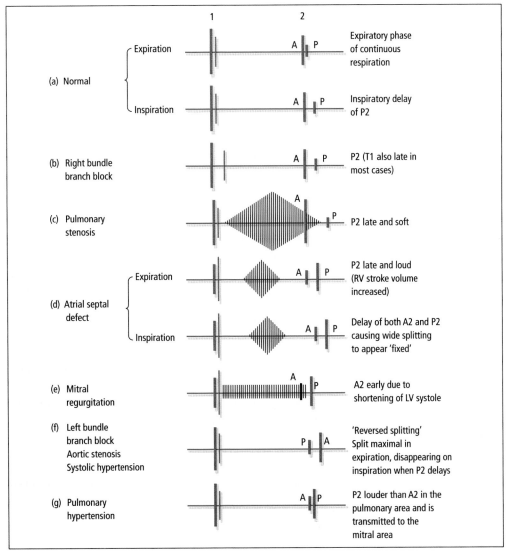

Fig. 2.6 S2 as heard in the pulmonary area.

but is usually loudest at the upper right sternal edge, whereas P2 is loudest at the upper left sternal border. Each coincides with its respective valve closure, which in turn coincides with the dicrotic notch on the pressure downstroke of its respective great vessel (aorta or pulmonary artery). Splitting of A2 and P2 is audible in normal individuals and may be increased (**inspiration, right bundle branch block**), decreased (**expiration, pulmonary hypertension**), fixed (**atrial septal defect**) or may move in a reverse direction (reverse splitting) in which splitting decreases on inspiration (**complete left bundle branch block, right ventricular pacing**). Either of the components of the second sound may be absent if the respective valve is immobile (aortic stenosis, pulmonary stenosis), or accentuated (systemic hypertension (A2), pulmonary hypertension (P2)).

Early diastolic sounds

The most common of these is the **opening snap** (OS) of MS. Normal left atrial pressure is low (around 5 mmHg) and even in severe MS may only rise to levels of 15–25 mmHg. Levels significantly above this predispose towards pulmonary oedema. Thus, even in severe MS, the pressure gradient between the left atrium and LV during diastolic emptying is small in absolute terms. Hence, the diastolic murmur and OS of MS are low-pitched sounds, best heard in expiration using the bell of the stethoscope positioned at the apex with the patient turned to the left. The OS is generated by the opening movement of the anterior leaflet of the mitral valve being abruptly halted in early diastole, the thickened valve being unable to open fully. A shuddering sound is generated which is accentuated by the elevated left atrial pressure. For an OS to be present the valve must retain some mobility, and hence it may disappear as the stenotic process becomes severe. The higher the left atrial pressure, the more severe the MS and the earlier the OS occurs after the second sound. The gap between S2 and the OS can therefore be used as an indicator of the severity of the MS.

Other rarer early diastolic sounds include a 'pericardial knock' (**pericardial constriction**) and a

'tumour plop' (**atrial myxoma**). An opening early diastolic sound will be heard when a mechanical mitral valve prosthesis (ball and cage or tilting disc) is present.

Mid and late diastolic sounds

Added sounds occurring after very early diastole coincide with the three phases of diastolic ventricular filling. The first phase is the so-called '**passive**' one when the ventricles fill as a result of a complex interaction of ventricular relaxation (causing an effect like suction) and the positive pressure gradient that exists between atria and ventricles. Rapid filling in this phase is associated with a **third sound** (S3). The second phase (**diastasis**) is short and relatively unimportant in terms of its contribution to ventricular filling. The third phase coincides with atrial contraction and, when ventricular filling is rapid during this period, a **fourth sound** (S4) may be heard.

All diastolic added sounds are best heard with the bell of the stethoscope, and may originate in either of the ventricles. Children and young adults may have a physiological S3 but not an S4, and in the elderly an S4 may be present, especially after exercise. An S3 in adults is usually pathological (ventricular dysfunction) and an S4 is usually associated with a fibrotic (coronary artery disease) or hypertrophic (hypertension) ventricle. Since these sounds reflect rapid rises in ventricular filling pressure, their presence implies an unobstructed AV valve on the corresponding side of the heart. When present, an S3 or S4 will create a **triple or gallop rhythm**. When both S3 and S4 occur the rhythm is described as **quadruple** and, as the heart rate increases, S3 and S4 may merge to form a **summation sound**.

Murmurs (see Table 2.6 and Fig. 2.7)

Introduction

Murmurs represent the audible flow of blood between vascular structures, and are characterized according to the seven features in Box 2.1. Some may be innocent, due to flow turbulence, but when pathological usually imply that a pressure gradient exists between the chamber from which

Table 2.6 Cardiac murmurs.

Murmur	Cause
Ejection (mid-) systolic	AS, PS, HOCM or innocent flow turbulence
Holosystolic	MR or TR, VSD
Late systolic	MV prolapse
Systolic arterial	Increased flow, arterial tortuosity or innocent turbulence, arteriosclerosis, coarctation of aorta
Early diastolic	AR or PR
Mid-diastolic	MS or TS, high diastolic flow
Late diastolic	MS in sinus rhythm, Austin Flint murmur of severe AR
Continuous	Patent ductus arteriosus
	Ruptured aortic sinus of Valsalva
	Aortopulmonary collaterals
	Arteriovenous fistulae
	Anomalous origin of coronary arteries
	Pulmonary arteriovenous malformations

AR, aortic regurgitation; AS, aortic stenosis; HOCM, hypertrophic obstructive cardiomyopathy; MR, mitral regurgitation; MS, mitral stenosis; MV, mitral valve; PR, pulmonary regurgitation; PS, pulmonary stenosis; TR, tricuspid regurgitation; TS, tricuspid stenosis; VSD, ventricular septal defect.

blood is flowing to the chamber or vessel to which it is directed. When the pressure gradient is large, the murmur will be high pitched and best heard with the diaphragm of the stethoscope. Examples of these include the systolic murmurs of **aortic stenosis, mitral regurgitation and ventricular septal defect**, and the diastolic murmur of **aortic regurgitation** (AR). Conversely, when the pressure gradient is relatively small, the murmur is lower pitched and best heard with the bell of the stethoscope. Examples of these include the diastolic murmurs of **mitral stenosis and tricuspid stenosis**. The pitch of the murmurs associated with pulmonary stenosis (systolic) or regurgitation (diastolic) will depend on the level of right ventricular and pulmonary artery pressures.

A murmur will disappear when the pressure in the two chambers has equalized and flow between them therefore ceases. For example, in severe AR, a large volume of blood will reflux from the aorta into the LV from the time when the aortic valve attempts to close (A2). By mid-diastole the combination of this gross regurgitant flow, and forward flow through the mitral valve, may raise left ventricular pressure to the point where it is equal

Box 2.1 Characterization of murmurs

- **Intensity (loudness)**: graded 1–6 (murmurs of grades 4–6 are usually palpable as well as audible)
- **Quality**: descriptive terms such as blowing, harsh, musical, etc.
- **Frequency (pitch)**: graded high to low
- **Duration**: short to long
- **Configuration**: for systolic murmurs this is crescendo, decrescendo, crescendo–decrescendo (diamond-shaped), plateau (even) and variable (uneven). Diastolic murmurs are usually decrescendo
- **Timing**: in relation to the cardiac cycle
- **Radiation**: direction in which the murmur radiates

to the lowered aortic diastolic pressure (a consequence of the AR). At this point, further filling of the LV ceases and the aortic regurgitant murmur disappears. In this situation, therefore, a short diastolic murmur suggests severe valvular disease. In contrast, in severe MS, left atrial pressure will remain higher than left ventricular pressure throughout diastole and hence a long diastolic murmur exists. Here it is a long, rather than short, diastolic murmur that is suggestive of a severe valve problem.

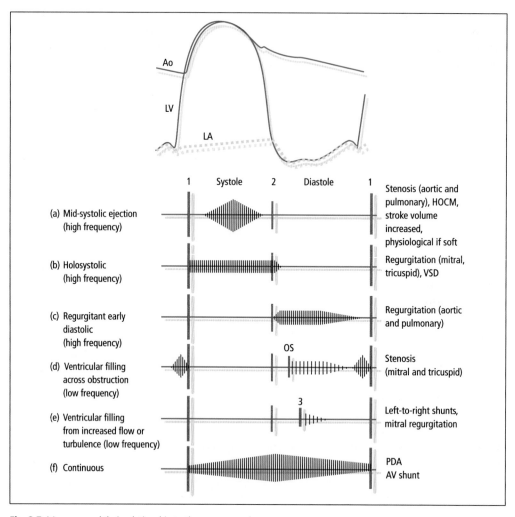

Fig. 2.7 Murmurs and their relationship to the pressure pulses.

Timing the murmur in relation to the cardiac cycle is crucial and forms the basis of its classification as: (i) **systolic** (starting at or after S1 and ending at or before the corresponding S2 on its side of origin); (ii) **diastolic** (starting at or after S2 and ending before the corresponding S1 on its side of origin); or (iii) **continuous** (starting in systole and continuing without interruption into all or part of diastole). Pericardial rubs will be included here although they are not strictly murmurs.

Systolic murmurs

Ejection (mid-) systolic murmurs do not start at the very beginning of ventricular systole (S1) because contraction occurs before the aortic or pulmonary valves (**termed semilunar valves**) open, during which no movement of blood occurs (isovolumetric phase of systole). Once the semilunar valves open, the murmur gradually increases in intensity and then declines, ending just before A2 or P2. Causes include **aortic and pulmonary stenosis, ventricular outflow tract obstruction** (e.g. HOCM), **high flow situations** (flow across the pulmonary valve in left-to-right shunting, fever, pregnancy, thyrotoxicosis) or **innocent flow murmurs** (vibratory mid-systolic murmurs especially in those with narrow anteroposterior chest diameter).

Holosystolic murmurs start at the beginning of ventricular systole (S1) and end of or very soon after S2. In other words, they occupy the whole (Gr. *Holos* = entire) of systole. The term holosystolic is preferable to pansystolic because the latter tends to imply pan-intensity (same intensity throughout systole) and, while murmurs caused by **mitral or tricuspid regurgitation or ventriculoseptal defects** are typically holosystolic, they are not always pan-intensity. Indeed, the murmur of mitral regurgitation, which is the one most commonly termed 'pansystolic', may sometimes occur mainly in early systole (severe mitral regurgitation), or in mid- to late systole depending on factors determined by the prolapsing valve leaflet, and in these cases is neither holosystolic nor pan-intensity.

Late systolic murmurs begin in mid- to late systole and end at or very soon after S2. The most typical example of this is the murmur of mitral valve prolapse, which often starts after a mid- to late systolic click.

Systolic arterial murmurs may occur in normal arteries in the presence of increased flow or vessel tortuosity, or in abnormal arteries due to narrowing. They are usually diamond-shaped and are often heard innocently in the supraclavicular fossa in children and young adults, when they can frequently be made to disappear by extension of the shoulders. In older subjects they usually indicate atherosclerosis. **Aortic coarctation** produces a systolic murmur best heard in the interscapular region.

Diastolic murmurs

Early diastolic murmurs begin immediately after S2 and are usually decrescendo in configuration. The most common cause is AR. **Pulmonary regurgitation** is less common but may occur in severe MS (**Graham Steell murmur**) when secondary pulmonary hypertension has developed.

Mid-diastolic murmurs begin a clear interval after S2, and the most common example is the decrescendo low-pitched '**rumbling**' diastolic murmur of MS with atrial fibrillation. In sinus rhythm,

a mitral stenotic murmur often has a late diastolic (presystolic) crescendo accentuation due to the onset of atrial contraction, giving an overall decrescendo–crescendo pattern. TS produces similar murmurs but is rare. Mid-diastolic murmurs may occur in the presence of an unobstructed atrioventricular valve due to high blood flow across it (e.g. mitral regurgitation or ventriculoseptal defect causing high diastolic flow across the mitral valve, and tricuspid regurgitation or large atrioseptal defect causing high diastolic flow across the tricuspid valve).

Late diastolic murmurs occur immediately before S1 and follow atrial contraction. Consequently, they occur rarely in patients with atrial fibrillation, in which atrial contraction is lost. Typically, they are mitral in origin and usually due to MS in sinus rhythm (see above). However, mitral late diastolic murmurs may occur in severe AR when the large volume of refluxing blood causes such a rise in left ventricular diastolic pressure that partial closure of the mitral valve occurs before the onset atrial contraction. When atrial contraction then occurs, it is against a partially closed mitral orifice, resulting in a late diastolic murmur (**Austin Flint murmur**).

Continuous murmurs

These begin in systole and continue through S2 into all or part of diastole. They are uncommon and usually best heard with the diaphragm of the stethoscope. Examples include **patent ductus arteriosus, ruptured aortic sinus of Valsalva, aortopulmonary collaterals in pulmonary atresia, the anomalous origin of a coronary artery from the pulmonary trunk, arteriovenous fistulae including iatrogenic shunts created for haemodialysis, and pulmonary arteriovenous malformations.**

Pericardial rubs

These are 'scratchy' sounds produced by inflamed visceral and parietal layers of pericardium rubbing on one another (pericarditis—see Chapter 12). They are frequently heard after **cardiac surgery**, and commonly occur with **viral pericarditis** or following **myocardial infarction**. Rubs usually have systolic and diastolic components and are most easily heard using the diaphragm of the stethoscope. They may be positional, sometimes disappearing when the patient leans forward.

Examination of the lungs

The posterior chest wall should be inspected, particularly for thoracotomy scars which might suggest previous cardiothoracic surgery. Left posterolateral surgical approaches, as opposed to the more common median sternotomy (**valvular, coronary or ascending aortic surgery**), are used for operations on the distal aortic arch (**coarctation**) or descending thoracic aorta (**aneurysms, aortic dissection**), and were used in the past for surgical mitral valvotomy (**mitral stenosis**).

Lung expansion should be assessed by palpation, observing any discrepancy between the two sides. Dullness on percussion of the lung bases may suggest pleural effusions, which are not uncommon in advanced heart failure or in the early postoperative period following cardiac surgery. On auscultation, fine crackles (crepitations) may be heard, due to fluid in the bronchioles that arises when pulmonary venous pressure is elevated above plasma oncotic pressure. This generally implies left-sided cardiac disease (**mitral or aortic valve disease, left ventricular dysfunction**). Crepitations tend to be heard mainly in late expiration at the lung bases, but as pulmonary oedema worsens they are heard more extensively and may be associated with a wheeze due to peribronchial oedema causing bronchoconstriction. Reduced breath sounds and bronchial breathing may be heard in association with a pleural effusion. Because the pleural veins drain into the systemic as well as the pulmonary venous circulation, venous hypertension in one system will not result in pleural fluid collection as frequently as hypertension in both. Hence, pleural effusions due to cardiac disease are most commonly seen in congestive (right and left) heart failure.

Examination of the abdomen

Apart from any general abdominal abnormalities

Box 2.2 Abdominal examination

- **Liver**: for enlargement and tenderness (right heart failure, tricuspid regurgitation, pericardial constriction) and pulsatility (tricuspid regurgitation)
- **Ascites**: (right heart failure)
- **Spleen**: for enlargement (infective endocarditis, infiltrative disorders)
- **Kidneys**: because renal failure and renovascular causes of hypertension are relevant to the cardiovascular system. The kidneys may be enlarged (polycystic disease), there may be renal arterial bruits (atherosclerosis, fibromuscular dysplasia, aortic dissection) or the patient may have undergone renal transplantation
- **Abdominal aorta**: should be palpated (aortic aneurysm) and auscultated for bruits (atherosclerosis), and the abdomen inspected for scars suggesting abdominal aortic or ilio-femoral arterial surgery

---

that might be sought as a consequence of the patient's history, the liver, presence of ascites, spleen, kidneys and abdominal aorta should be examined because of their particular relevance to the cardiovascular system. See Box 2.2 for details.

Examination of the legs

This is the final part of the cardiovascular examination, and the following should be specifically assessed.

Femoral pulses should be palpated to confirm their presence and, if absent or reduced, should suggest **atherosclerosis** or, less commonly, **aortic coarctation**. If coarctation is suspected, the presence of any **radio-femoral delay** should be sought by comparing the radial and femoral pulses simultaneously. The femorals should also be auscultated for **systolic bruits**, which are most commonly due to atherosclerotic disease. Femoral arterial abnormalities are of relevance if the patient is to undergo cardiac catheterization, which is most commonly undertaken via a femoral approach. Also, femoral arterial (false) aneurysms may occur following catheterization and may be palpable and cause a bruit.

Peripheral pulses (popliteal and foot) should be palpated, their weakness or absence suggesting **peripheral vascular disease**.

Peripheral oedema is usually pitting in nature and occurs in **right heart failure** and **deep venous thrombosis**, as a side-effect of using **calcium antagonist drugs** (especially nifedipine or amlodipine) and where the long saphenous vein has been harvested for **coronary artery bypass graft surgery**. Other causes include the effects of gravity in patients who are relatively immobile, varicose veins, hypoproteinaemia or lymphatic obstruction.

Toes should be examined for the presence of **clubbing** and **splinter haemorrhages**, both of which have the same associations as with their respective finger abnormalities.

Chapter 3

The electrocardiogram

Electrocardiogram (ECG)

This is a graphical representation of the electrical activity of the heart and is recorded using 10 electrodes placed in specific locations on the body (Fig. 3.1). This electrical activity is displayed as 12 traces (12-lead surface ECG; see Fig. 3.2). Each deflection of the electrogram represents a particular activity in the cardiac cycle. Very minor changes to the structure or function of the heart can produce quite marked changes of the ECG, which can therefore be a powerful diagnostic tool. It is important to understand the principles behind the ECG so as to understand normality and thereafter recognize abnormality.

Electrical activity of the normal heart

The start of electrical activity in the heart occurs in an area of the right atrium where specialized pacemaker cells form the sinoatrial node (SA node). Electrical discharges from these cells produce depolarization that spreads through the atrial muscle from right to left. The only route by which electrical activity can then reach the ventricles is via further specialized pacemaker cells; the atrioventricular node (AVN). From the AVN, electrical activity then spreads rapidly down the His bundle, which subsequently divides into right and left branches; the left bundle further divides into anterior and posterior fascicles (Fig. 3.3).

Recording the ECG

The ECG is recorded with the patient lying down and relaxed. Cardiac electrical activity that is directed towards an electrode produces a positive deflection, and when directed away produces a negative deflection, on the ECG.

- Standard leads I, II and III are bipolar and oriented in the coronal plane.
- Leads aVR, aVL and aVF ('a' for augmented as instrumental augmentation is necessary because of the low potential at the extremities) are unipolar leads oriented in the coronal plane.
- Leads V_1–V_6 are unipolar leads oriented in the horizontal plane.

The vectorial orientation of these leads is illustrated in Fig. 3.1.

Components of the normal ECG (Fig. 3.4)

- **P wave.** This represents atrial depolarization. The deflection arising as a result of repolarization is so small that it is not seen in the P wave.
- **PR interval.** This represents the time taken to conduct from the atria to the ventricles, and is taken from the onset of the P wave to the first deflection of the QRS.
- **QRS complex.** This represents ventricular depolarization. Q is the first negative deflection, R the first positive deflection and S is the first negative deflection following a positive deflection. As the left ventricle contributes most of the mass of

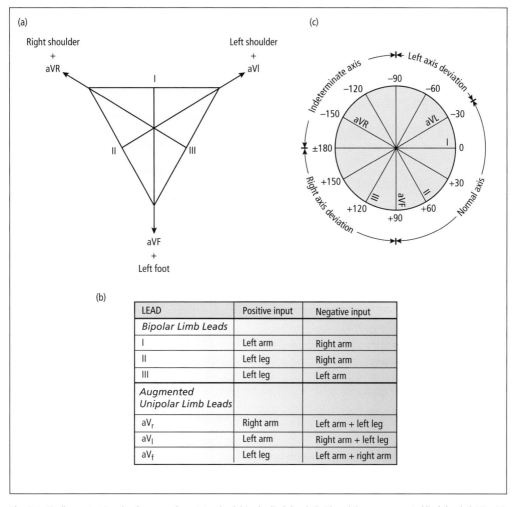

(a)

Right shoulder
+
aVR

Left shoulder
+
aVl

I

II

III

aVF
+
Left foot

(c)

Indeterminate axis

Left axis deviation

-120

-90

-60

-150

aVR

aVL

-30

±180

I

0

Right axis deviation

+150

III

aVF

II

+30

Normal axis

+120

+90

+60

(b)

LEAD	Positive input	Negative input
Bipolar Limb Leads		
I	Left arm	Right arm
II	Left leg	Right arm
III	Left leg	Left arm
Augmented Unipolar Limb Leads		
aV$_r$	Right arm	Left arm + left leg
aV$_l$	Left arm	Right arm + left leg
aV$_f$	Left leg	Left arm + right arm

Fig. 3.1 Eindhoven's triangle: there are three 'standard' bipolar limb leads (I–III) and three augmented limb leads (aVR, aVF and aVL).

myocardium, it also contributes most of the electrical activity of the QRS component. Its duration is measured from the first deflection to the end of the QRS.

• **ST segment.** This is defined as the component of the ECG that occurs from the end of the QRS complex to the start of the T wave. The QT interval is measured from the onset of the QRS to the end of the T wave. The QT interval is affected by heart rate and so the 'corrected' QT interval (QTc) is more clinically useful.

$$QTc = QT/\sqrt{R-R'} \text{ interval}$$

Where the QT is the measured QT in seconds, and R–R' is the interval between the R waves of consecutive QRS complexes, measured in seconds.

• **T wave.** This represents ventricular repolarization.

• **U wave.** This is usually a small deflection or 'hump' seen in the end portion or after the T wave. It is not always present and the exact cause of it is unknown.

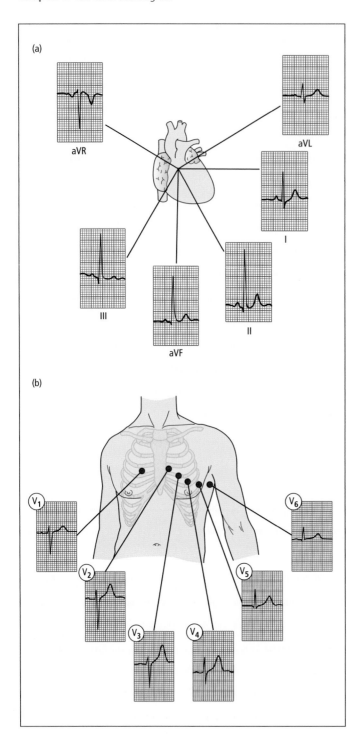

Fig. 3.2 Normal 12-lead ECG. (a) Limb lead electrode positions and ECG complexes. (b) Chest lead electrode positions and ECG complexes.

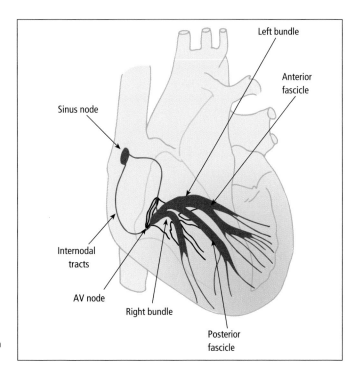

Fig. 3.3 The cardiac conduction system.

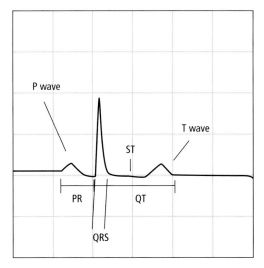

Fig. 3.4 ECG of a single cardiac cycle illustrating the different components of the ECG and relevant intervals.

Normal intervals

Each small square on the ECG paper represents 0.04 s (40 ms) and each large square 0.20 s (200 ms).

The following are normal ranges (Fig. 3.1):
- PR interval = 0.12–0.20 s
- QRS duration = <0.12 s
- QT interval = 0.35–0.45 s
- QTc interval = 0.38–0.42 s

  (the QTc normal value for females is slightly longer than that for males)

Analysing the ECG

The key to accurate ECG diagnosis is to have a methodical approach to the ECG that you can apply to every ECG (Fig. 3.5). The following section identifies aspects of the ECG that require particular attention.

Cardiac rate and rhythm

In addition to the 12 leads of the ECG, most machines will display a rhythm strip. Use this to determine the rate and rhythm. The **heart rate** can quickly be calculated by counting the number of large squares between each R–R' interval and dividing into 300:

- 1 square = 300 beats/min (bpm)
- 2 squares = 150 bpm
- 3 squares = 100 bpm
- 4 squares = 75 bpm

- 5 squares = 60 bpm
- 6 squares = 50 bpm

The heart rate can then be roughly defined as:

- Bradycardic <60 bpm
- Normal 60–100 bpm
- Tachycardic >100 bpm

The **cardiac rhythm** is determined by looking at the regularity or irregularity of QRS complexes and their association with each P wave. A regular rhythm where each QRS complex is preceded by a P wave (with a normal PR interval) is defined as normal sinus rhythm. If the rhythm is irregular, then this should be further qualified by identifying whether there is any regularity to the irregularity or whether it is irregularly irregular (usually atrial fibrillation (AF) or frequent ectopic beats). If the electrical baseline does not appear flat and has a 'chaotic' appearance to it, then it is most probably AF (Fig. 3.6).

Extrasystoles

A premature depolarization of the atrium or ventricles will produce extrasystoles (ectopic beats). If they originate from the atrium, they will appear as a premature P wave which may have a different morphology and may be lost in the preceding T wave of the normal beat (Fig. 3.7a). If they originate from the ventricle, they will appear as a premature abnormal looking QRS complex (Fig. 3.7b). When normal sinus beats alternate with extrasystoles, the rhythm is called bigeminy (Fig. 3.7c).

Bradycardias/conduction abnormalities

Abnormalities of the conduction system at any level may cause bradycardias. Careful analysis of the rhythm strip should allow you to determine the level at which the abnormality exists.

Sinus bradycardia

A P wave precedes each QRS complex with a normal PR interval but the rate is slow (Fig. 3.8). This suggests abnormal sinus node function.

Junctional bradycardia

No P wave is seen before a normal QRS. The level of abnormality may be just above the level of the

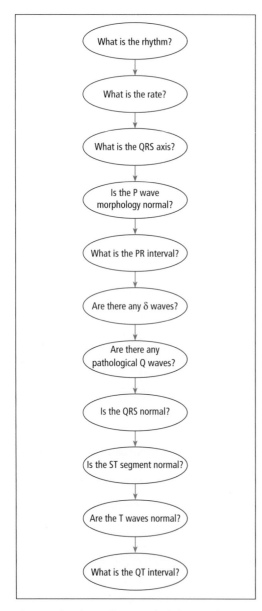

Fig. 3.5 Algorithm to illustrate a logical approach to ECG analysis.

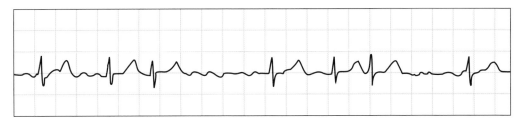

Fig. 3.6 Atrial fibrillation (note the irregular rhythm and chaotic baseline with no evidence of P waves).

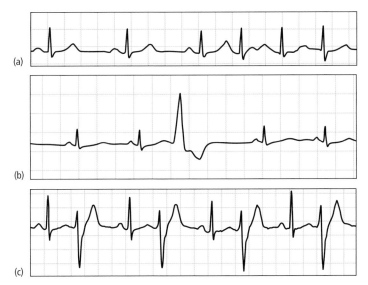

Fig. 3.7 Rhythm strips demonstrating: (a) three sinus beats followed by three atrial extrasystoles; (b) two sinus beats followed by a ventricular extrasystole; and (c) ventricular bigeminy with alternating sinus and ventricular extrasystoles.

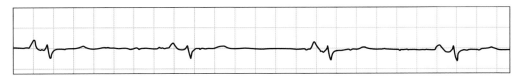

Fig. 3.8 Sinus bradycardia.

AVN and thus the P wave may be 'buried' within the QRS complex (Fig. 3.9).

Atrioventricular block

Disease of the AVN will produce differing relationships of the P waves and QRS complexes as the degree of disease and speed with which the AVN conducts (Fig. 3.10a–e). First degree block results in prolongation of the PR interval (Fig. 3.10b). Second degree block is divided into Mobitz Type I (Wenckebach) where there is progressive PR prolongation followed by a non-conducted P wave (Fig. 3.10c), and Mobitz Type II where the PR interval is more constant but P waves intermittently fail to be conducted (Fig. 3.10d). Third degree, or

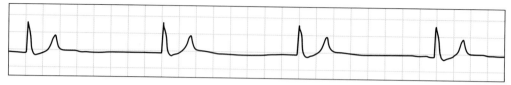

Fig. 3.9 Junctional bradycardia with no evidence of P waves.

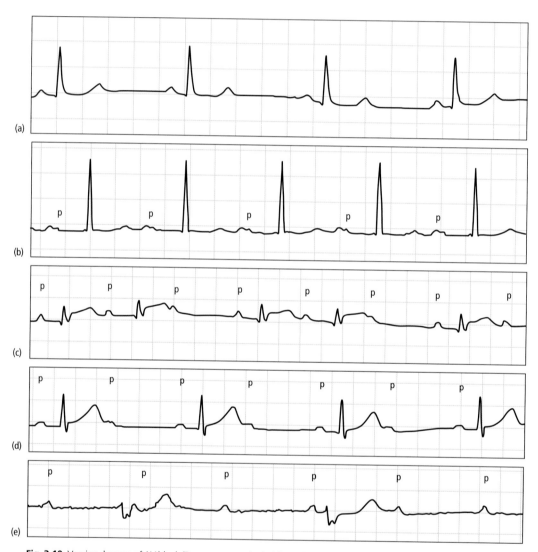

Fig. 3.10 Varying degrees of AV block (P waves are marked with a 'p'). (a) Normal sinus rhythm. (b) First degree heart block. (c) Mobitz I (Wenckebach). (d) Mobitz II. (e) Complete heart block with broad QRS complexes and no association with the P waves.

complete, heart block results in failure of any P waves to be conducted, resulting in independent and dissociated P and QRS rhythms (Fig 3.10e).

Bundle branch block

If the abnormality exists in the His bundles, then there will be classical abnormal appearances of the QRS complexes depending on whether the right (RBBB; see Fig. 3.11) or left (LBBB; see Fig. 3.12) bundle is affected. Delay in one bundle causes the QRS to be prolonged (>0.12 s) and to appear fractionated into an imperfect 'M' or 'W' configuration. Identifying the 'M' or 'W' in leads V_1 and V_6 will provide the diagnosis (see Box 3.1).

Tachycardias

If the QRS complexes are wide (>0.12 s), then the tachycardia is defined as a broad complex tachycardia; if it is narrow, then it is a supraventricular tachycardia.

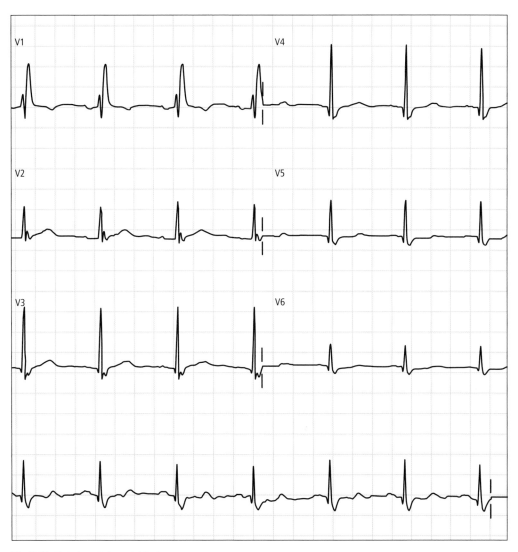

Fig. 3.11 Right bundle branch block.

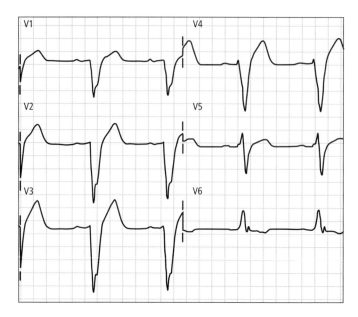

Fig. 3.12 Left bundle branch block.

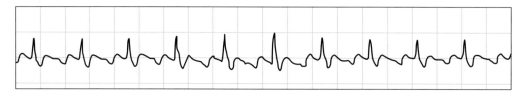

Fig. 3.13 Atrial flutter (note the saw-tooth appearance of the baseline).

Box 3.1

Mnemonic to remember whether conduction abnormality is left bundle branch block (LBBB) or right bundle branch block (RBBB).

V_1 V_6

*W*i**LL**ia*M* = LBBB

*M*o**RR**o*W* = RBBB

Supraventricular tachycardias (SVTs)

These may be further defined:
- Atrial fibrillation — irregularly irregular with chaotic baseline (Fig. 3.6).
- Atrial flutter — tends to be regular with classic flutter waves that appear as a saw-tooth baseline

(Fig. 3.13). The rate of the flutter waves is usually around 300 bpm giving a QRS rate of 150/min (if 2 : 1 ventricular conduction) or 100/min (3 : 1 conduction), etc.
- Atrial tachycardia, AV nodal re-entry tachycardia and AV re-entry tachycardia — all appear as a regular narrow complex tachycardia (Fig. 3.14).

Ventricular tachycardia (VT)

This is usually a regular broad complex tachycardia (Fig. 3.15). Occasionally an SVT may appear broad complex if there is associated bundle branch block. However, it is always safer in this situation to assume that a broad complex tachycardia is VT. Certain features may help distinguish one from the other (see Box 3.2).

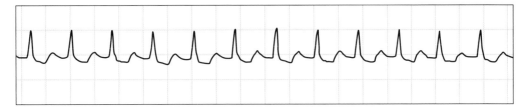

Fig. 3.14 Supraventricular tachycardia producing a narrow complex tachycardia.

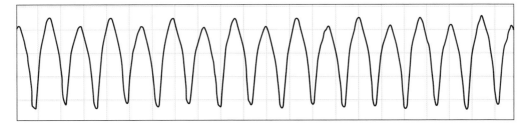

Fig. 3.15 Broad complexes of ventricular tachycardia.

Box 3.2

Features that suggest a broad complex tachycardia is VT, rather than SVT with bundle branch block:
- AV dissociation (P waves seen in the tachycardia unrelated to the QRS complexes)
- Significant axis deviation compared with a pre-arrhythmia ECG
- Concordance of the chest leads (all chest lead QRS complexes are either negatively or positively directed)
- Very broad QRS complexes (>0.14 s)
- Fusion beats (occur when a P wave and QRS occur together producing a different shaped QRS)
- Capture beats (occur when a P wave transmits in the normal way to the ventricle producing a normal QRS complex)

QRS axis

The direction of spread of depolarization through the ventricles can be determined by the QRS complexes in leads I, II and III (Fig. 3.16a–c). The normal axis is defined as 0 to +90°, a leftward axis as 0 to −30° (may be normal), left axis deviation as less than −30°, and right axis deviation as more than +90°.

A change in the axis from normal to right usually occurs when strain is placed on the right side of the heart. A change from normal to left may occur as a result of left ventricular strain, but more commonly occurs with conduction abnormalities, particularly LBBB or block of the left anterior fascicle.

To calculate the direction of the QRS axis, use a 12-lead ECG as an example and refer to the vectorial diagram in Fig. 3.1. By using only the three standard limb leads (I, II, III) and the augmented unipolar limb leads (aVR, aVL, aVF), identify the lead in which the QRS is closest to having the same amount of positive and negative deflection compared with the isoelectric baseline. Having done so, the axis is 90° to this lead, being in either a rightward or leftward direction. For instance, if aVL is the 'isoelectric' lead, the direction of the QRS axis is either −120° or +60° (i.e. 90° to the left or right of aVL, which itself is positioned at −30°). If, in this example, the QRS were positive in aVR then the axis would be −120° (unusual), whereas if lead II has a positive QRS then the axis will be +60° (normal).

Abnormalities of particular components of the ECG

P wave

If P waves are absent, then consider heart block, atrial fibrillation or other abnormal rhythm as

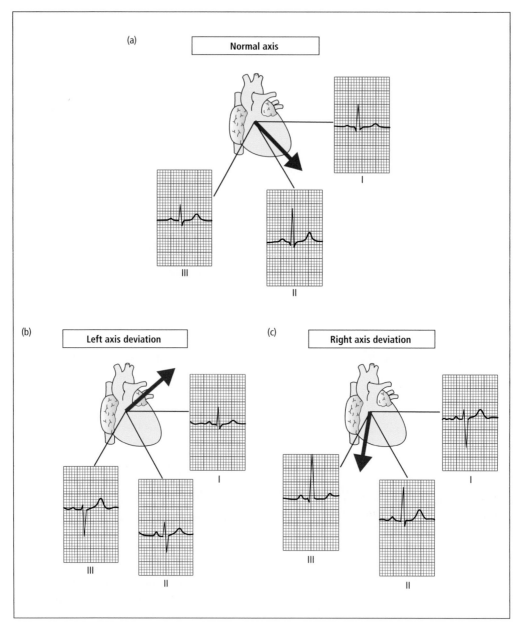

Fig. 3.16 (a) Normal axis with dominant component of QRS in I and II. (b) Left axis deviation with dominant component in lead I. (c) Right axis deviation with dominant component in II and III.

above. Tall P waves (>2.5 mm) that are peaked indicate right atrial enlargement (Fig. 3.17), whereas broad P waves (>0.08 s) that are bifid suggest left atrial enlargement (Fig. 3.18).

QRS complexes

A Q wave is the first downward deflection after a P wave. Some leads may have small Q waves that are

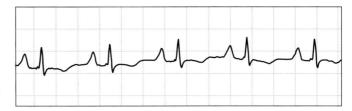

Fig. 3.17 Tall P wave of right atrial enlargement.

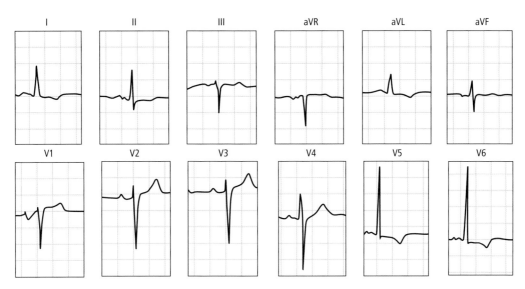

Fig. 3.18 Bifid P wave of left atrial enlargement.

normal, such as occurs in lead V_6 due to ventricular septal depolarization (Fig. 3.19). 'Pathological' or abnormal Q waves are defined as >2 small squares deep, or >25% of the height of the following R wave, or >1 small square wide (Fig. 3.20). Pathological Q waves are seen particularly after myocardial infarction, but also with left ventricular hypertrophy, and in bundle branch block.

Large amplitude complexes in the chest leads may indicate left ventricular hypertrophy. This is defined as an R wave in V_5 or V_6 plus the S wave in V_1 or V_2 which exceeds 35 mm (Fig. 3.21). However, in some young, thin individuals these criteria may be met but without left ventricular hypertrophy. A dominant R wave in V_1 (i.e. greater than the S wave) may indicate right ventricular hypertrophy (Fig. 3.22).

Small amplitude QRS complexes are seen in obesity, chronic obstructive pulmonary disease (COPD), pericardial effusion and severe heart failure.

ST segment

This lies between the end of the S wave and the beginning of the T wave. It is usually on the isoelectric line (baseline). However, it can be elevated (in acute myocardial infarction or pericarditis) or depressed (in ischaemia, drugs, left ventricular hypertrophy) (Fig. 3.23a–c).

T waves

These may be taller than normal (hyperkalaemia, myocardial ischaemia) (Fig. 3.24), smaller than normal (hypokalaemia, pericardial effusion, hypothyroidism) or inverted (myocardial ischaemia, myocardial infarction, ventricular hypertrophy and digoxin toxicity).

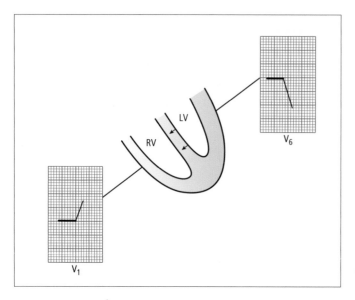

Fig. 3.19 Q wave in V$_6$ as a result of normal ventricular depolarization.

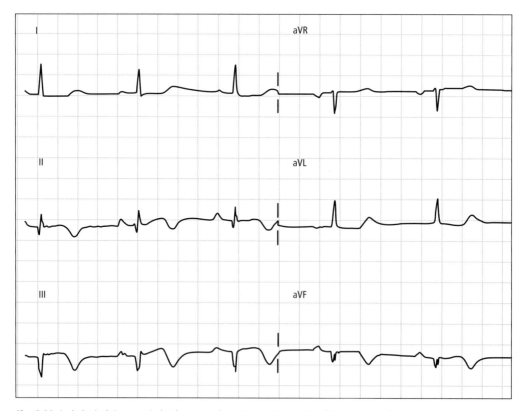

Fig. 3.20 Pathological Q waves in leads II, III and aVF in a patient 4 days following an inferior ST elevation myocardial infarction.

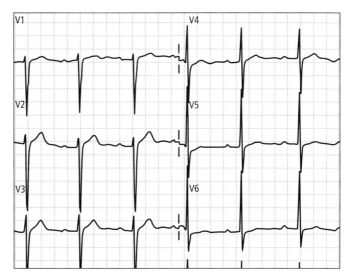

Fig. 3.21 Left ventricular hypertrophy with large QRS complexes across all of the chest leads.

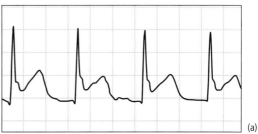

(a)

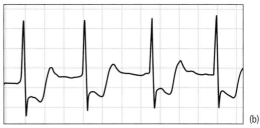

(b)

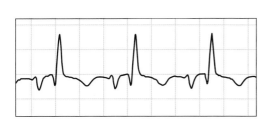

Fig. 3.22 Right ventricular hypertrophy with dominant R wave in V₁.

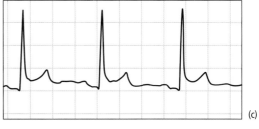

(c)

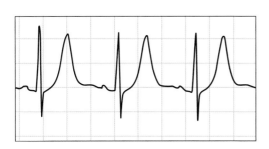

Fig. 3.24 Tall T waves associated with acute myocardial ischaemia.

Fig. 3.23 ST segment changes: (a) elevation associated with acute myocardial infarction; (b) depression seen with myocardial ischaemia; (c) elevation associated with acute pericarditis (note the saddle-shaped ST elevation in comparison with Fig. 3.16a).

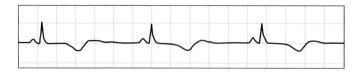

Fig. 3.25 Prolonged QT interval in patient with inherited long QT syndrome.

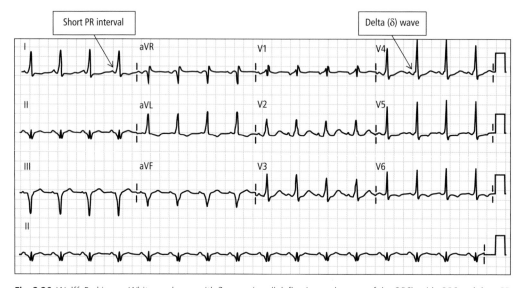

Fig. 3.26 Wolff–Parkinson–White syndrome with δ waves (small deflection at the start of the QRS), wide QRS and short PR interval.

QT interval

The QTc can be shorter than normal (hypercalcaemia and digoxin effect) or prolonged (drug induced, hypocalcaemia, inherited long QT syndrome) (Fig. 3.25).

δ Waves

These are small deflections seen at the start of the QRS complex in patients with Wolff–Parkinson–White syndrome. An accessory pathway connects the atria to the ventricles leading to a short PR interval, δ wave and a broad QRS complex (Fig. 3.26).

Chapter 4

Imaging

Introduction

Imaging has become a major part of modern cardiac diagnosis and includes a wide range of investigative procedures, the optimum choice depending on clinical circumstances. See Box 4.1 for a summary of cardiac imaging techniques. It is important to understand the strengths and limitations of these various imaging techniques.

The chest radiograph

Although the chest radiograph remains valuable, much of its importance has been superseded by cross-sectional imaging techniques such as two-dimensional echocardiography and magnetic resonance imaging (MRI). Nevertheless, a good quality chest radiograph can be very helpful for

---

Box 4.1 Cardiac imaging techniques

- Chest radiograph
- TTE
- TOE
- Cardiac catheterization
- Coronary arteriography
- CT scanning
- MRI
- Radionuclide ventriculography
- Myocardial perfusion nuclear scanning
- Positron emission tomography

---

diagnosis and for serial monitoring of the effects of treatment.

The cardiac silhouette

An example of a normal posterior–anterior (PA) chest radiograph is shown in Fig. 4.1. The cardiovascular structures that make up the cardiac silhouette are illustrated. It is important to recognize that the right ventricle does not contribute to the cardiac silhouette of a PA radiograph, but is readily seen on a lateral film immediately behind the sternum (Fig. 4.2). Interpretation of the chest radiograph should include an assessment of overall heart size, evidence of specific chamber enlargement, and any changes in the lung fields. The overall heart size should be less than 50% of the cardiothoracic diameter and should be measured from the widest point of the cardiac silhouette. Enlargement of the left ventricle (LV) produces a more spacious, rounded appearance to the lower left heart border, but the evidence of left ventricular enlargement may be quite subtle. The radiographic appearances of left atrial dilatation include a double shadow at the right heart border, filling in and later bulging of the bay below the main pulmonary artery due to enlargement of the left atrial appendage (LAA), and an increase in the angle of the carina at the tracheal bifurcation. Left atrial dilatation is often associated with enlargement of the main pulmonary arteries due to secondary

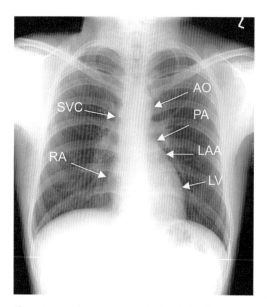

Fig. 4.1 Normal PA chest radiograph with the structures of the cardiac silhouette illustrated. SVC, superior vena cava; RA, right atrium; LV, left ventricle; LAA, left atrial appendage; PA, pulmonary artery; AO, aorta.

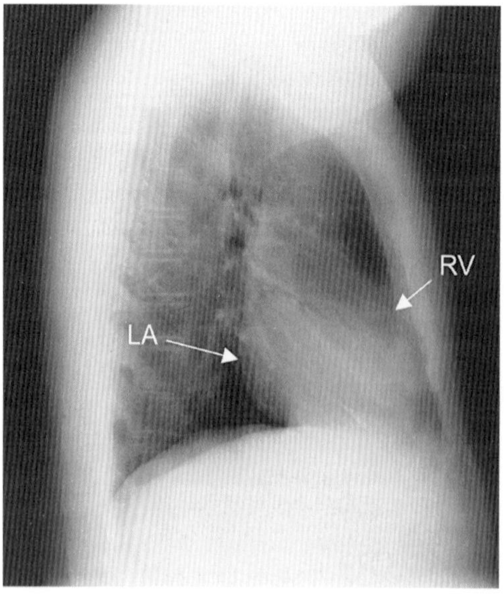

pulmonary arterial hypertension. This combination causes straightening of the left heart border, a sign often associated with significant mitral valve disease.

Right ventricular enlargement can only be appreciated from a lateral chest radiograph where the cardiac shadow is more fully apposed to the sternum. The lateral chest radiograph is also useful for identifying the presence of pericardial calcification or calcification of the mitral and aortic valves, which can be easily missed on a standard PA chest radiograph. Valvular calcification is readily appreciated by echocardiography, but pericardial calcification is much more difficult to appreciate and a lateral chest radiograph can be particularly helpful in selected cases.

The lung fields

There are no valves between the pulmonary veins and the left atrium (LA), and therefore an increase in the left atrial pressure will cause distension of the pulmonary veins and an increase in the pulmonary capillary pressure. This will result in upper lobe venous distension and subsequently pulmonary oedema (Fig. 4.3) (recognized by diffuse bilateral opacification of the lung fields), and lymphatic distension, the so-called Kerley B lines. Cardiomegaly is present and there may be associated small pleural effusions. Pulmonary oedema can

Fig. 4.2 Normal lateral chest radiograph with the structures of the cardiac silhouette illustrated. LA, left atrium; RV, right ventricle.

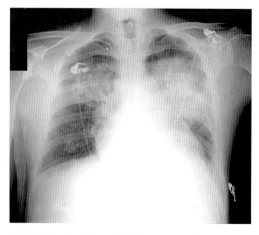

Fig. 4.3 Chest radiograph of pulmonary oedema.

also result from non-cardiac causes, such as hypo-albuminaemia and the so-called 'shock lung' (adult respiratory distress) syndrome, or the appearances may be mimicked by other conditions such as bronchopneumonia, pulmonary fibrosis or lymphangitis carcinomatosis. Thus, pulmonary oedema on a chest radiograph does not always imply left heart failure, and when it is due to a cardiac cause it is often difficult to determine the underlying cardiac pathology from a plain film. Serial chest radiograph appearances may be useful for monitoring the progress of disease and the success of therapeutic interventions.

Echocardiography

Echocardiography has revolutionized non-invasive cardiac diagnosis by providing high-resolution, real-time, two-dimensional and, more recently, three-dimensional images of cardiac structure and function. Not only is the investigation painless, but it can be repeated as often as necessary, so it is ideally suited to serial assessment of patients with a wide range of cardiac disorders. There are a number of different imaging modalities that combine to provide a comprehensive cardiac ultrasound examination:

- M-mode echocardiography;
- two-dimensional echocardiography;
- three-dimensional imaging;
- spectral Doppler ultrasound;
- colour Doppler flow mapping.

M-mode echocardiography

Ultrasonic waves will be reflected from any tissue interface and this reflected signal can be used to build up a picture of cardiac structures. If a single beam of pulsed ultrasound is used and the reflected signal recorded on moving paper, then a picture can be constructed from one line through the heart extending from the chest wall through to the posterior heart structures such as the LA and the posterior pericardium deep within the chest. This is known as M-mode echocardiography and, by angling the ultrasound transducer in different directions from the base of the heart towards the apex, M-mode echocardiographic images can be ob-tained at the level of the aortic valve with the LA behind, at the level of the mitral valve and at a level which transects the right and left ventricles (Fig. 4.4). The structural information is displayed over time so a number of cardiac cycles can be displayed on a single tracing. M-mode echocardiography has largely been superseded by two-dimensional imaging but remains useful for measuring chamber dimensions, most usefully made for clinical purposes at end-diastole and at peak systole. A reasonably accurate assessment of left ventricular function can be obtained by visualizing the contraction of the ventricular myocardium and from the change in ventricular dimension during systole.

Two-dimensional echocardiography

The limitations of M-mode echocardiography should be immediately apparent. Imaging a single point within the heart is less than ideal, particularly as abnormalities of both structure and function can often be quite complex, especially in patients with congenital heart disease. Two-dimensional echocardiography overcomes this by providing a real-time cross-sectional image of the heart and great vessels (Fig. 4.5). This allows a more comprehensive appreciation of the cardiac structures in a dynamic format and is useful for assessing global and regional myocardial function, chamber dimensions and valve pathology. Echocardiography images the cardiac structures with a high level of accuracy. Additional Doppler imaging techniques are required to provide functional information in valve disease and congenital heart disease.

Three-dimensional echocardiography

Real-time three-dimensional echocardiography is a relatively recent advance in imaging and provides a greater spatial appreciation of complex cardiac anatomy and function such as are found in congenital heart disease. It can also allow structural and functional images to be viewed from any direction, allowing the cardiac surgeon to view cardiac pathology from a similar perspective to that observed in the operating theatre (Fig. 4.6).

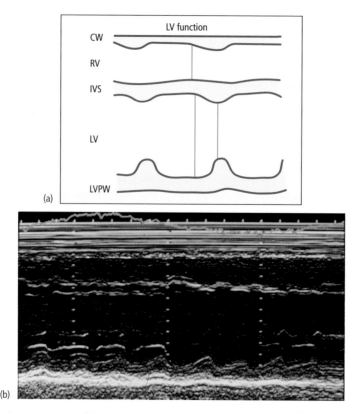

Fig. 4.4 (a) Schematic representation of M-mode echo at the level of the left ventricle. (b) Clinical image in a patient with left ventricular dysfunction. CW, chest wall; RV, right ventricle; IVS, interventricluar septum; LV, left ventricle; LVPW, left ventricular posterior wall.

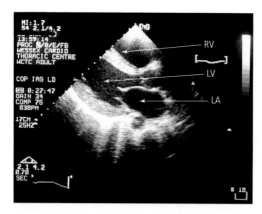

Fig. 4.5 Two-dimensional echocardiographic image in the long axis of the heart.

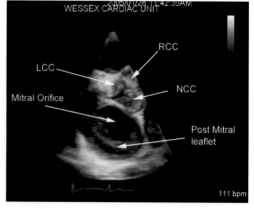

Fig. 4.6 Three-dimensional echocardiographic image viewed from the left atrial direction, showing the surgical view of the mitral and aortic valves. LCC, left coronary cusp; NCC, non-coronary cusp; RCC, right coronary cusp.

Spectral Doppler and colour flow mapping

The structural information provided by echocardiography is further complemented by Doppler ultrasound techniques which allow a qualitative and quantitative assessment of normal and abnormal blood flow within the heart and great vessels. The Doppler effect is well known to all of us, even though we may not recognize it. As a train or car approaches, the pitch of the noise it creates increases and, when it is going away from the observer, it decreases. This is because the sound waves are compressed in one direction and stretched out in the other direction, resulting from the motion of the train or car. The faster it is moving, the more the pitch of the sound is altered. Because the change in frequency is proportional to the velocity of the moving structure, in this case the bloodstream, the velocity of blood can be accurately measured. In the normal heart, velocities are usually around 1 m/s, well within the resolution of pulsed wave Doppler, but in heart disease and particularly valve disease, velocities may exceed 6 m/s. Doppler ultrasound information is displayed in a format as illustrated in Fig. 4.7. This **spectral** display indicates the velocity value on the *y*-axis and time on the *x*-axis, with the phase of the cardiac cycle apparent from the displayed electrocardio-

gram. The intensity of the signal is proportional to the number of blood cells travelling at that particular velocity. Because it is also possible to determine the direction of blood flow from Doppler ultrasound, the spectral signal can be displayed above the zero-velocity line, when blood flow is directed towards the ultrasound transducer, and below it when blood flow is away from the transducer. By colour encoding Doppler information for both direction of blood flow and velocity, and overlaying this display onto the two-dimensional structural echocardiogram, a composite image which includes structural and flow velocity information can be produced, blood flow towards the transducer being displayed as increasing intensities of red, and flow away from the transducer as increasing intensities of blue. Turbulent or disturbed flow such as associated with valve stenosis or regurgitation produces characteristic multicoloured, mosaic patterns on a colour flow map easily distinguishable from normal (Fig. 4.8).

Clinical applications

Echocardiography and Doppler ultrasound techniques have gained widespread clinical application in modern cardiac diagnosis. They are of particular value in the assessment of ventricular function, valvular heart disease and congenital heart disease,

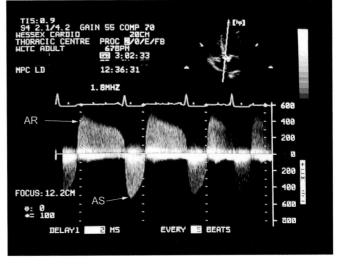

Fig. 4.7 Spectral display of Doppler ultrasound information with the velocity on the *y*-axis and time on the *x*-axis. The intensity of the spectral display indicates the strength of the signal. Direction away from the transducer is indicated by the signal shown below the zero-velocity line (as seen in systole) rather than toward the transducer indicated as signal above the zero-velocity line (as seen in diastole).

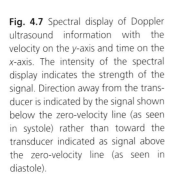

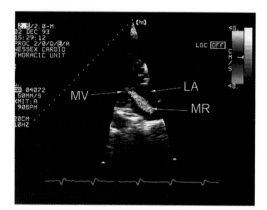

Fig. 4.8 Colour Doppler flow map image of mitral regurgitation. LA, left atrium; MR, mitral regurgitiation; MV, mitral valve.

assessment of valvular heart disease falls into two main categories: (i) confirmation of diagnosis; and (ii) quantification of the severity of individual valve lesions. Quantification of the severity of valve pathology, particularly valve stenosis, by Doppler ultrasound relates to the principle that velocity increases through a narrowed orifice and that this increase in velocity is directly proportional to the severity of the obstruction. It is possible to estimate fairly accurately the pressure gradient across a stenotic valve from the following modified Bernoulli equation:

$$\Delta P = 4V^2$$

where ΔP is the pressure gradient in mmHg across the stenotic valve, and V is the maximum velocity measured by continuous wave Doppler.

providing a comprehensive assessment of cardiac structure and function. Echocardiography tends to be more useful in assessing ventricular function, whereas Doppler techniques may provide more quantitative information in patients with valvular heart disease.

Assessment of ventricular function

Echocardiography can provide accurate, quantitative assessment of ventricular function, in patients with both global dysfunction, such as dilated cardiomyopathy, and regional ventricular dysfunction associated with myocardial infarction. Appreciation of the global nature of the myocardial dysfunction is apparent on two-dimensional imaging and it is the technique of choice for assessing ventricular dysfunction in patients with regional defects where more of the LV can be imaged simultaneously.

Valvular heart disease

It is in the area of valvular heart disease that echocardiography and Doppler techniques have had their greatest impact on adult cardiology. Prior to their introduction, much of the information now gained by cardiac ultrasound could only be obtained by cardiac catheterization. The role of echocardiography and Doppler ultrasound in the

Mitral stenosis

The diagnosis of mitral stenosis (MS) is usually suspected clinically, but echocardiography confirms the presence of a thickened, often calcified valve with reduced opening on both M-mode echocardiography and two-dimensional imaging. Quantification of the severity of MS is more difficult to define using echocardiography alone. Spectral Doppler can accurately estimate the severity of MS from the increase in velocity across the mitral valve and the reduced rate at which this velocity returns to the baseline (Fig. 4.9). The rate at which mitral velocity decreases during diastole can be measured in milliseconds as the **mitral pressure half-time**. This is the time taken for the initial peak velocity of mitral flow to fall to a velocity value that is half the initial mitral pressure drop, calculated by the modified Bernoulli formula shown above. Mitral pressure half-time is particularly valuable because it is not significantly affected by changes in cardiac output and therefore provides an accurate reflection of the actual degree of stenosis rather than simply the gradient across the valve, which is dependent on blood flow across it. As a result, it is possible to estimate the mitral valve area (MVA) in cm^2 from the mitral pressure half-time using the formula MVA = 220/pressure half-time.

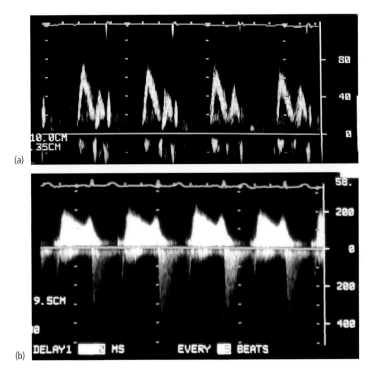

Fig. 4.9 (a) Spectral Doppler of normal mitral flow and (b) mitral stenosis. In the normal flow, the peak velocity is only 0.8 m/s and falls towards zero rapidly with a late diastolic increase due to atrial contraction, whereas in mitral stenosis the initial peak velocity is higher, almost 2 m/s, and reduces more slowly, sustaining a high velocity throughout diastole prior to the secondary increase associated with atrial contraction.

Aortic stenosis

The presence of a thickened, calcified valve is usually seen on echocardiography, but the degree of obstruction may not be clear from imaging alone. Doppler ultrasound can estimate the severity of aortic stenosis (AS) from the increase in velocity through the stenotic aortic valve. Figure 4.10 illustrates the appearance on Doppler ultrasound from a normal aortic valve and from a valve from a patient with severe AS. As with MS, the modified Bernoulli equation can be used to estimate the pressure gradient across the aortic valve. Colour Doppler flow mapping provides little if any useful additional information in the majority of patients with AS.

Valve regurgitation

Doppler ultrasound is extremely sensitive in detecting valve regurgitation, and even trivial valve lesions can be easily detected. In fact, a small degree of regurgitation can even be detected in normal individuals through the tricuspid and pulmonary valves, and occasionally through the mitral valve, particularly in children. This is not apparent clinically, is often known as 'physiological' regurgitation and is of no clinical or haemodynamic significance. Both mitral (Figs 4.8 and 4.11) and aortic regurgitation (AR) (Figs 4.7 and 4.12) are readily apparent on spectral Doppler and colour Doppler flow mapping. When using colour Doppler flow mapping, it is important not to assume that the size of the colour flow jet directly reflects the severity of regurgitation as it can be affected by many instrumentation and haemodynamic factors, although, particularly in mitral regurgitation, a larger jet generally reflects more severe regurgitation.

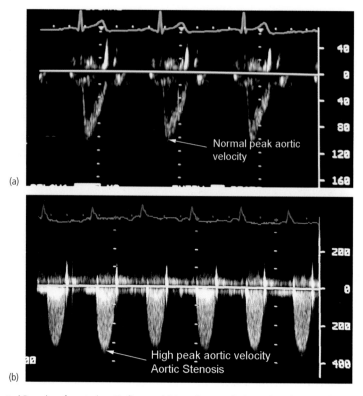

Fig. 4.10 (a) Spectral Doppler of normal aortic flow and (b) aortic stenosis. Note that the normal peak velocity is around 1 m/s compared with almost 4 m/s in the patient with significant aortic stenosis.

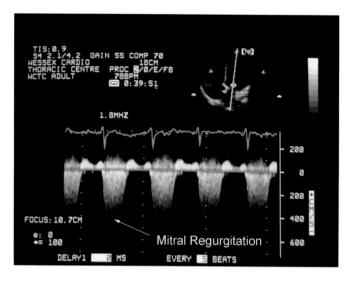

Fig. 4.11 Spectral Doppler recording of mitral regurgitation. Note the high velocity pansystolic jet below the zero-velocity line.

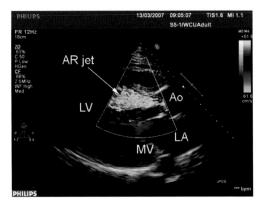

Fig. 4.12 Colour Doppler flow map image of aortic regurgitation. LA, left atrium, LV, left ventricle, Ao, aorta, MV, mitral valve, AR, aortic regurgitation.

Limitations of echocardiography

Although echocardiographic imaging through the chest wall has revolutionized the evaluation of cardiac anatomy and function, it does have a number of limitations. Ultrasound does not penetrate air-filled cavities such as lung tissue, and this limits the available imaging 'windows'. This can be overcome by using transoesophageal echocardiography (see below). In addition, there is a considerable learning curve in acquiring high-quality echo images as well as some subjectivity in their interpretation. Doppler ultrasound can underestimate the true velocity of flow through a stenotic or regurgitant valve if the ultrasound beam is at a significant angle to the blood flow or if the narrow jet is not interrogated by the Doppler signal. Overestimation of flow velocity is much less common, but the instantaneous valve gradient obtained by Doppler ultrasound may be significantly higher than the gradient obtained by comparing peak pressures after withdrawing a catheter across the valve (peak-to-peak gradient) at cardiac catheterization. Measurements taken at different times and/or under different physiological conditions will often vary significantly.

Transoesophageal echocardiography (see Box 4.2)

Transoesophageal echocardiography (TOE) over-comes many of the limitations of transthoracic imaging, particularly the problems of acoustic penetration through lung tissue, but at the expense of being a more invasive technique similar to endoscopy, performed under intravenous sedation and with topical pharyngeal local anaesthetic. As with transthoracic echocardiography (TTE), transoesophageal imaging combines two-dimensional, real-time imaging of cardiac structures with flow velocity information from spectral Doppler ultrasound and spatial velocity information from the addition of colour Doppler flow mapping.

Transoesophageal images are considerably clearer than their transthoracic counterparts due to higher frequency transducers and the fact that the ultrasound does not have to penetrate the chest wall structures. The best images are obtained from structures that lie close to the oesophagus: the LA, pulmonary veins, mitral and aortic valves and the interatrial septum. The right atrium (RA) is generally well seen, but the tricuspid valve, right ventricle, pulmonary valve and the right ventricular outflow tract are quite distant from the oesophagus and are often seen better from the transthoracic approach. So sensitive is the transoesophageal technique that it can also identify very sluggish blood flow as a smoke-like contrast effect within the affected cardiac chamber, most often the LA. Commonly, the underlying cause is MS, though it is also seen in a dilated LA secondary to left ventricular dysfunction, particularly dilated cardiomyopathy.

Box 4.2 Indications for TOE

- Poor transthoracic echo images
- Cardiac source of embolism
- Suspected thoracic aortic dissection
- Aortic regurgitation
- Assessment for mitral reconstructive surgery
- Hypotension following cardiac surgery
- Mitral regurgitation
- Intracardiac tumours
- Infective endocarditis
- Adult congenital heart disease
- Prosthetic valve function

Source of cardiac embolism

In the vast majority of patients with a cerebrovascular accident or transient ischaemic attack (TIA), the heart is not implicated. However, in young patients in whom one may not anticipate cerebrovascular disease, or in those who have TIA in more than one cerebral arterial territory, the search for a source of embolism may be indicated. TTE is generally unhelpful in the investigation of these patients unless they have overt heart disease such as MS or severe left ventricular dysfunction due to dilated cardiomyopathy. Even here, TTE may detect the major cardiac pathology but it will still be insensitive to the presence of thrombus within the LV or atrium, particularly the LAA which often harbours thrombus but is rarely seen using conventional transthoracic imaging. TOE (Fig. 4.13) is therefore essential in this group of patients in whom a source of embolism is sought.

A patent foramen ovale between the right and left atria is a common finding on TOE, being present in as many as 25% of normal individuals. The importance of this finding in patients with TIA or stroke is uncertain, but the ability to shunt across the foramen from right to left can allow venous thrombus to pass into the left side of the heart and hence cause systemic embolization. This is rare, but in patients with no other source of embolism this possibility should be considered, particularly if the patient has high right heart pressures or a tendency to venous thrombosis. Because transoesophageal imaging can visualize virtually all the thoracic aorta, it can demonstrate the presence of aortic atheroma. This is a potential source of embolism particularly if the atheroma is mobile and pedunculated.

Suspected aortic dissection

TOE can visualize virtually all of the thoracic aorta, the first third of the aortic arch being partially obscured by the left main bronchus passing between the aorta and the oesophagus. Dissection confined to this part of the aorta is rare, and most commonly occurs in the ascending aorta or at the upper descending aorta just distal to the origin of the left subclavian artery, both areas well visualized on TOE. Aortic dissection is seen as an intimal flap within the aorta, dividing it into a true and a false lumen (Fig. 4.14). The major advantage of TOE is the rapidity of diagnosis, in that it takes only a few minutes to perform the investigation once a transthoracic echocardiogram has been completed. Additionally, the investigation can be performed within the confines of the intensive care unit and does not require the patient to be moved from a specialist care area into the scanner. If the clinical suspicion of aortic dissection involving the ascending aorta is high, or has been seen using TTE, transoesophageal imaging can even be performed in the anaesthetic room as the patient is being prepared for surgery.

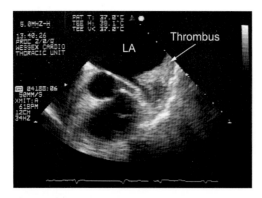

Fig. 4.13 Transoesophageal echo image of thrombus in the left atrial appendage. LA, left atrium.

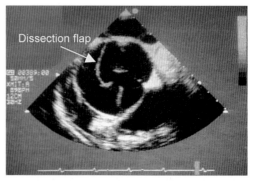

Fig. 4.14 Transoesophageal echo image of a patient with dissection of the ascending aorta.

Mitral valve surgery

Mitral reconstructive surgery rather than mitral valve replacement is now commonly used for patients with isolated mitral regurgitation. TOE has two main roles to play in the evaluation of these patients. Firstly, preoperative TOE can provide high-resolution images of the structural abnormalities of the mitral valve. This is usually prolapse of one or both of the mitral leaflets with or without chordal rupture, and TOE can precisely define the valve morphology, the severity of regurgitation and the suitability for mitral valve repair surgery (Fig. 4.15). Secondly, TOE is now commonly used within the operating theatre to evaluate the success of mitral valve reconstruction immediately following surgery, so that if significant regurgitation remains, the patient can undergo mitral valve replacement at the same operation.

Transoesophageal echocardiography in the intensive care unit

Pre- and particularly postoperative patients who are lying prone and who are ventilated are notoriously difficult to image using conventional TTE. Additionally, precordial dressings over a sternotomy scar further limit the accessibility of transthoracic imaging. In comparison, TOE is extremely

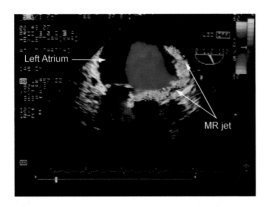

Fig. 4.15 Transoesophageal echo image of a patient with mitral valve prolapse and significant mitral regurgitation prior to mitral valve repair. Note the jet of regurgitation swirling around the lateral wall of the left atrium.

easy to perform in a ventilated patient providing high-resolution, dynamic imaging of cardiac anatomy and function.

Contrast echocardiography

Contrast echocardiography has been a standard part of echocardiographic examination for many years, but since the introduction of colour Doppler flow mapping it has been less commonly used. An intravenous injection of agitated normal saline or commercially available contrast agents will cause echo reflections from the microbubbles in the right heart chambers. These microbubbles do not normally pass through the pulmonary circulation, so any opacification of the left heart structures implies the presence of a shunt. It is useful in patients with congenital heart disease or embolic stroke, and in commercial or recreational divers it can establish the presence of a patent foramen ovale by detecting the presence of right-to-left shunting during a Valsalva manoeuvre at the time of contrast injection. More recently, contrast agents which cross the pulmonary circulation and allow opacification of left heart structures from an intravenous injection have led to an increase in contrast echocardiographic imaging. This can be used to better define the endocardial borders of the LV for functional assessment or aid the detection of left ventricular thrombus.

It is also possible to image myocardial perfusion with contrast-enhanced echocardiography. This is likely to improve further the non-invasive assessment of the functional significance of coronary artery lesions and may allow a simple, non-invasive method for identifying viable myocardium in patients with coronary artery disease who would gain particular benefit from coronary revascularization or for detecting coronary reperfusion in patients treated with thrombolysis.

Stress echocardiography

Exercise or pharmacological stress can be combined with echocardiographic assessment of regional and global LV function in an attempt to improve the sensitivity and specificity for the detection of significant coronary artery disease and has largely superseded functional nuclear imaging in the majority of cases. The left and right ventricles are divided into 16 segments, with each segment being visually assigned a number based on the presence of wall motion abnormalities, where normal = 1, hypokinesis = 2, akinesis = 3, dyskinesis = 4. A wall motion score index achieved by dividing the total by the number of segments provides a semi-quantitative assessment of global left ventricular function. Individual segments are examined at rest and during stress to identify new wall motion abnormalities, implying the presence of ischaemia in that particular territory.

• Anterior wall motion abnormalities usually imply significant disease in the left anterior descending (LAD) artery.

• Lateral wall motion abnormalities relate to the circumflex coronary artery and inferior.

• Inferior wall and right ventricular abnormalities indicate disease in the right coronary artery (RCA) though there is significant overlap, particularly in the myocardial territories supplied by the circumflex and right coronary arteries.

Cardiac catheterization and coronary angiography

(see Boxes 4.3 and 4.4)

Although the vast majority of patients undergo cardiac catheterization to determine the presence and severity of coronary artery disease, it remains an important investigation for those patients in whom non-invasive information is inadequate, for

---

Box 4.3 Indications for coronary angiography

• Diagnosis of coronary artery disease
• Angina uncontrolled by medication
• Assessment of suitability for coronary intervention
• Recurrence of angina following coronary angioplasty or bypass grafting
• Strongly positive exercise test and/or poor blood pressure response to exercise
• Preoperative assessment in patients undergoing surgery for valvular heart disease

---

Box 4.4 Indications for cardiac catheterization

• Assessment of left ventricular function
• Haemodynamic assessment of valvular heart disease
• Aortic trauma
• Massive pulmonary embolism
• Constrictive pericarditis
• Post-myocardial infarction ventricular septal defect
• Acute ischaemic mitral regurgitation
• Congenital heart lesions

---

example in patients with valvular heart disease who are poor echo subjects. Also, in the assessment of left ventricular dysfunction or the severity of valve disease, clinical evaluation and the non-invasive investigations are not always concordant, and cardiac catheterization may be necessary to establish more precise diagnostic information.

Although the indications for invasive cardiac investigation are wide and varied they fall into three basic categories:

1 haemodynamic assessment;
2 angiography; and
3 coronary arteriography.

Haemodynamic assessment and angiography can be performed on both the right and left side of the circulation, whereas coronary arteriography is obviously performed only from the systemic circulation. All these procedures carry minimal risk in experienced hands, serious complications of death, stroke and myocardial infarction being in the order of only 1 in 5000 cases.

Right heart catheterization

Right heart catheterization is the safest of the cardiac catheterization procedures as the systemic circulation is not entered unless the patient has a congenital communication between the systemic and pulmonary circulations, such as an atrial septal defect. It is usually performed either via the femoral vein, via a cephalic or brachial vein in the antecubital fossa or by subclavian vein puncture, and the term is generally used to indicate assessment that includes the heart and pulmonary arteries to distinguish it from central venous cannulation.

Femoral vein cannulation is performed by the Seldinger technique of direct venous puncture under local anaesthetic. Right heart catheters are available in a variety of different shapes. They are designed to allow passage through the right heart into the pulmonary arteries and to allow both pressure measurements and blood samples to be obtained. Blood samples are used to measure the oxygen saturation of the blood at each catheter position. Throughout the right side of the heart, blood is normally desaturated of oxygen (~70%) in comparison with that of the systemic circulation (~99%). Typical pressures measurements in the heart and great vessels are indicated in Fig. 4.16.

The pulmonary capillary wedge position relates to the point at which the catheter is 'wedged' in a distal PA. Because there are no valves between this position and the LA, the pulmonary capillary wedge pressure is an indirect measurement of left atrial pressure. If a blood sample is taken at this point, it should be fully oxygen saturated as pulmonary capillary blood is withdrawn, in comparison with the desaturated blood samples obtained from the other venous positions. If there is an increase in oxygen saturation at any position in the pulmonary circulation, this implies there has been transfer or 'shunting' of systemic circulation blood into the pulmonary circulation. 'Shunting' of blood is usually from the left (heart) to right (heart) due to the higher pressures in the systemic as opposed to the pulmonary circulation. The position of this oxygen 'step-up' can be identified from the catheter position on radiograph screening and the pressure waveform.

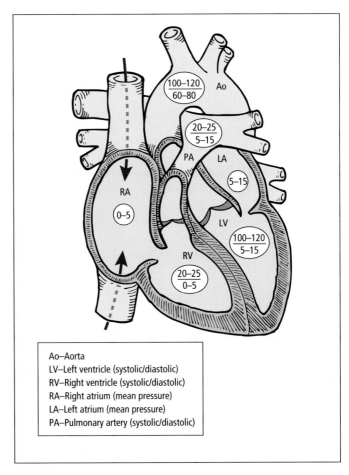

Ao–Aorta
LV–Left ventricle (systolic/diastolic)
RV–Right ventricle (systolic/diastolic)
RA–Right atrium (mean pressure)
LA–Left atrium (mean pressure)
PA–Pulmonary artery (systolic/diastolic)

Fig. 4.16 Schematic diagram of the normal range of pressure measurements (in mmHg) within the heart.

The amount of systemic blood entering the pulmonary circulation can be calculated from the degree of oxygen 'step-up'. Because a shunt from left to right will cause more blood to flow through the pulmonary circulation compared with the systemic circulation, the size of the shunt is traditionally expressed as a ratio of pulmonary to systemic flow, the so-called Qp:Qs ratio. The formula for calculation of the Qp:Qs ratio from the oxygen saturation results is as follows:

Arterial O_2 saturation – Mixed venous O_2 saturation Qp:Qs ratio = Pulmonary vein O_2 saturation – Pulmonary artery O_2 saturation

The mixed venous saturation reflects the oxygen saturation in the venous system proximal to the point of shunting and is usually estimated from an average of two SVC samples and one IVC sample. For example, if the systemic arterial saturation (usually sampled from aorta or left atrium) was 99%, the mixed venous saturation was 69%, pulmonary venous saturation was 99% and the PA saturation was 89%, the Qp:Qs ratio would be 3 : 1.

Common abnormalities from right heart pressure tracings

The most common abnormality of right heart catheterization encountered in adult practice is the presence of pulmonary hypertension. This is usually secondary to left heart abnormalities, particularly mitral valve disease or left ventricular dysfunction. It is also a common association with primary lung disease or with severe pulmonary embolism. Initially, the PA and right ventricular systolic pressure increases, but if the right ventricle begins to fail under the increased afterload, right ventricular diastolic and, hence, right atrial pressure rise. Dilatation of the right ventricle can cause functional tricuspid regurgitation with a resultant large 'v' wave in the right atrial tracing.

Obstruction to flow at any point in the right heart will cause a difference in pressure between the two sides of the obstruction. For instance, in pulmonary valve stenosis, the right ventricular systolic pressure will be higher than the PA systolic pressure, reflecting an obstruction at the level of the pulmonary valve. However, right heart obstruction is rare in adult practice. The most common obstruction is mild residual pulmonary valve stenosis as a consequence of congenital pulmonary valve stenosis. Pulmonary and/or tricuspid valve stenosis from rheumatic heart disease or carcinoid syndrome are extremely rare.

Left heart catheterization

Entry to the systemic circulation for the purposes of left heart catheterization is performed from the femoral artery, radial artery or brachial artery. Femoral artery cannulation is generally performed with an arterial sheath, usually 6 or 7 French in size, being inserted into the femoral artery. The sheath is removed at the end of the procedure and haemostasis is secured either by direct compression of the femoral artery over the site of arterial puncture or by the use of a percutaneous femoral artery closure device such as a collagen plug or a direct suturing device. Left heart catheterization usually involves combined angiography (aortography and/or left ventricular angiography) and coronary arteriography.

Direct access to the arterial circulation allows pressure measurement within the aorta and, if a catheter is passed retrogradely across the aortic valve, measurement of left ventricular pressure. Using this method, any systolic pressure difference between the LA and the aorta indicates a degree of obstruction to flow as a result of AS, with the degree of pressure difference representing a measure of its severity (Fig. 4.17). Although a pressure gradient of 50 mmHg or greater is indicative of significant AS likely to merit surgical intervention, one should be careful to interpret the pressure gradient in the context of left ventricular function, as patients with severe AS and poor left ventricular function may be unable to generate such a high pressure gradient. This potential error can be overcome by assessing left ventricular function by echocardiography, or at the time of left heart catheterization using left ventricular angiography. In addition, cardiac output can be measured and

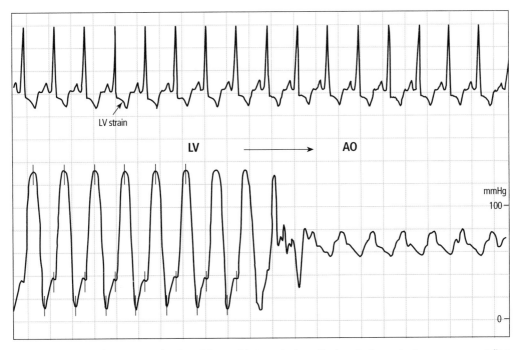

Fig. 4.17 Withdrawal pressure tracing from left ventricle to aorta in aortic stenosis demonstrating a pressure gradient across the aortic valve, with single lead ECG above showing the LV strain pattern (ST-T wave inversion) of LV hypertrophy.

combined with the aortic pressure gradient to provide an assessment of the functional area of the aortic valve, with an area of $0.8 \, cm^2$ or less indicating the presence of significant AS. Pressure gradients can be measured within the LV itself as a result of hypertrophy, particularly in patients with hypertrophic cardiomyopathy. Supravalve AS is rare but produces a pressure gradient within the ascending aorta immediately above the aortic valve, and coarctation of the aorta can similarly produce a pressure gradient usually located at the distal aortic arch and upper part of the descending thoracic aorta.

Cardiac output (Box 4.5)

Cardiac output can be measured invasively, either at the time of cardiac catheterization or as a separate procedure, or non-invasively. Invasive techniques are more accurate, particularly for measurement of absolute cardiac output, whereas

---

Box 4.5 Cardiac output — measurement techniques

Invasive measurement techniques
- Fick principle
- Dye dilution
- Thermodilution
- Left ventricular angiography

Non-invasive measurement techniques
- Echocardiography and transoesophageal echocardiography
- Oesophageal Doppler velocity
- Aortovelography
- Transthoracic impedance
- Non-invasive Fick application
- Pulse contour analysis

---

non-invasive techniques vary in their accuracy but provide valuable serial or continuous estimates particularly of relative changes in cardiac output, often useful for assessing the effect of therapeutic interventions.

Invasive cardiac output estimation

There are three main methods of measuring cardiac output invasively:

1 dilution techniques — thermodilution and dye dilution;

2 Fick cardiac output estimation; and

3 angiographic cardiac output.

Dilution techniques

Thermodilution is probably the most commonly used method of cardiac output estimation and one of the most reliable. A known volume (usually 10 ml) of cold saline (or dextrose) is rapidly injected into the RA via the proximal port of a Swan–Ganz catheter. A temperature probe at the distal end of the catheter situated in the PA monitors the change in temperature, and a computer-generated curve of changing temperature against time can be used to calculate cardiac output. In essence, the more rapidly the temperature drops and returns to baseline in the PA, the greater the cardiac output. Continuous monitoring of cardiac output can be achieved by emitting thermal energy from a thermal filament incorporated into the pulmonary artery catheter and using the thermodilution principle to estimate cardiac output on a continuous basis. A similar dilution effect can be obtained by injecting a known amount of dye (indocyanine green) into a peripheral vein and sampling from a systemic artery, to produce a dye dilution curve based on the appearance and disappearance of the dye against time rather than a temperature change as with the thermodilution technique.

Fick cardiac output

By measuring the oxygen saturation in systemic arterial (aorta) and venous (vena cava) blood, the amount of oxygen consumed by tissue metabolism can be calculated. If the rate of tissue oxygen consumption (a reflection of metabolic rate) is known, then the amount of blood passing through the tissue (cardiac output) can be calculated. The most difficult aspect of the Fick technique is the accurate estimation of oxygen consumption. Traditionally, this is done by measuring expired gases over a period of time, but this is rarely undertaken and

most centres use an 'assumed' value for oxygen consumption, calculated from age, sex and body surface area, and assuming a basal metabolic rate. The Fick technique is subject to a number of inaccuracies but has generally been regarded as more useful at very low cardiac outputs, in atrial fibrillation or in the presence of significant tricuspid regurgitation, where thermodilution techniques can be unreliable.

Angiographic cardiac output

Stroke volume can be estimated from a left ventricular angiogram, taking end-diastolic and end-systolic images, and estimating volumes from these images assuming a geometric shape to the LV. Cardiac output is then calculated from the product of stroke volume and heart rate. Significant errors can arise in patients with segmental abnormalities of left ventricular function, as commonly occurs in coronary artery disease. The technique is rarely used in preference to the other techniques described above, unless there is significant valvular heart disease with aortic or mitral regurgitation, where errors can occur with the Fick technique.

Non-invasive cardiac output estimation

Non-invasive estimation of cardiac output is generally based on ultrasound assessment of flow velocity, non-invasive application of established invasive technique, or other specific non-invasive techniques.

Ultrasound assessment of cardiac output

Doppler ultrasound can measure blood flow velocity in the aorta. This, combined with the aortic dimensions, can provide an estimate of cardiac output and is more readily used to determine changes in cardiac output from the aortic velocity alone, measured intermittently from the suprasternal notch or continuously with an oesophageal Doppler ultrasound probe. Cardiac output can be calculated from transthoracic or transoesophageal echocardiography by volume estimation of the LV at end-diastole and end-systole, similar to that described for angiography, but measurement errors and difficulty in obtaining good images have not led to its use in routine clinical practice.

Other non-invasive methods of cardiac output assessment

Cardiac output can be estimated by measuring transthoracic impedance from externally applied electrodes. Changes in thoracic blood volume with cardiac contraction alter thoracic impedance, and the rate of change is related to cardiac output. However, impedance only changes by around 0.5% throughout the cardiac cycle, introducing inherent inaccuracies. In ventilated patients, it is possible to use a modification of the Fick principle to estimate cardiac output by measuring CO_2 generation during a brief period of rebreathing. By utilizing only CO_2 production, inaccuracies can occur in situations of ventilation/perfusion mismatch. The pulse contour analysis of cardiac output is based on the fact that changes in cardiac output affect the distention and elastic recoil of the aorta and major arteries which is reflected in the pulse contour. Although this has been applied to finger pulse monitors, accurate recordings require an arterial line and calibration.

Angiography

Injection of radio-opaque dye into the circulation allows real-time dynamic appreciation of cardiovascular structures and the relationship of blood flow in a variety of pathophysiological situations. The two most common angiographic investigations in adult cardiology are left ventricular angiography and aortography, both performed via left heart catheterization as described above. A multi-hole catheter, usually of a 'pig-tail' design, is used to allow rapid injection of contrast without displacement of the catheter. Between 30 and 50 mL of contrast is typically injected over around 2 s for most angiography in the systemic arterial circulation.

Left ventricular angiography

Injection of contrast medium into the LV allows assessment of both global and regional left ventricular function, and left ventricular ejection fraction can be calculated from end-systolic and end-diastolic images (Fig. 4.18). Although echocardio-

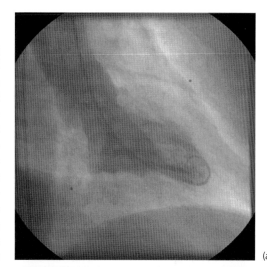

(a)

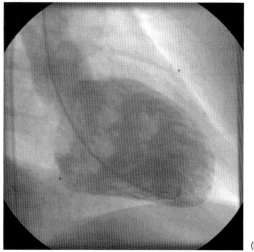

(b)

Fig. 4.18 (a) End-systolic and (b) end-diastolic frames from a normal left ventricular angiogram.

graphy is generally used for assessment of LV function, angiography is commonly performed in conjunction with coronary arteriography. Left ventricular angiography is usually performed in the right anterior oblique projection, though for a more thorough assessment of regional wall abnormalities, a further angiogram in the orthogonal left anterior oblique projection may also be used. The ejection fraction, an estimate of the percentage of the end-diastolic volume ejected with each beat, is a useful measurement of overall left ventricular function but, in patients with coronary artery disease, regional abnormalities are more common. The function of individual myocardial segments is often graded as normal, hypokinetic, akinetic or dyskinetic (aneurysmal). This regional assessment allows comparison of wall motion abnormalities with the extent and distribution of coronary artery disease, assessed at coronary arteriography.

In addition to the assessment of myocardial function in coronary artery disease, left ventricular angiography can provide information on primary muscle abnormalities, such as dilated cardiomyopathy where there is a dilated LV with globally poor function in the absence of coronary artery disease, or hypertrophic cardiomyopathy where obliteration of the left ventricular cavity can occur during systolic contraction. Left ventricular angiography is also useful for the assessment and quantification of mitral regurgitation. Injection of contrast into the LV with regurgitation through the mitral valve during systole opacifies the left atrial cavity to a varying degree, depending on the severity of regurgitation. Although much information on the severity of mitral regurgitation can be obtained clinically and from non-invasive imaging techniques, left ventricular angiography remains an important confirmatory investigation.

Aortography

Aortography is generally used for the assessment of aortic root pathology or AR. The presence and extent of aortic root dilatation can be accurately visualized, and in patients with suspected aortic dissection an intimal flap may be seen. However, the superb resolution of modern imaging techniques such as TOE, CT scanning and MRI have largely superseded aortography in these conditions. The inherently volumetric nature of contrast angiography preserves a role for aortography in the quantification of AR. As with left ventricular angiography and mitral regurgitation, aortography allows assessment of the severity of regurgitation through the aortic valve. Again, much information on regurgitation severity can be obtained clinically and from the other available and less invasive imaging techniques, but aortography remains a

valuable confirmatory and diagnostic investigation in doubtful or difficult cases.

Pulmonary angiography

In adult cardiology, pulmonary angiography has been used for the diagnosis of acute massive pulmonary embolism but has been superseded by cross-sectional imaging techniques particularly helical CT scanning. Right ventricular and pulmonary angiography is occasionally used in the assessment of adult congenital heart disease, particularly if previous surgical reconstruction of the right ventricular outflow tract has been performed. In addition, right ventricular angiography may be indicated in patients with ventricular arrhythmias where right ventricular dysplasia is the suspected arrhythmic substrate, but again cross-sectional imaging with MRI and CT generally provide superior information in a non-invasive manner.

Coronary arteriography

Coronary arteriography, although invasive, is a low-risk procedure usually performed in conjunction with left heart catheterization as described above, via the femoral, radial or occasionally brachial routes, using catheters shaped specifically to access the ostia of the left and right coronary arteries. Once positioned within the ostium of the coronary artery, 5–10 mL of radiograph contrast medium is injected by hand through the catheter to opacify the coronary artery lumen. Different angulations allow a comprehensive analysis of the coronary anatomy (Fig. 4.19).

The severity of stenoses within the coronary vessels can be assessed visually by an experienced operator, or quantitative angiography can be used to provide computer assessment of lesion severity, in comparison with a normal segment of artery. The severity of coronary lesions is described using the percentage stenosis, with >50% usually being regarded as significant. The first segment of the left coronary artery, the left main stem, is a common trunk which arises from the aortic sinus of the left coronary cusp of the aortic valve and soon divides into its two main branches, the LAD artery and the

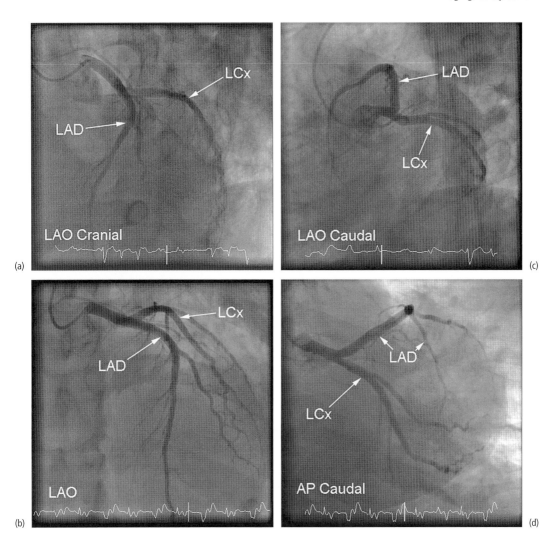

Fig. 4.19 Normal angiograms of the left (LCA) and right (RCA) coronary arteries, from different projections including cranial and caudal angulations. LAD, left anterior descending artery; LCx, left circumflex artery; LAO, left anterior oblique projection; RAO, right anterior oblique projection; AP, antero-posterior projection (continued overleaf).

circumflex (Cx) coronary artery. The LAD traverses the front of the heart in the interventricular groove, and supplies the majority of the anterior surface of the heart and approximately the anterior two-thirds of the interventricular septum (IVS). The Cx traverses the left lateral aspect of the heart in the atrioventricular groove and supplies the lateral wall of the heart, and is usually the smallest of the three main coronary vessels. The RCA has a separate origin from the aortic sinus of the right coronary cusp of the aortic valve. It follows the atrioventricular groove on the right and supplies the inferior surface of the heart and the right ventricle. In around 90% of patients, the RCA is described as 'dominant' because it supplies the artery to the AV node and gives off the posterior descending artery which runs in the posterior interventricular groove and supplies the posterior one-third of the IVS. In the remaining 10%, the posterior descending artery arises from the Cx

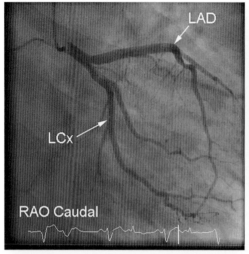

(e)

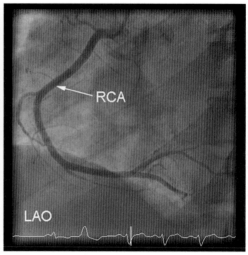

(f)

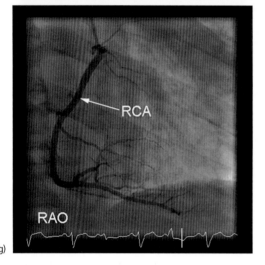

(g)

Fig. 4.19 *Continued*

artery (left dominant anatomy). The RCA supplies the whole of the inferior left ventricular myocardium, but in some cases the circumflex coronary artery is the dominant vessel and the RCA is relatively small and non-dominant.

An example of a severe lesion in the LAD is shown in Fig. 4.20. Coronary artery disease is often classified as one-vessel, two-vessel or three-vessel disease, depending on the distribution of significant lesions in the three major coronary vessels. This classification is useful as patients with multivessel disease have a poorer prognosis, and the recommendations for treatment are often based on

the extent and severity of coronary artery disease and left ventricular function as well as on symptomatic grounds.

Endomyocardial biopsy

Biopsy of the ventricular myocardium is occasionally performed at the time of cardiac catheterization, either to assist the diagnosis of cardiomyopathy, particularly infiltrative myopathies such as cardiac amyloid, or in patients who have undergone cardiac transplantation where regular biopsies are required to monitor tissue rejection. Biopsy

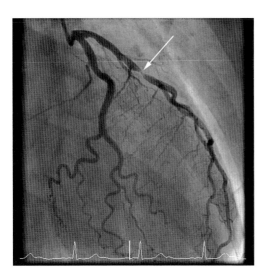

Fig. 4.20 Severe stenosis of the left anterior descending coronary artery (arrowed).

is performed through a long outer sheath inserted into the right or left ventricle, with the biotome introduced through the sheath to obtain a small piece of endomyocardium. Several biopsies are usually taken and although the risks are small they include ventricular arrhythmias, chest pain, pericardial effusion and cardiac perforation with tamponade.

CT scanning and MRI (see Box 4.6)

Cross-sectional imaging of the heart using either CT scanning or MRI has gained an increasingly important role in cardiac imaging particularly with the introduction of helical, ultra-fast CT scanning. Using ECG gating to allow for cardiac motion during the cardiac cycle, high-resolution cross-sectional images of the heart can be obtained. CT scanning and MRI are not affected by body habitus, unlike TTE, although it may not be possible physically to fit grossly obese patients into the scanner. Static images are produced, usually in the axial, sagittal or coronal views, though off-axis imaging can also be performed, usually to enhance imaging of the great vessels. Three-dimensional reconstruction can be performed to provide a better appreciation of the spatial relationship between cardiac structures, and a cine-loop format of images constructed throughout the cardiac cycle can provide dynamic appreciation of cardiac function and flow.

Magnetic resonance imaging

MRI uses extremely powerful magnets (usually 0.5–1.5 Tesla) which have to be located in a protected environment for safety reasons, excluding ferro-magnetic objects and credit cards which are easily damaged. The strong magnetic field 'lines up' the body's protons, and a radio-frequency signal applied to the required cross-section allows construction of an image from the received signal. Different radio-frequency pulse sequences can be used to highlight or enhance certain types of tissue or blood flow. Conventional ECG-gated images, or spin-echo imaging, produce a static cross-sectional image with cardiac tissues displayed at varying intensity, and blood, which produces no signal, is displayed as black (Fig. 4.21). In the cine-loop format, or gradient-echo imaging, which displays dynamic cardiac motion and flow throughout the cardiac cycle, blood has a high signal and is displayed as white, with cardiac tissues shown at lower intensity (Fig. 4.22). Image quality can be adversely affected by the presence of cardiac arrhythmias because of the need for ECG gating. The presence of vascular clips in the brain and cardiac pacemakers are absolute contraindications to performing MRI. Prosthetic heart valves, cardiovascular clips and sternal wires are not contraindications to performing MRI but may cause significant artefacts, usually seen as black holes in the image, when using the flow-enhanced cine-loop imaging techniques. Flow velocities within the heart and great vessels can be measured accu-

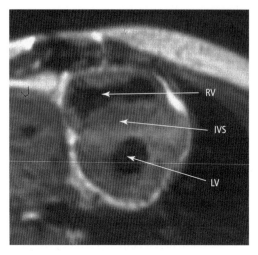

Fig. 4.21 MRI of the heart in a patient with hypertrophic cardiomyopathy showing the left ventricle (LV) in cross-section with marked thickening of the interventricular septum (IVS). Note that blood within the ventricle is displayed as black, with no signal.

rately by some magnetic resonance scanners, though this information is often more readily obtained by echocardiography and Doppler ultrasound techniques. Using pharmacological stress and gadolinium contrast agents, stress MRI imaging can now provide information on myocardial perfusion in addition to the assessment of myocardial function, allowing detection of regional ischaemia and myocardial hibernation.

CT scanning

CT scanning uses ionizing radiation to construct cross-sectional imaging of the heart. Ultra-fast, helical CT scanning now provides high-resolution imaging much more rapidly, with the total scan being performed within a single breath hold, to minimize respiratory artefact. CT scanning detects the presence of calcification much better than MRI and, for example, may be more useful in patients with pericardial disease where calcification may occur without much pericardial thickening or effusion (Fig. 4.23). High-resolution CT scanning is also gaining value as a screening tool for detecting

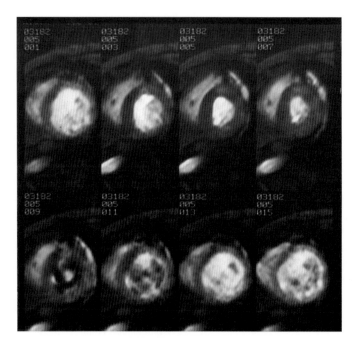

Fig. 4.22 Cine-loop flow-enhanced MRI showing a cross-section of the left ventricle at different time periods throughout the cardiac cycle from diastole in the top left-hand image through systole and diastole to the bottom right-hand image. Note that with flow-enhanced MRI blood produces a high-intensity signal.

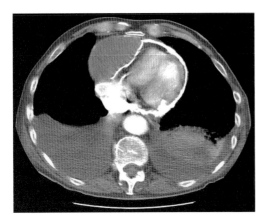

Fig. 4.23 Helical CT scan from a patient with pericardial disease. The calcified pericardium is clearly seen as a white band surrounding the heart.

coronary artery calcification, as a method of detecting early, developing coronary artery disease.

Aortic disease

CT scanning and MRI can provide images of the whole of the thoracic and abdominal aorta, which may be helpful in patients with extensive aortic dissection. In a haemodynamically unstable patient, TOE may be a more appropriate investigation as it can be performed in the intensive care unit or anaesthetic room. However, in a stable patient or one in whom immediate surgical intervention is not necessary, CT or MRI may be a better investigation as these can often provide additional information, particularly if the dissection extends beyond the thoracic aorta.

Pericardial disease

Pericardial effusion is readily identified by echocardiography, but evaluation of pericardial thickening and/or calcification is notoriously difficult and both CT scanning and MRI can be useful. CT scanning has the advantage of more readily identifying the presence of calcification (Fig. 4.23). Tumour involvement of the pericardium, usually from carcinoma of the lung or breast, can also be delineated, whereas this can easily be missed by echocardiography.

Pulmonary hypertension/ pulmonary embolism

Pulmonary hypertension has a wide spectrum of aetiology, and CT/MRI can be helpful in diagnosis when this is either primarily cardiac or respiratory in origin. Many cardiac causes such as chronic left ventricular failure or mitral valve disease may be apparent using echocardiography, but CT scanning is particularly valuable when evaluating a respiratory aetiology or in patients with suspected primary pulmonary hypertension, where not only is it helpful in excluding many pathologies, but it can also demonstrate the effects of pulmonary hypertension on the pulmonary vasculature and right heart. Ultra-fast, helical CT scanning is now proving valuable for the diagnosis of pulmonary embolism, both acute and chronic. The high resolution of the pulmonary vasculature from the central main pulmonary vessels into the periphery of the lung allows accurate diagnosis of even relatively small pulmonary embolism, and it is the imaging method of choice for suspected pulmonary embolism, having largely superseded radionuclide V/Q scanning.

Nuclear cardiology

There are a number of nuclear techniques, both established and developing, that play a role in cardiac diagnosis. They fall into four main categories:
1 blood pool imaging;
2 infarct imaging;
3 myocardial perfusion imaging; and
4 positron emission tomography.

Blood pool imaging

The basis of blood pool imaging is to 'tag' red blood cells with a radionuclide isotope so that imaging can be performed as the labelled red cells initially pass through the cardiac chambers, so-called 'first pass' imaging, or once the labelled blood cells are in equilibrium with the rest of the circulation. Because the value of this technique is in the investigation of global and regional ventricular function, it is often known as radionuclide

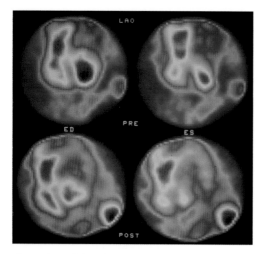

Fig. 4.24 End-diastolic and end-systolic image from a radionuclide ventriculogram using technetium-99 m imaging. The patient has a left ventricular aneurysm, and the diastolic and systolic images are shown before (top) and after (bottom) surgical resection.

ventriculography (RVG). Technetium-99 m is the radioactive tracer used for red blood cell labelling. Gamma camera imaging over the heart allows acquisition of images throughout the cardiac cycle so that end-systolic and end-diastolic images (Fig. 4.24) can be used to measure ejection fraction (EF) from the difference between the number of nuclear 'counts' obtained as:

$$EF(\%) = \frac{End\text{-}diastolic - End\text{-}systolic\ counts}{End\text{-}diastolic\ counts} \times 100$$

Although this technique has the advantage over echocardiography of being unaffected by factors such as ultrasound penetration and body habitus, as echocardiographic and MRI techniques have advanced, the need for nuclear blood pool imaging has significantly reduced. It is now only used where other imaging techniques are either difficult, unavailable or contraindicated.

Imaging of myocardial infarcts

Technetium pyrophosphate is a radionuclide tracer used for bone scan imaging. Myocardial cell death allows this agent access to intracellular calcium in areas of myocardial necrosis and can

potentially be used to diagnose, localize and assess the extent of myocardial infarction. However, this is almost never used in clinical practice for several reasons.

- A substantial area of myocardial damage is required for a positive scan, residual blood flow to the necrotic area is required in order to allow delivery of the tracer, and the optimal scan time is 24 h after the onset of infarction, by which time the major potential advantages of thrombolytic and other reperfusion techniques have disappeared.
- Also, newer biochemical markers of myocardial damage such as troponin T and troponin I more easily and rapidly provide information on myocardial damage. As such, although myocardial infarct imaging is possible using nuclear imaging techniques, it is largely of historical interest.

Myocardial perfusion imaging

Unlike infarct imaging, myocardial perfusion imaging is a well-established and widely used clinical imaging technique, although again it is being largely superseded by stress echocardiography and stress MRI. There are a number of different isotopes that can be used, most commonly thallium-201 or technectium-99 m 2-methoxy-isobutyl isonitrile (MIBI). Different imaging techniques are used, including multiple, single-plane imaging and tomographic imaging using single photon emission computed tomography (SPECT), but the basic technique is identical. These isotopes accumulate in viable myocardium with normal perfusion. Ischaemic muscle or infarct territory does not demonstrate isotope accumulation to the same extent and is indicated on the scan as areas of reduced isotope uptake. In order to induce ischaemia, scans are performed under stress conditions, either exercise-induced or pharmacological stress (dobutamine, arbutamine, adenosine or dipyridamole). Scans are then later repeated under resting conditions in order to detect areas of 'reversible ischaemia' (see Chapter 6). 'Non-reversible' defects which occur both at rest and during stress usually reflect the presence of myocardial infarction, though it is possible that an area of infarction may also be surrounded by or adjacent to another area of myocardium demonstrating reversible ischaemia.

Positron emission tomography

PET scanning is not widely available as it requires the presence of a linear accelerator to generate the appropriate isotopes, often glucose- or oxygen-related analogues, which have such a short half-life that they need to be generated in the immediate proximity of the scanner. PET scanning is a method of performing radioactive tagging of intracellular metabolites within the myocardium so that imaging is obtained dependent solely on the presence of living or viable muscle. The ability to provide information on true myocardial viability, irrespective of myocardial perfusion, or muscle function is of considerable clinical potential. PET scanning is the current 'gold standard' for determining the presence of viable myocardium in non-functioning segments of the heart, but expense and practical difficulties combined with the advances in surrogate viability assessment techniques of stress echocardiography, stress MRI and SPECT imaging has largely precluded its use in routine clinical practice.

Chapter 5

Hypertension

Introduction

In Western societies, blood pressure (BP) rises with age, and the distribution of BP readings within societies is a continuous variable, making it somewhat arbitrary where the normal range is defined as ending and where an abnormally elevated range (hypertension) begins. The importance of defining hypertension, and distinguishing normal and raised levels, arises out of the morbidity associated with its natural history if uncontrolled. A diagnosis of hypertension carries with it a likelihood of drug treatment for life, and implications regarding life assurance risk analysis, so its definition is important. BP varies enormously depending on circumstances, rising with exercise, emotion and stress and falling during sleep. Multiple readings on at least three occasions over 4–6 weeks should therefore be taken before the diagnosis of hypertension is made. Home measurements can be undertaken by patients with the use of proprietary sphygmomanometers so as to increase the number of readings available for analysis. Because 24-hour ambulatory BP has been shown to correlate better with subsequent end-organ damage than measurements made by physicians, and is a better predictor of cardiovascular outcome, this technique is employed where doubt remains concerning the diagnosis and in the assessment of response to treatment. The number of patients with hypertension is likely to grow as the population ages and the prevalence of obesity increases.

The contents of this chapter draw on the recommendations of the British Hypertension Society, which published its most recent guidelines in 2004, together with their update on management of hypertension which appeared as a report from the National Institute for Health and Clinical Excellence (NICE) in 2006.

Measuring blood pressure

The patient should be allowed to **rest** in a quiet room for 5–10 min. **Stimulants** such as tea, coffee and caffeine-containing soft drinks should be avoided in the preceding hour. The patient should be **seated** with tight clothing removed and the arm supported at the level of the heart; standing BP should be recorded at least once in the elderly, and in diabetics to assess postural drop (orthostatic hypotension). Palpate the radial pulse on the ipsilateral side and inflate the sphygmomanometer cuff gradually to a systolic pressure 20 mmHg above the point where the radial pulse is felt to disappear. Auscultate over the brachial artery and allow the cuff to deflate at approximately 2 mmHg/s, recording the point at which the first pulsation is heard (phase 1, or first Korotkoff sound); this is the **systolic BP**. The point at which the pulsatile sound disappears (phase V, or fifth Korotkoff sound) is the **diastolic** pressure. The point at which the sound becomes muffled (fourth Korotkoff), before disappearing should only be used as the diastolic if pulsatile sound continues to be audible down to

Table 5.1 British Hypertension Society (BHS) classification of blood pressure levels.

	Systolic (mmHg)	Diastolic (mmHg)
Optimal	<120	<80
Normal	<130	<85
High-normal	130–139	85–89
Mild hypertension (grade 1)	140–159	90–99
Moderate hypertension (grade 2)	160–179	100–109
Severe hypertension (grade 3)	≥180	≥110
Isolated systolic hypertension (grade 1)	140–159	<90
Isolated systolic hypertension (grade 2)	≥160	<90

zero pressure, which can occur in some patients. Measure the BP **at least twice**, separated by as long a period as possible (at least 5–10 min). Ensure there is no difference between arms and, if there is, use the arm with the higher pressures for future readings.

The standard adult sphygmomanometer cuff is 12 cm wide and 26 cm in length. Smaller cuffs with less coverage may give spuriously high readings. In obese patients, it may be necessary to use a large cuff (12 × 40 cm) or a wide thigh cuff (20 × 42 cm) on the upper arm instead of the standard cuff. Intra-arterial cannulation allows the direct measurement of BP to be made but is rarely undertaken outside research studies. All adults should have their BP measured routinely at least every 5 years until the age of 80. If found to be borderline, measurements should be every 3–12 months. Whilst it can be helpful to have home self-monitored readings recorded by the patient, care should be taken to ensure the device used is accurate and properly calibrated. Wrist monitors are less accurate than upper arm devices. For the classification of blood pressure levels see Table 5.1.

Primary hypertension

Also termed 'essential' or 'idiopathic', this accounts for >95% of all cases of hypertension. Its aetiology has been the subject of considerable research over the last 75 years. BP is related to the product of cardiac output and vascular resistance, so for BP to rise either cardiac output must be increased or peripheral vascular resistance must be elevated, or both. Although the mechanisms involved in generating

hypertension must involve these changes, hypertension as a clinical condition is usually diagnosed some years after any tendency towards it has started. By this time, many secondary compensatory physiological mechanisms have been initiated so these fundamental abnormalities of cardiac output or peripheral resistance may not be clearly identifiable. In early established hypertension, cardiac output is usually normal or only slightly increased, and peripheral resistance is normal. In the later stages of hypertension, cardiac output tends to fall and vascular resistance to increase. Also, the presence of hypertension will cause arterial and arteriolar wall thickening, perhaps partly mediated by factors known to stimulate vascular hypertrophy and vasoconstriction (insulin, catecholamines, angiotensin II, endothelin, growth hormone), creating secondary reasons why an elevation of BP will be perpetuated. The presence of these complex compensatory mechanisms and secondary consequences of established hypertension has made research into its aetiology difficult and observations made open to a variety of interpretations. It is likely to be due to a complex interplay between factors, which may be different among individuals. Some of the factors that have been suggested as being relevant to the mechanisms resulting in hypertension are as follows.

Genetic. Western blacks are more predisposed to hypertension, have generally higher BP levels and have greater morbidity and mortality due to their hypertension than whites, suggesting possible genetic differences. Some have postulated abnormalities in the region of the angiotensinogen gene, but the mechanisms are probably polygenic.

Geographic and environmental. Marked population differences exist, with economically less developed races, such as certain South American Indians, having significantly lower BP which rises less with age than in Western societies.

Fetal. These factors may exert an influence because low birthweight appears to predispose to hypertension later in life, perhaps due to a lower number of nephrons and ability to excrete a sodium load in low birthweight babies.

Sex. Hypertension is less common in premenopausal women than in men, suggesting hormonal influences.

Sodium. Much evidence supports a role for sodium in the genesis of hypertension, perhaps due to a genetic or acquired inability to excrete a sodium load efficiently.

Renin–angiotensin system. Renin stimulates the production of angiotensin (a pressor agent) and aldosterone (which promotes sodium and consequent water retention). Some studies have shown a proportion of patients with primary hypertension to have elevated renin levels, but the majority have been normal or low, a finding which has been attributed to the homeostatic effects of negative feedback because volume overload and an increase in BP would both be expected to suppress renin production.

Sympathetic hyperactivity. This may be seen in young hypertensives. Catecholamines will stimulate renin production, constrict arterioles and veins, and increase cardiac output.

Insulin resistance/hyperinsulinaemia. The association of primary hypertension with insulin resistance has been noted for years, especially in obese subjects. Insulin is a pressor agent itself and increases levels of catecholamines and renal sodium reabsorption.

Endothelial cell dysfunction. Hypertensives may have reduced vasodilatory responses to nitric oxide, and endothelium contains local vasoconstrictor substances, such as endothelin-1, although their relevance to hypertension is uncertain.

Natural history

Individuals with hypertension are usually asymptomatic, an elevated BP being detected during medicals for screening, employment or life assurance purposes. Symptoms commonly attributed to hypertension (headache, dizziness, tinnitus, fainting) are just as common in the normotensive population. In particular, the presence of headaches has been found to correlate poorly with the level of BP. Organ damage, principally cardiac, cerebral and renal, is related to the severity of the hypertension. The principal organ changes seen include the following.

Cardiac

Left ventricular hypertrophy (LVH) results in increased wall stiffness to diastolic filling and a prominent 'a' wave (atrial systole) on echocardiography. Left ventricular failure (systolic and diastolic dysfunction) may ensue, often with a ventricle that is not dilated. Treatment with most antihypertensive agents, and especially the angiotensin-converting enzyme (ACE) inhibitors, has been shown to reduce left ventricular hypertrophy if BP is reduced. Coronary artery disease is common in hypertensives, and this, together with left ventricular dysfunction, probably accounts for their higher cardiac mortality. The risk of cardiac events (death, myocardial infarction, heart failure, ventricular arrhythmias) is reduced if BP is lowered.

Renal

The gradual development of renal impairment and failure is frequently seen in long-standing hypertension, especially where control has been poor, and is more common in black individuals. Loss of urinary concentrating ability may cause nocturia to develop. Microalbuminuria progresses to more severe proteinuria, and creatinine clearance declines. Eventually, end-stage renal failure may occur and dialysis may be necessary. In accelerated severe hypertension (see later, p. 73), acute renal failure is common and is a major cause of mortality if the hypertension is left inadequately treated. Such an occurrence is a medical emergency.

Cerebral

Strokes and transient ischaemic attacks are more common in hypertensives. During a stroke, BP may increase acutely, and caution must be taken in lowering it too rapidly or too vigorously. Cerebral vascular resistance will be increased due to the long-standing effects of hypertension, as well as to the possible acute effects of cerebral oedema, and too great a reduction in cerebral arterial perfusion pressure may increase cerebral ischaemia. An indication of end-organ damage can be gained by examining the fundi for changes associated with hypertension (see Box 5.1 and Fig. 5.1). Grades 3 and 4 are more commonly seen in accelerated severe hypertension, whereas grades 1 and 2 correlate more closely with other target organ damage in chronic hypertension.

Assessment

All patients with suspected or established hypertension should have a thorough history taken and a full examination, but only a few routine investi-

gations are necessary (see Box 5.2); in the majority even these will be normal. Some patients will need more complex investigations and specialist referral, such as those with:
- accelerated (malignant) hypertension (see later, p. 73);
- suspected secondary hypertension (see later, p. 71);
- therapeutic problems or failures;
- special circumstances (e.g. pregnancy, p. 72).

Indications for treatment

From numerous trials it has become clear that the morbidity and mortality associated with hypertension progressively rise as its severity increases, with systolic elevations carrying at least as much risk as diastolic. Also, the benefits achieved by lowering BP are greatest for those with the highest pressures. Meta-analysis of trials involving a total of over

---

Box 5.1 Retinopathy associated with hypertension

- **Grade 1**: mild narrowing or sclerosis of the retinal arteriolar lumen producing a 'silver wiring' effect
- **Grade 2**: moderate to marked sclerosis of the arterioles, visible as arteriovenous 'nipping'
- **Grade 3**: progressive retinal changes resulting in oedema, 'cotton wool' spots and haemorrhages
- **Grade 4**: all of the above with papilloedema (see Fig. 4.1)

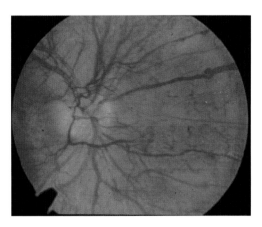

Fig. 5.1 Fundal changes of grade 4 hypertensive retinopathy.

Box 5.2 Investigations for hypertension

Test	Reason
• Urinalysis for blood and protein, blood electrolytes and creatinine	May indicate renal disease either causing or caused by the hypertension, or rarely may suggest adrenal (secondary) hypertension
• Blood glucose	To exclude diabetes or glucose intolerance
• Serum total and high-density lipoprotein (HDL) cholesterol	To help assess future cardiovascular risk
• ECG	May suggest left ventricular hypertrophy

0.5 million patients has shown a continuous and independent association of BP with both stroke and coronary heart disease. Prolonged elevation of diastolic pressure by >10 mmHg appears to increase the risk of stroke by 56% and coronary heart disease by 37%. Once the diastolic pressure rises above 95–100 mmHg, the risks of future cerebral and cardiac events are significant, and drug therapy should be given if satisfactory control cannot be achieved by lifestyle changes. Treatment is clearly not required for those with diastolics less than 80–85 mmHg where the risk is acceptably low. Between these two levels, 85–95 mmHg, borderline and mild hypertension may still double the relative risk of future adverse events, though the frequency of these events will still be low in absolute terms. As many as 60% of hypertensives fall into these categories, amounting to a large number of individuals.

The massive Framingham study and other epidemiological data have demonstrated a number of independent risk factors for the development of premature vascular disease (see Box 5.3). The 2005 Joint British Societies guidelines have created risk charts based on several risk factors (age, gender, smoking habits, systolic BP and the ratio of total to high-density lipoprotein (HDL) cholesterol. (See Joint British Societies' guidelines on prevention of cardiovascular disease in clinical practice (2005)). It has been calculated that a man aged 55 years, with a systolic BP of 160 mmHg, may have a risk of a vascular event over the next 10 years of around 14%, whereas the same man with the same BP, but with all the risk factors in Box 5.3, will have a 60% risk. The higher the overall risk, the more vigorous one should be at lowering BP, and in patients with mild hypertension the lower the BP threshold at which treatment should be considered.

The BHS have published an algorithm with recommended thresholds for intervention (see Fig. 5.2). In summary, the following patients should receive drug treatment:

- All with sustained systolic BP ≥160 mmHg or diastolic BP ≥100 mmHg.
- Those with systolic BP 140–159 mmHg or diastolic BP 90–99 mmHg if:
  - end-organ damage is present;
  - evidence of existing cardiovascular disease is present;
  - diabetic; or
  - if calculated 10-year cardiovascular risk is ≥20%.

For most patients, a target of systolic BP <140 mmHg and diastolic BP <85 mmHg is recommended. For patients at high risk (diabetics, renal impairment or established cardiovascular disease), a lower target of <130/80 mmHg is recommended.

National surveys continue to show that hypertension in the UK remains underdiagnosed, undertreated and inadequately controlled, at least in part because of the tendency to use monotherapy despite the fact that the majority of hypertensive patients will require the use of more than one drug.

Box 5.3 Independent risk factors in the development of premature vascular disease

- Advancing age
- Elevated serum total cholesterol
- Reduced levels of serum high-density lipoprotein (HDL) cholesterol
- Elevated serum glucose
- Cigarette smoking
- Left ventricular hypertrophy on electrocardiographic voltage criteria

---

Hypertension in the elderly

Both men and women are living longer, and >50% of those above the age of 60 years will have isolated systolic hypertension (systolic BP 160 mmHg and diastolic 90 mmHg). Because cardiovascular risk rises with age, elderly patients with these levels of BP are more likely to require treatment than younger ones. Lowering BP has been shown to decrease the incidence of heart failure, may reduce dementia and may help preserve cognitive function, and trial data have shown that this treatment benefit

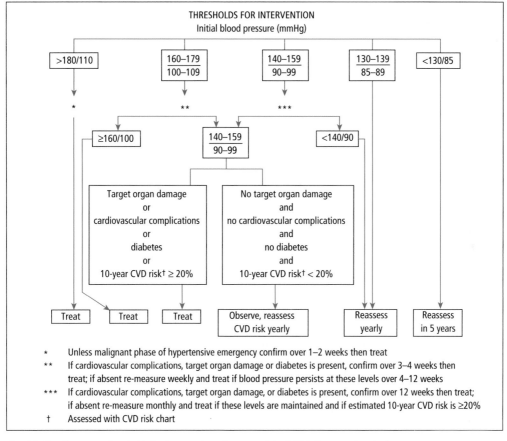

THRESHOLDS FOR INTERVENTION
Initial blood pressure (mmHg)

| >180/110 | 160–179
100–109 | 140–159
90–99 | 130–139
85–89 | <130/85 |

* ** ***

≥160/100   140–159
90–99   <140/90

Target organ damage
or
cardiovascular complications
or
diabetes
or
10-year CVD risk† ≥ 20%

No target organ damage
and
no cardiovascular complications
and
no diabetes
and
10-year CVD risk† < 20%

| Treat | Treat | Treat | Observe, reassess
CVD risk yearly | Reassess
yearly | Reassess
in 5 years |

*   Unless malignant phase of hypertensive emergency confirm over 1–2 weeks then treat
**   If cardiovascular complications, target organ damage or diabetes is present, confirm over 3–4 weeks then
     treat; if absent re-measure weekly and treat if blood pressure persists at these levels over 4–12 weeks
*** If cardiovascular complications, target organ damage, or diabetes is present, confirm over 12 weeks then treat;
     if absent re-measure monthly and treat if these levels are maintained and if estimated 10-year CVD risk is ≥20%
†   Assessed with CVD risk chart

Fig. 5.2 Blood pressure thresholds for intervention. Courtesy of the British Hypertension Society.

extends up to at least the age of 80 years. There are few trial data on patients older than 80 years, but if treatment has been started at an earlier age it should be continued in these elderly patients. Decisions regarding treatment of those presenting at over 80 years need to be made in the light of co-morbidities and overall cardiovascular risk.

Secondary hypertension

Defined causes of hypertension account for <5% of cases and may be grouped as follows.

Renal parenchymal disease (3%)

Any cause of renal failure (glomerulonephritis,

pyelonephritis, obstructive causes) that involves parenchymal damage will tend to cause hypertension, and hypertension itself will cause renal damage.

Renovascular disease (1%)

This encompasses conditions affecting renal blood supply and can be broadly divided into **atherosclerosis**, which affects mainly the proximal third of the renal artery and is most common in older patients, and **fibrodysplasia**, which mainly affects the distal two-thirds and is most common in younger individuals, especially women. Reduced renal blood supply stimulates ipsilateral production of renin and hence elevation of BP. It should be suspected if the hypertension is abrupt in onset, refractory to treatment generally but appears to normalize with ACE inhibitors, is severe or accelerated, and if an abdominal bruit is detected.

Endocrine (1%)

Consider **primary aldosteronism** (**Conn syndrome**) when hypokalaemia, high normal serum sodium and metabolic alkalosis are associated with hypertension. High aldosterone and low renin levels result in sodium and water overload. This is usually due to a solitary benign adenoma or bilateral adrenal hyperplasia. Diagnosis is helped by CT or MRI scanning, and treatment is by tumour resection or use of the aldosterone antagonist spironolactone. **Cushing syndrome** is due to bilateral adrenal hyperplasia caused by an adrenocorticotrophic hormone (ACTH)-secreting pituitary adenoma in two-thirds of cases, and a primary adrenal tumour in one-third. Suspect if hypertension is associated with obesity, thin skin, muscle weakness and osteoporosis. Diagnosis is by 24-hour urinary cortisol and dexamethasone suppression test, then pituitary and adrenal CT or MRI scanning if cortisols are abnormal. **Congenital adrenal hyperplasia** is a rare cause of hypertension in childhood. **Phaeochromocytoma** is due to a cathecholamine-secreting tumour of chromaffin cells of neural origin, 90% arising in the adrenals. Approximately 10% occur elsewhere in the sympathetic chain, 10% of all tumours are malignant and 10% of adrenal adenomas are bilateral. Suspect phaeochromocytoma if BP fluctuates widely, and is associated with tachycardia, sweating or sometimes pulmonary oedema due to cardiac failure. Diagnosis is by 24-hour or spot urine measurement of total metanephrine (cathecholamine metabolite), although levels may be affected by certain antihypertensive drugs, especially labetalol. If metanephrines are equivocal, measure plasma norepinephrine (noradrenaline) after a dose of clonidine (adrenergic inhibitor). Once diagnosed, attempt to locate the secreting tumour using CT, MRI or radioisotope scanning. Optimum treatment is to resect the tumour if possible.

Coarctation of the aorta (see Chapter 18)

This most commonly affects the aorta at or just distal to the left subclavian artery and results in hypertension in the arms and lower pressures in the legs, with weak or absent femoral arterial pulses. Systemic arterial vasoconstriction occurs due to stimulation of the renin–angiotensin system (due to low renal arterial perfusion pressure) and sympathetic hyperactivity. Diagnosis is by CT or MRI scanning and/or contrast aortography. Hypertension may often persist even after successful surgical resection or percutaneous intervention, especially if the hypertension has been longstanding preoperatively.

Pregnancy related

Gestational hypertension occurs in up to 10% of first pregnancies, is more common in younger mothers, is thought to be due to poor uteroplacental blood flow and generally occurs in the last trimester or early in the post-partum period. It is associated with increased serum urate levels, and when severe causes the syndrome of pre-eclampsia (systolic BP >140 mmHg or diastolic BP >90 mmHg after 20 weeks in previously normotensive woman associated with proteinuria >300 mg in 24 h). Delivery of the fetus results in resolution of the hypertension. Pregnancy may also worsen pre-existing primary hypertension, and this 'acute-on-chronic' variety is more common in older, multigravid mothers and reveals itself usually before 20 weeks' gestation. Antihypertensive drugs should be avoided in pregnancy where possible and the hypertension should be treated by bed rest and fetal monitoring, with delivery where appropriate. However, when drug therapy has to be used, methyldopa, hydralazine, nifedipine and labetalol are suitable agents.

Drug-induced

The most common medication associated with hypertension is the oral contraceptive pill (OCP), with around 5% of women developing hypertension within 5 years of starting. Older women (>35 years) are more predisposed, as are women who have had hypertension in pregnancy. BP will fall to normal in 50% within 3–6 months of stopping the OCP. It is uncertain whether the hypertension is caused by the OCP or whether taking it merely reveals an underlying predisposition. Other drugs associated with hypertension include cyclosporine, erythropoietin and cocaine.

Accelerated hypertension

Also known as malignant hypertension, this condition arises when the BP rises rapidly to diastolic levels above 130–140 mmHg. It occurs in <1% of patients with primary hypertension, but more commonly in cases of secondary hypertension, especially phaeochromocytomas and conditions causing rapidly progressive renal failure. Retinal haemorrhages and exudates are common, and papilloedema will ensue. Initially the cerebral vessels constrict with increasing hypertension (autoregulation) but, in accelerated cases, the vessels eventually cannot withstand the rapidly rising pressure and they dilate, resulting in cerebral hyperperfusion and cerebral oedema (hypertensive encephalopathy), with symptoms of headache, irritability and alterations in consciousness. If left untreated, accelerated hypertension results in progressive renal damage, hyperaldosteronism due to renal ischaemia, microangiopathic haemolytic anaemia and disseminated intravascular coagulation (DIC). In these advanced cases, the mortality rate is high.

Management of hypertension

Potential benefits of treatment

Trials have been conducted over long time periods to assess the benefits of treatment and, hence, most data relate to the use of the earlier antihypertensive agents and, in particular, β-blockers and diuretics. Meta-analyses of the larger treatment trials suggest an overall 40% reduction in stroke and 16% reduction in coronary events. The importance of systolic hypertension is strongly emphasized, as it is at least as important as diastolic BP as a predictor of cardiovascular risk.

Lifestyle modifications

All hypertensive patients and individuals with borderline or high normal BP should be advised regarding lifestyle changes.
- Achieving ideal body weight (body mass index 20–25 kg/m^2).
- Reducing salt intake to <100 mmol (<2.4 g of Na$^+$, or 6 g of NaCl) per day.
- Limit alcohol consumption; maximum 3 units/day (men), 2 units/day (women).
- Aerobic exercise (>30 min/day at least three times per week, preferably daily).
- Consume at least five portions per day of fresh fruit and vegetables.
- Reduce intake of total and saturated fat (http://www.eatwell.gov.uk).
- Avoid smoking.

Lifestyle changes can reduce the age-associated rise in BP and therefore reduce the number of individuals requiring drug therapy. Effective implementation requires knowledge, enthusiasm, patience, considerable time spent with patients and other family members, and reinforcement. It is best undertaken by well-trained health professionals, such as practice or clinic nurses.

Drug therapy

When drug therapy is felt necessary, use the lowest dose initially and increase incrementally depending on the response to treatment, allowing at least 4 weeks to see the effect, unless more urgent reduction in BP is needed. In general, medication should be taken in the morning rather than at night, to try to avoid exacerbating the usual early morning drop in BP which may be a contributing factor towards the observation of a higher incidence of cardiovascular events during the hours 5.00–8.00 am.

Diuretics

All diuretics will lower BP acutely by salt and water loss, but over 4–6 weeks equilibrium is restored and

BP returns towards previous levels. However, the thiazides have a direct vasodilatory effect on arterioles which results in a sustained hypotensive effect. Thiazides reduce serum potassium and tend to increase blood glucose, urate, insulin, cholesterol and calcium. Nearly 25% of men suffer impotence as a side-effect. For treatment of hypertension, use the longer-acting thiazides, such as hydrochlorothiazide (12.5–50 mg/day) or bendrofluethiazide (2.5–5.0 mg/day), perhaps with the addition of a potassium-sparing agent such as amiloride, unless an ACE inhibitor is also being used. Indapamide is a sulphonamide diuretic with actions similar to thiazides but with little effect on glucose or cholesterol.

Adrenergic inhibitors

These may act centrally on the vasomotor centre in the brainstem, peripherally on neuronal catecholamine release, or by blocking α- or β-receptors, or both. Examples of each of these agents are given in Table 5.2, with those agents in parentheses rarely being used nowadays. In vascular smooth muscle, alpha stimulation causes vasoconstriction and beta stimulation causes relaxation. In the vasomotor centre, sympathetic outflow is inhibited by alpha stimulation. The effects of β-blockers centrally are less certain. β-Blockers have been widely used antihypertensives. All seem about equally effective at lowering BP, but some have greater selectivity towards cardiac β-receptors (see Table 5.2) than others

which are non-cardioselective. Also, some β-blockers have some intrinsic sympathomimetic activity (ISA) (pindolol, oxprenolol, acebutalol and celiprolol), a characteristic that results in a smaller fall in heart rate, cardiac output and renin for a similar change in BP when compared with β-blockers without ISA. β-Blockers may worsen bronchospasm, claudication and untreated congestive cardiac failure, and are relatively contraindicated in these conditions. Symptoms of hypoglycaemia in diabetics may be blunted and glucose control may be worsened due to interference with insulin sensitivity. Side-effects may include fatigue, insomnia, nightmares, hallucinations, depression and impotence. They are relatively ineffective in the elderly hypertensive.

Direct vasodilators

These lower BP by reducing peripheral vascular resistance. The most common examples of this group of drugs are the oral agents hydralazine, prazosin and minoxidil, and the intravenous agents diazoxide and nitroprusside. All tend to cause a reflex tachycardia, hydralazine may be associated with a lupus syndrome if used in high doses, and minoxidil commonly results in hirsutism.

Calcium antagonists

These are now commonly used antihypertensives. The choice of agent depends partly on their differ-

Table 5.2 Adrenergic inhibitor agents.

Vasomotor centre	Neurone	α-Receptor	β-Receptor	α- and β-Receptors
Methyl dopa	(Reserpine)	Prazosin	Acebutalol*	Labetalol
(Clonidine)	(Guanethidine)	Doxasocin	Atenolol*	Carvedilol
	(Bethanidine)	Terazosin	Bisoprolol*	
	(Debrisoquine)	(Phenoxybenzamine)	Metoprolol*	
		(Phentolamine)	Esmolol*	
			Celiprolol*	
			Nadolol	
			Pindolol	
			Timolol	
			Propranolol	

*β-blockers with greater selectivity towards cardiac β-receptors.

Table 5.3 Relative effects of calcium antagonists.

	Negative chronotropism	Negative inotropism	Flushing/Oedema	Constipation
Nifedipine	0	0	++	0
Verapamil	++	++	+	++
Diltiazem	+	+	+−	+

ent effects with regard to slowing the heart rate (negative chronotropism), reducing myocardial contractility (negative inotropism) and their propensity to cause side-effects such as flushing, peripheral oedema and constipation. Examples of the oldest agents are given in Table 5.3, but others include nisoldipine, nicardipine, amlodipine and felodipine. The calcium antagonists have little adverse effect on lipids or glucose.

Renin–angiotensin inhibitors

Adrenergic receptor blockers inhibit renal production of renin from the juxtaglomerular apparatus and it is possible to block the conversion of renin substrate to angiotensin. However, the most widely used of this group of agents in treating hypertension are the ACE inhibitors, such as captopril, enalapril, lisinopril and ramipril, and the more recently developed angiotensin II receptor blockers such as losartan and valsartan. Angiotensin II is a vasoconstrictor and stimulates the production of aldosterone, so blocking its production (ACE inhibitors) or binding to its receptor (AII receptor blockers) will reduce peripheral vascular resistance, with little or no effect on heart rate, cardiac output or body fluid volumes. ACE inhibitors may cause loss of taste, skin rashes and commonly cause an irritating dry cough, probably due to elevation of bradykinin levels. Cough and other side-effects are seen less frequently with the AII receptor blockers. The ACE inhibitors are particularly useful for diabetic nephropathy, where efferent arteriolar dilatation slows the progressive loss of renal function and may reduce proteinuria. They may also improve insulin sensitivity. They have no effect on serum lipids or urate.

Choice of drug agent

The most recent meta-analysis of large-scale morbidity and mortality trials that have compared anti-hypertensive agents (see Blood Pressure Lowering Treatment Triallists' Collaboration (2003)) included 29 trials and over 700 000 years of patient follow-up. The principal conclusion is that the main driver of benefit is from lowering of BP; little evidence exists of additional benefits specific to a class of drug with regard to major cardiovascular outcomes. However, this generalization needs to be expressed with a few caveats.
- Calcium antagonists may be less protective than other agents against the development of heart failure.
- Previous concerns over the safety of calcium antagonists are unfounded.
- Calcium antagonists may have a small, and angiotensin receptor blockers an even greater, benefit with regards to stroke reduction compared with other agents.
- Specific drug classes may have compelling indications in certain clinical situations (see below).

Most hypertensive patients will require drug combinations to achieve adequate BP control. Drug classes generally have additive effects on BP when prescribed together, so submaximal doses of two drugs result in larger BP responses. This approach may be associated with fewer side-effects than maximal doses of a single drug.

Each hypertensive patient needs to be considered separately when considering the choice of therapy (see Table 5.4), the choice being determined by factors such as age, co-morbidity (e.g. diabetes, coronary heart disease, asthma) and

Table 5.4 The choice of drug class for treating hypertension (adapted from British Hypertension Society Guidelines, 1999).

Class of drug	Compelling indication	Possible indication	Possible contraindication	Compelling contraindication
α-Blockers	Prostatism	Dyslipidaemia	Postural hypotension	Urinary incontinence
ACE inhibitors	Heart failure Left ventricular dysfunction Type I diabetic nephropathy	Chronic renal disease* Type II diabetic nephropathy	Renal impairment* Peripheral vascular disease†	Pregnancy Renovascular disease
Angiotensin II receptor antagonists	ACE inhibitor-induced cough	Heart failure Intolerance of other antihypertensive drugs	Peripheral vascular disease†	Pregnancy Renovascular disease
β-Blockers	Myocardial infarction Angina	Heart failure‡	Heart failure‡ Dyslipidaemia Peripheral vascular disease	Asthma/chronic obstructive pulmonary disease Heart block
Calcium anatgonists (dihydropyridine)	Elderly isolated systolic hypertension	Elderly angina	—	—
Calcium antagonists (rate-limiting)	Myocardial infarction Angina	—	Combination with β-blockade	Heart failure Heart block
Thiazides	Elderly	—	Dyslipidaemia	Gout

* ACE inhibitors may be beneficial in chronic renal failure but should be used with caution and under specialist supervision.
† Caution with ACE inhibitors and angiotensin II receptor antagonists in peripheral vascular disease because of possible coexistence of renovascular disease.
‡ β-Blockers may acutely worsen heart failure, but with specialist guidance are used in the long-term treatment of heart failure.

the drug's pharmacological profile and side-effects. However, when no other drug is particularly indicated or contraindicated, the British Hypertension Society proposed an AB/CD algorithm (2004 guidelines) where A = ACE inhibitor or angiotensin receptor blocker, B = β-blocker, C = calcium channel blocker and D = diuretic (thiazide and thiazide-like) (see Fig. 5.3). The basis of this algorithm is broadly that hypertension can be classified as being either 'high renin' or 'low renin' varieties. People **under 55 years** of age **and white** have **higher renin** levels, whereas those who are **older, or of black African descent**, tend to have **lower renin** levels. Therefore, A + B drugs are more effective in younger white patients, and C + D drugs more effective in those who are older or black people of any age. If two drugs are required, logical combinations are (A or B) + (C or D). If three drugs are needed, the combination (A or B) + C + D is recommended, and if hypertension remains resistant A + B + C + D or the addition of an α-blocker or low-dose spironolactone are options.

The AB/CD algorithm should be regarded as a useful template for guidance and not an inflexible directive. More recently (2006), the 'B' in the algorithm, which was referred to in parentheses, has been removed altogether as a result of further data from outcome trials, which have suggested:

- an increased incidence of diabetes in patients with B or D drugs, compared with A + C, particularly when B + D are combined; and
- inferiority of β-blockers in reducing major cardiovascular events (particularly stroke) when compared with other drugs.

Most recent guidance (NICE, 2006) has therefore concluded that, in the absence of other compelling indications for β-blockade (e.g. angina), β-blockers should not be a preferred **initial** treatment for hypertension. NICE also recommends, where possible, that treatment is with drugs taken only once per day and, where there is equivalence of efficacy, the least costly option should be chosen.

Hypertensive crisis

When the BP rises over a few days to levels above around 180/120 mmHg, renal failure and hypertensive encephalopathy may follow. It is important to lower BP, but to do so in as controlled and gradual manner as possible because too rapid

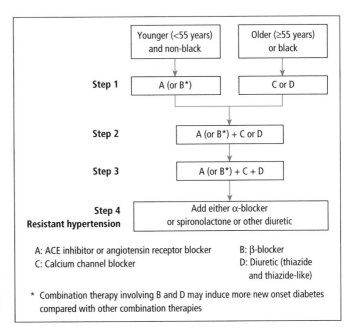

Fig. 5.3 Recommendations for combining blood pressure-lowering drugs (AB/CD rule). Courtesy of the British Hypertension Society.

reduction can result in cerebral and renal under-perfusion. Intravenous agents such as labetalol, diazoxide, esmolol, nicardipine and sodium nitroprusside are used, although use of the last should be limited to a few days because of the risk of thiocyanate accumulation.

Additional drug therapy

Aspirin

Guidance remains the same as given in the BHS 2004 guidelines, namely that aspirin 75 mg should be given:
• as **primary prevention** in hypertensive patients aged 50 years or over, with controlled BP (<150/90 mmHg) and:
  – target organ damage and/or
  – diabetes and/or
  – a calculated 10-year cardiovascular risk ≥20% (Joint British Societies' guidelines on prevention of cardiovascular disease in clinical practice, 2005)
• as **secondary prevention** for **all** hypertensive patients who have evidence of existing cardiovascular disease (e.g. angina, myocardial infarction) or diabetes.

Statins

In keeping with European guidelines (Guidelines for Management of Hypertension, 2004), the British Hypertension Society recommends that statins should be used at appropriate doses to achieve ideal target cholesterol levels (total cholesterol <4.0 mmol/L or low-density lipoprotein (LDL) cholesterol <2.0 mmol/L):
• as **primary prevention** in hypertensive patients (up to at least the age of 80 years) with a baseline total cholesterol ≥3.5 mmol/L and a calculated 10-year cardiovascular risk of ≥20% (Joint British Societies' guidelines on prevention of cardiovascular disease in clinical practice, 2005);

• as **secondary prevention** for **all** hypertensive patients (up to at least the age of 80 years), who have evidence of existing cardiovascular disease (e.g. angina, myocardial infarction) or diabetes. This is irrespective of baseline cholesterol levels.

Further reading

Blood Pressure Lowering Treatment Triallists' Collaboration. Effects of different blood-pressure lowering regimens on major cardiovascular events: results of prospectively-designed overviews of randomized trials. *Lancet* 2003; 362: 1527–45.

British Hypertension Society Guidelines for Hypertension Management (BHS-IV): Summary. *British Medical Journal* 2004; 328: 634–40.

European Society of Hypertension/European Society of Cardiology guidelines for the management of arterial hypertension. *Journal of Hypertension* 2003; 21: 1011–53.

Guidelines for management of hypertension. Report of the fourth working party of the British Hypertension Society, 2004 — BHS IV. *Journal of Human Hypertension* 2004; 18: 139–85.

Joint British Societies' guidelines on prevention of cardiovascular disease in clinical practice. *Heart* 2005;91:1–52. http://heart.bmj.com/cgi/content/full/91/suppl_5/v1

National Institute for Health and Clinical Excellence (NICE) Clinical Guideline 34. *Management of Hypertension in Adults in Primary Care.* June 2006 (and see http://www.nice.org.uk/guidance/CG34/guidance/pdf/English). Update of previous Clinical Guideline 18 (see http://www.nice.org.uk/CG018).

Seventh Report of the Joint National Committee on Prevention, Detection, Evaluation, and Treatment of High Blood Pressure: the JNC 7 report. *Journal of the American Medical Association* 2003; 289: 2560–72.

Chapter 6

Coronary heart disease

Epidemiology

Since the last edition of *Lecture Notes: Cardiology* (published in 2002), there have been further significant improvements in the cardiovascular disease-related mortality and morbidity in the UK. Cardiovascular disease now kills just over one in three of the population (39%), and accounted for 216 000 deaths in 2004: one in five men and one in six women who die annually do so from coronary heart disease (CHD), which represents approximately half of all deaths attributable to cardiovascular disease. There is a misconception that CHD occurs rarely in women: in fact, there is little difference in the incidence of the disease taking into account the longer life expectancy of women compared with men.

Although CHD remains the main cause of premature mortality in the UK, death rates have been falling progressively over the last 30 years. This is particularly true for the older age groups, where, for example, there has been a 49% fall for men aged 55–64 years compared with a 30% fall for men aged 35–44 years. For women, the equivalent figures are 56 and 20% for older and younger women, respectively. A number of other countries including Norway, Australia and New Zealand have exceeded the UK's fall in mortality. Death rates for CHD in the UK used to be one of the highest in the world but are now exceeded by many other countries, particularly those from the former Eastern bloc, together with Ireland. In the UK, there are marked regional, socio-economic and ethnic differences in the prevalence of CHD, rates being higher in the north of England and Scotland, in manual workers and in the Asian population.

A reduction in death rate from CHD was one of the ambitious targets in *The Health of the Nation* paper (Department of Health, 1996); the target set for 2005 had already been exceeded by 2002. In the UK there are approximately 338 000 new cases of angina each year, of which 178 500 are in men and 159 500 are in women. Currently in the UK there are approximately 2 million people who have or have had angina, of whom 1 million are men and 920 000 are women. In the UK there are approximately 268 000 heart attacks each year, of which 147 000 are in men and 121 000 are in women. Within the UK there are over 1.2 million people who have had a heart attack, of whom around 838 000 are men and 394 000 are women.

Overall, there were approximately 421 000 inpatient cases treated for CHD in National Health Service hospitals in 2004/2005; these represent 5% of all inpatient cases in men and 2% in women; the number of inpatient cases treated for CHD has increased by almost 11% in the last 4 years. CHD cost the health care system in the UK approximately £3500 million in 2003, which represents a cost per capita of approximately £60. The cost of hospital care for people who have CHD accounted for about 79% of these costs, that of drugs and of dispensing them about 16%.

In 2003, production losses due to mortality and morbidity associated with CHD cost the UK over £3100 million, with around 70% of this cost (£2173 million) due to death and 30% (£961 million) due to illness in those of working age. The cost of informal care for people with CHD in the UK was around £250 million in 2003.

The *National Service Framework for Coronary Heart Disease* (Department of Health, 2000) set a series of targets for the investigation and treatment of the patient with CHD, from primary through to tertiary care; the document also attempted to standardize access to facilities across the UK. The provision for the investigation and treatment of patients with CHD in the UK falls far behind Europe, with a significant minority of the population not having immediate access to a specialist cardiologist in their local hospital. However, since the publication of the *National Service Framework* in 2000, the number of cardiologists working in the NHS increased by just under 50% between September 1999 and March 2004, from 467 to 685. Over the same period, the number of consultant cardiothoracic surgeons increased by 19%, from 182 to 217: it is estimated that 1200–1500 consultant cardiologists will be needed by 2010.

Risk factors (see Box 6.1)

Lipids and diet

The percentage of food energy derived from fat in the British diet has fallen gradually over the last 30 years, from 40% to 37%. More impressive has been the shift away from saturated fat intake, from 19% to 14%. The significant regional differences in fat intake are matched by the increase in fresh fruit and vegetable consumption in the south, particularly amongst the professional classes. There is a direct relationship between the risk of CHD and levels of blood cholesterol. In the UK, cholesterol levels are high: in men the mean blood cholesterol is 5.6 mmol/L; in women it is 5.7 mmol/L. Sixty-six per cent of the UK population have levels in excess of 5.0 mmol/L, which would be regarded as high.

Cholesterol is transported in the blood in the form of lipoproteins, 75% as low-density lipopro-

> **Box 6.1 Selected risk factors for CHD**
>
> - Elevated cholesterol
> - Smoking
> - Obesity
> - Diabetes mellitus
> - Systemic hypertension
> - Male gender
> - Family history (CHD)
> - Personality
> - Physical activity
> - Clotting disorders

tein (LDL) and 20% as high-density lipoprotein (HDL). Low levels of LDL cholesterol are implicated in CHD, and there is an inverse relationship between HDL levels and the incidence of CHD.

The role of triglycerides as a risk factor for CHD is controversial. Grossly elevated triglyceride levels are associated with pancreatitis and should be treated. Similarly, combined hyperlipidaemia (e.g. in patients with diabetes) warrants intervention, but the power of an elevated triglyceride as an isolated risk factor once cholesterol has been normalized is weak.

Increased levels of lipoprotein (a) are an independent risk factor for CHD. The function of this protein is unclear, but it has been implicated in familial CHD risk and can be found in atherosclerotic plaque in association with fibrinogen.

Smoking

Approximately 24% of deaths from CHD in men and 11% in women are due to smoking. Although there has been a progressive decline in the proportion of the population who smoke since the 1970s, in 2003 28% of UK men and 24% of women still smoked. Of particular concern is the prevalence of smoking in teenagers, which is increasing, especially in young girls. Non-smokers who live with smokers (i.e. passive smokers) have a 25% increase in risk compared with those living with other non-smokers. The risk of developing CHD from smoking is dose-related, with those smoking 20 or more cigarettes daily having a risk of two to three times that of the general population of developing a major coronary event.

The role of smoking in the pathogenesis of CHD is complex and includes:

- promotion of atherosclerosis;
- increase in thrombogenesis;
- increased vasoconstriction (including coronary artery spasm);
- increase in blood pressure (BP) and heart rate;
- provocation of cardiac arrhythmias;
- increase in myocardial oxygen demand;
- reduction in oxygen-carrying capacity.

The risk of developing CHD from smoking falls to 50% at 1 year after smoking cessation, and to normal within 4 years of quitting the habit. Smoking is also a major risk factor in the development of:

- lung cancer;
- chronic airflow obstruction (chronic bronchitis and emphysema);
- cerebral and peripheral vascular disease;
- abdominal aortic aneurysm;
- recurrent angina following coronary revascularization procedures (coronary artery bypass grafting (CABG) and coronary angioplasty).

Obesity

There is an inter-relationship between weight, an elevated BP, raised blood cholesterol, non-insulin-dependent diabetes mellitus (NIDDM) and low levels of physical activity. The proportion of the population who are classified as obese (body mass index (BMI) >30 kg/m^2) in the UK has increased progressively in the last 20 years. Approximately 23% of men and 24% of women are obese, and an additional 44% of men and 35% of women are judged to be overweight (BMI 25–30 kg/m^2).

Diabetes mellitus

Patients with diabetes have more severe, more aggressive, more complex and more diffuse CHD than do age-matched controls. In general, coronary disease develops at a younger age than in the non-diabetic patient. In insulin-dependent diabetes, premature coronary disease is detectable in population studies from the fourth decade, and by the age of 55 years up to one-third of patients have died from the complications of CHD: the presence of microalbuminaemia or diabetic nephropathy increases the risk of CHD significantly.

The risk of developing CHD in the patient with NIDDM is 2–4 times higher than in the general population and does not appear to relate to either the severity or the duration of the diabetes, possibly because the presence of insulin resistance may pre-date the onset of clinical symptoms by 15–25 years. Diabetes, although an independent risk factor for CHD, is also associated with the presence of abnormalities of lipid metabolism, obesity, systemic hypertension and an increase in thrombogenesis (increased platelet adhesiveness and elevated levels of fibrinogen). Late results of CABG are less favourable in patients with diabetes, and diabetics have both an increased early mortality and a higher risk of restenosis following coronary angioplasty.

Systemic hypertension (see Chapter 5)

The risk of CHD is directly related to BP: for each 5 mmHg reduction in diastolic BP the risk of CHD is reduced by approximately 16%. BP values for the UK population are generally high: approximately 34% of men and 30% of women are hypertensive, defined as a systolic BP of >140 mmHg and a diastolic pressure of >90 mmHg.

Gender and sex hormones

Morbidity from CHD in males is twice that in females, and the condition occurs approximately 10 years earlier in men compared with women. Endogenous oestrogen is protective in women, but after the menopause the incidence of CHD rises steeply and parallels that seen in men. Smokers have an earlier menopause than non-smokers. Symptoms from CHD in women may be atypical: this, coupled with gender bias and difficulties with interpretation of standard investigations (e.g. treadmill exercise test), leads to the under-investigation of females compared with males. Furthermore, the results of revascularization procedures are more beneficial in men and are associated with a higher perioperative complication rate in women.

The use of oral contraceptives increases the risk of CHD approximately threefold, with some evidence that the risk with the newer, third generation preparations may be less. There is a synergistic relationship between oral contraceptive use and smoking, with a relative risk for myocardial infarction of >20:1.

Family history

A family history of CHD in a first-degree relative aged less than 70 years is an independent risk factor for the presence of CHD, with an odds ratio of 2–4 times that of a control population. Family aggregation of CHD suggests a genetic predisposition to the condition. There is some evidence that a positive family history may influence the age of onset of CHD in near relatives.

Race

Asians living in the UK have a higher incidence of premature death from CHD than the indigenous population, which is matched by a lower rate for Afro-Caribbeans.

Geography

Death rates from CHD are higher in Northern Ireland, Scotland and the north of England, and may reflect in part differences in diet, water hardness, smoking, the socio-economic structure and urban living.

Social class

Socio-economic gradients in CHD mortality are widening, such that premature death rates from CHD are three times higher for male unskilled workers compared with members of the professions (e.g. doctors, lawyers). Furthermore, the wives of manual workers are at least twice as likely to die prematurely from CHD as the wives of non-manual workers. Other risk factors are inter-related, including diet, cigarette consumption, obesity and exercise, etc.

Personality

Stress, either physical or mental, is a risk factor for CHD. In the present era, the work environment has become a major cause of stress, and there is an inter-relationship between stress and abnormalities of lipid metabolism. Coronary-prone behaviour (Type A personality) includes aggression, competitiveness, hostility, cynicism, desire for recognition and achievement, sleep disturbance, road rage, etc. Both anxiety and depression are important predictors of CHD.

Physical activity

Regular aerobic activity reduces the risk of CHD, although only 11% of men and 4% of women meet government targets for exercise. It is estimated that one-third of men and two-thirds of women cannot sustain a normal walking pace up a gradual slope (3 mph up a 5% gradient). Regular exercise may be associated with a 20–40% reduction in the incidence of CHD.

Clotting

A number of thrombogenic elements may influence the incidence of CHD, including levels of fibrinogen, endogenous fibrinolytic activity, blood viscosity and the levels of factors VII and VIII. Inhibitors of plasminogen activators (e.g. plasminogen activator inhibitor PAI-1) appear to be increased in some patients with CHD. The increased incidence of CHD in patients with the rare autosomal recessive disorder of homocystinuria may be manifest through altered clotting.

Infection

Infection with *Chlamydia pneumoniae*, an intracellular Gram-negative organism and a common cause of respiratory disease, may be linked to the presence of atherosclerotic coronary disease.

Alcohol

Although there is a theoretical basis for the protective effect of low to moderate doses of alcohol, this is controversial. Alcohol in low dose increases endogenous thrombolysis, reduces platelet adhesion and increases circulating levels of HDL, but the literature is not uniformly supportive of the concept. Increasing doses of alcohol are associated with an increase in cardiovascular mortality due to arrhythmias, systemic hypertension and dilated cardiomyopathy.

Pathophysiology

Angina pectoris occurs as a consequence of myocardial ischaemia. Oxygen supply fails to meet oxygen demand, due invariably to a reduction in supply as a consequence of impaired coronary artery flow. Major determinants of myocardial oxygen consumption (MVO_2) include systolic wall tension, contractile state and heart rate. The subendocardium is particularly sensitive to ischaemia, and the redistribution of myocardial perfusion in the presence of coronary stenoses may account for susceptibility to subendocardial infarction. The presence of ventricular hypertrophy is an additional factor affecting the likelihood of subendocardial ischaemia.

Fixed obstruction

The effect of an atherosclerotic stenosis on coronary flow dynamics is complex and may be affected by numerous variables including lesion severity, complexity, length, coronary vascular tone, pressure drop across the lesion, branch points, turbulence, etc. At rest, luminal diameter must be reduced by >75% to affect flow, but maximal flow (e.g. during exercise) may be reduced when the lumen is impaired by as little as 30%. In clinical practice, a lesion of >50% on a coronary arteriogram is judged 'significant'.

Coronary artery spasm

Alterations in coronary vascular tone via endogenous nitric oxide production may account for much of the variation in 'angina threshold' between one patient and another, and one day and the next. Many factors modulate coronary artery

tone including hypoxia, endogenous catecholamines, and vasoactive substances, which may be derived from platelets (e.g. serotonin, adenosine diphosphate) or endothelium (e.g. endothelium-derived relaxing factor, EDRF).

Collaterals

The presence of collateral vessels may offer alternative routes of myocardial perfusion when a major epicardial coronary artery is either stenosed or occluded. These channels are dormant in normal circumstances, but within a few hours existing collaterals dilate and go on to develop the characteristics of a mature vessel. Numerous factors determine the collateral response to myocardial ischaemia, but it is clear that collateral blood flow can develop very rapidly, for example during balloon occlusion of a vessel during coronary angioplasty.

Plaque-fissure

A sudden change in the pattern of angina from stable to unstable or the occurrence of an acute myocardial infarct is usually related to the presence of a plaque-fissure. At points of high shear stress (e.g. on the acute margin of the right coronary artery), and often in association with a minor atherosclerotic plaque, the wall of the artery (the internal elastic lamina) is breached and the thrombogenic constituents of the arterial wall are exposed to the lumen (Fig. 6.1). This results in platelet deposition,

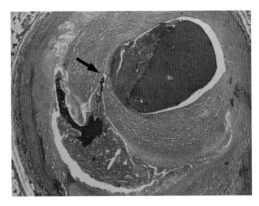

Fig. 6.1 Plaque-fissure.

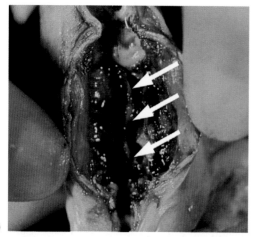

(a)

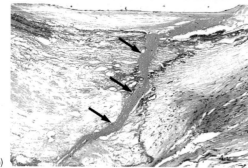

(b)

Fig. 6.2 (a) Coronary artery dissection. (b) Histology of the early stages of a coronary dissection with blood tracking deep into the arterial wall.

thrombus formation and a rapid reduction in coronary blood flow: thus, a minor lesion may over a period of a few minutes progress to coronary dissection (Fig. 6.2a and b) and acute occlusion.

Angina: clinical syndromes

(see Box 6.2)

Stable angina

Having a clinical diagnosis of chest pain with other symptoms provoked by a number of stimuli (see below), stable angina is relieved by rest or removal of the stimulus. Symptoms are provoked by myocardial ischaemia, usually occurring as a result of impaired myocardial blood supply as a consequence of a significant (>50%) stenosis (either fixed

---

or dynamic) of an epicardial coronary artery. In stable angina, symptoms are reversible and not progressive.

Acute coronary syndromes (ACS)

It was clear that the World Health Organization (WHO) definition of acute myocardial infarction dating from 1979 was too restrictive, therefore the term acute coronary syndromes (ACS) was defined by a joint committee of the European Society of Cardiology and the American College of Cardiology in 2000. Within this spectrum of patients with ischaemic chest pain at rest, three categories were defined: unstable angina (UA); non-ST segment elevation (non-Q wave) myocardial infarction (NSTEMI); and ST segment elevation (Q-wave) myocardial infarction.

The term unstable angina (UA) should be restricted to describing a subgroup of patients who exhibit angina of increasing frequency and severity, with attacks that are often prolonged and only partially relieved by sublingual nitrates. The history is usually short (days or weeks) and the prognosis is poor, with a significant likelihood of progression to established myocardial infarction or sudden death. In that the key discriminatory test for diagnosing an NSTEMI is elevation of troponin, which may not be significantly raised for up to 12 h after the onset of chest pain, it is not always possible to differentiate between UA and NSTEMI at the time of initial presentation on the basis of symptoms alone. Furthermore, it is important to introduce the appropriate treatment for NSTEMI (including clopidogrel) early, often before the troponin levels are available. The change in definition occurring in 2000 has resulted in 10–20% of patients who would originally have been diagnosed as UA being reclassified as NSTEMI on the basis of an isolated troponin rise. Two large surveys (Euro Heart Survey and the GRACE Registry) have determined the relative frequency of the three ACS categories as STEMI 30–33%, NSTEMI 25% and UA 38–42% (see also Acute myocardial infarction, page 104).

Silent ischaemia

Ambulatory (Holter) monitoring in patients with CHD frequently demonstrates episodes of prolonged and significant (>1 mm) ST segment depression. These episodes may occur with or without associated symptoms, and there is evidence that reversible abnormalities of myocardial metabolism (confirmed on PET scanning) and function (both diastolic and systolic) may occur, even in the absence of symptoms. It has been suggested that asymptomatic episodes of ST segment depression ('silent ischaemia') may be the harbinger of symptomatic episodes that occur later in the natural history of the disease. Silent ischaemia appears to show a diurnal variation, with higher frequencies in the early hours, and may occur in the setting of autonomic dysfunction (e.g. in patients with diabetes) or following myocardial infarction.

Syndrome X

This syndrome should be reserved to describe the patient with symptoms of typical angina, often not exercise-related, but provoked by emotion and anxiety, and being diurnal in character, in the setting of normal epicardial coronary arteries on coronary arteriography. The condition is probably heterogeneous in aetiology, but should not be used to include the patient with atypical symptoms. In the absence of large vessel coronary artery disease, the microvasculature is likely to be abnormal, in terms of either structure or functional integrity. There would appear to be an association with ventricular hypertrophy, systemic hypertension, glucose intolerance and insulin resistance. Myocardial scintigraphy and PET scanning may be abnormal in the patient with syndrome X.

Prinzmetal's variant angina

Described by Prinzmetal in 1959, variant angina describes symptoms of angina at rest in association with ST segment elevation on the electrocardiogram (ECG) indicating transmural ischaemia. This uncommon condition appears to relate to the presence of augmented coronary artery tone, which is rapidly relieved by nitroglycerine and may be provoked by acetylcholine. Variant angina may occur in structurally normal coronary arteries, in the presence of mild 'fixed' coronary disease or in the setting of severe occlusive coronary stenoses.

Clinical history

Eliciting a good clinical history in the patient suffering from angina pectoris is fundamental to making an accurate diagnosis of possible CHD. This is especially true as physical examination is frequently non-contributory due to the paucity of physical signs. The hallmark is the presence of chest pain. The patient with chest pain presenting to the general practitioner is likely to have a cardiac cause 20% of the time, but this increases to 70% in a patient who calls an ambulance.

Chest pain

Many patients favour a description of their symptoms that does not include the word 'pain': 'tightness', 'heaviness', 'pressure' and 'ache' are all descriptors of the sensation which is frequently localized to the midline, in the retrosternal region. The use of non-verbal clues, for example a clenched fist or the flat of the hand applied firmly to the chest, is helpful as an additional pointer to the diagnosis. Very well-localized pain, superficial pain and chest wall discomfort that is tender to the touch are not typical of myocardial ischaemia. Symptoms may be localized to the arm (most commonly on the left side), the jaw or neck, and less commonly to the epigastrium. Angina tends to radiate from the axilla down the inside of the arm rather than down the lateral aspect of the arm, which is more typical of musculoskeletal pain originating from the cervical spine. Sensory symptoms in the arms (numbness, heaviness and loss of use) are common.

Anginal pain is short lived, lasting less than 5 min, and is usually provoked by exertion, emotion, food, anxiety, change in ambient temperature or smoking a cigarette. Exercise with the arms (e.g. shaving, brushing teeth) appears to be particularly potent in provoking angina. Exercise tolerance may be abbreviated when walking after a meal (postprandial pain) because of the necessary increase in cardiac output required for digestion. Typically, attacks are relieved by rest, removal of the emotional stimulus or by the administration of sublingual nitrates. More prolonged attacks suggest the presence of unstable angina or impending myocardial infarction. In women, attacks may be more atypical, occurring at rest or at night, with, at other times, a normal exercise tolerance. Angina on lying down (decubitus angina) occurs as a result of an increase in venous return and cardiac output, and pain at night is more common during REM (rapid eye movement) sleep or in association with dreaming. Some patients can 'walk through' their pain (second wind phenomenon) due to the recruitment of collaterals.

Breathlessness

Apprehension, sweating and breathlessness may occur in association with chest pain. Occasionally, breathlessness without chest pain may occur in the patient with severe coronary disease or associated left ventricular dysfunction, as a result of a raised left ventricular end-diastolic pressure (LVEDP) and a transient reduction in pulmonary compliance.

Altered consciousness

Syncope is rare in angina, although it may be provoked by nitrate ingestion, and should alert the clinician to an alternative diagnosis. Dizziness or presyncope in association with palpitation may indicate the presence of an arrhythmia.

Physical signs

Whereas the clinical history in the patient with angina is the key to diagnosis, physical examination is often unrewarding unless symptoms are

---

> **Box 6.3 Disease associated with angina pectoris**
>
> - Atherosclerotic coronary artery disease
> - Coronary artery spasm
> - Coronary arteritis (e.g. SLE, Kawasaki)
> - Coronary artery ectasia
> - Aortic stenosis
> - Aortic regurgitation
> - Hypertrophic cardiomyopathy
> - Primary pulmonary hypertension
> - Pulmonary stenosis (rare)
> - Mitral stenosis (rare)

occurring as a result of a condition other than CHD (Box 6.3). It can be helpful to examine the patient during an episode of chest pain, which may reveal the presence of transient added heart sounds (third sound (S3) or fourth sound (S4)) or murmurs (e.g. secondary to mitral regurgitation (MR)).

Stigmata of hyperlipidaemia

A corneal arcus senilis may be significant in younger patients, but can be a normal finding in patients over the age of 40 years and not necessarily indicative of hyperlipidaemia. Xanthelasma (intracellular lipid deposits, usually around the eye) are correlated with levels of triglyceride but are often seen in patients with normal lipid levels. Tuberous, tendinous and eruptive xanthomas should be sought on the elbows, knees, Achilles tendon, dorsum of the hand and elsewhere, as they are indicative of hyperlipidaemia.

Systemic blood pressure

An elevated BP is an important risk factor for CHD.

Pulse

The pulse is frequently normal in the patient with stable angina. During an acute attack, a tachycardia or a transient arrhythmia (e.g. atrial fibrillation, ventricular tachycardia) may be evident. A resting tachycardia or pulsus alternans may indicate severe ischaemic myocardial dysfunction as a consequence of previous infarction.

Venous pressure

This is normal in uncomplicated angina, but venous pressure may be elevated as a result of previous myocardial infarction.

Precordial palpation

A dyskinetic or displaced apex may be indicative of previous myocardial infarction with ventricular dilatation or the presence of a left ventricular aneurysm, otherwise examination of the precordium is normal.

Auscultation

During attacks of angina, a reduction in ventricular compliance causes an increase in left atrial pressure with an audible S4. Prolonged ventricular ejection may result in paradoxical (reversed) splitting of second sound (S2). An S3 is unusual in patients with angina unless there is pre-existing myocardial damage. Papillary muscle ischaemia or abnormalities of papillary muscle alignment (which may be transient) may result in the late systolic murmur of mild MR. Of rare interest is the mid-diastolic murmur audible at the left sternal edge and apex from a proximal coronary artery stenosis.

Evidence of other vascular disease

Physical examination of the patient with coronary disease should include an examination of the peripheral and extra-cranial vasculature for the presence of bruits or absent pulses. Abnormal abdominal pulsation from an aortic aneurysm formation may also be present.

Differential diagnosis (see Box 6.4)

Having elicited an accurate clinical history, there is frequently little doubt that the patient is suffering from angina. The characteristic pain and radiation,

> **Box 6.4 Differential diagnosis of angina**
>
> - Chest wall pain
>   Da Costa syndrome
>   Tietze syndrome
> - Pleurisy
> - Pulmonary embolism
> - Aortic dissection
> - Diseases of the cervical spine
> - Gastrointestinal pathology

the temporal relationship to exercise or other provocative factors, and the relief by rest or sublingual nitrates are typical. Chest wall pain is usually well localized, sharp, fleeting, rarely in the midline and may be postural. This type of pain may also be associated with anxiety, dizziness, lassitude, sighing and hyperventilation (neurocirculatory asthenia or Da Costa syndrome). Pain and swelling of the costal cartilages (Tietze syndrome) is rare. Left-sided chest pain is more common, probably because most patients are aware that their heart is on the left side. Disease of the cervical spine may cause pain over the anterior chest, axilla and arm, but is usually associated with limitation of movement, clinical findings of reduced movement, muscle weakness and absent or attenuated reflexes in the upper limb.

Gastrointestinal pain may cause real difficulty as there are features shared with angina, and sublingual nitrates may relieve oesophageal spasm. The association of gastrointestinal pathology (e.g. hiatus hernia, gastritis, peptic ulceration, gall bladder disease and biliary colic) with eating certain foodstuffs, the presence of dyspepsia or acid reflux and the relief by antacids all help point to the gastrointestinal tract. Widespread availability of endoscopy and oesophageal motility testing can confirm the diagnosis in the majority of patients.

Investigations (see Box 6.5)

Resting electrocardiogram
(see Chapter 3)

A normal resting ECG does not exclude a diagnosis of angina, although there may be evidence of

Box 6.5 Investigations in stable sngina

- Resting ECG
- Chest radiograph
- Exercise ECG
- Echocardiogram
- Radionuclide scan
- Coronary arteriography

Box 6.6 Indications for exercise testing

- Assessment of objective exercise tolerance
- Nature of symptoms limiting exercise (chest pain, fatigue, breathlessness, etc.)
- Evaluation of haemodynamic response to exercise
- Document ST segment changes occurring with exercise or during the recovery period
- Evaluation of exercise-induced arrhythmias
- Document beneficial effects of surgical procedures, PCI or medical therapy
- Risk stratification following acute myocardial infarction
- Guide to rehabilitation following acute myocardial infarction
- Risk stratification in patients with hypertrophic cardiomyopathy

pre-existing myocardial infarction (Q waves, T wave inversion, LBBB). Conversely, the presence of minor ST segment (repolarization) abnormalities is common in the population at large and they are not necessarily indicative of underlying coronary disease. The sensitivity of the resting ECG (when compared with coronary arteriography) is approximately 50% and the specificity approximately 70%. Reversible changes in the baseline ECG occurring with episodes of chest pain (ST segment shift, T wave inversion) are indicative of occlusive coronary disease. Widespread ECG changes are associated with a poor prognosis as they are commonly associated with severe and diffuse coronary disease.

Box 6.7 Contraindications to exercise testing

- Unstable angina
- Acute pericarditis
- Acute myocarditis
- Uncontrolled blood pressure
- Heart failure
- Critical aortic stenosis
- Sustained ventricular arrhythmia
- High grade atrioventricular block
- Acute systemic illness

Chest radiograph

Chest radiography is usually normal in the patient with angina. Cardiac enlargement and/or an elevation in venous pressure may indicate previous myocardial infarction or left ventricular dysfunction. Occasionally, the presence of a left ventricular aneurysm results in the characteristic bulge or calcification within the cardiac silhouette (Fig. 6.18), but these radiographic findings may be unreliable.

Exercise testing

The treadmill exercise test is pivotal in the investigation of the patient with chest pain. It should be viewed as a natural extension to the clinical examination, allowing firm decisions to be made regarding the need for further invasive investigation (coronary arteriography). A well-supervised, maximum, symptom-limited exercise test using one of the standard protocols allows the patient to be stratified for future risk of subsequent cardiac events.

A number of parameters are evaluated during the test and, although there is emphasis on ECG changes, the appearance of the patient, the occurrence of symptoms, blood pressure and heart rate response, and the amount of work achieved are all-important determinants of prognosis.

Indications and contraindications to exercise testing are listed in Boxes 6.6 and 6.7. Exercise tests should be supervised by a physician or technical personnel trained in advanced life support in an area equipped with full resuscitation facilities. An exercise protocol should be applicable to a wide variety of patient groups, including children and the elderly, and allow the aerobic threshold to be reached in the majority of patients within a few minutes. A number of protocols are available, but in practice the modified or full Bruce protocol is in use in the majority of centres (Table 6.1). In most exercise laboratories, a treadmill rather than bicycle ergometry is used as the stimulus to exercise. The treadmill has the advantage that it is under the control of the supervisor, resulting in a higher level of achieved exercise.

Table 6.1 Exercise stress test protocols.

Stage	Speed (mph)	Gradient (%)	Duration (min)
Full (standard) Bruce protocol			
I	1.7	10	3
II	2.5	12	3
III	3.4	14	3
IV	4.2	16	3
V	5.0	18	3
VI	5.5	20	3
VII	6.0	22	3
Modified Bruce protocol			
I	1.7	0	3
II	1.7	5	3
III	1.7	10	3
IV	2.5	12	3
V	3.4	14	3
VI	4.2	16	3
VII	5.0	18	3

Physical exercise results in an increase in myocardial oxygen requirement (MVO_2), which will provoke angina in the patient with significant CHD. During dynamic exercise, increasing MVO_2 is linearly related to increasing cardiac output that is mainly brought about by an increase in heart rate. BP increases during exercise, and an increase in systolic BP is particularly marked. The 'double product' (peak heart rate × peak systolic BP) correlates well with peak MVO_2. A full 12-lead ECG should be recorded during exercise and following completion of the test at intervals until the heart rate and BP have fallen to pre-test levels. ECG changes occurring during the recovery period (coinciding with the time of oxygen debt) are a sensitive indicator of the presence of CHD, as is the time taken for normalization.

In patients with CHD, myocardial ischaemia is reflected as ST segment depression, which is seen most frequently in the lead with the tallest R wave (usually V_5). Criteria for 'significant' ST segment depression represent a compromise between sensitivity and specificity (Fig. 6.3). Most series define positivity as >1 mm planar (horizontal) or downsloping ST segment depression measured 80 ms after the J point (Fig. 6.4). Changes in T wave morphology may be provoked by respiration or changes in posture and do not reliably indicate myocardial ischaemia. Similarly, J point depression accompanies a tachycardia due to

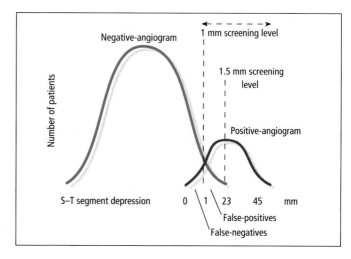

Fig. 6.3 Relationship between sensitivity and specificity of ST segment depression on exercise testing.

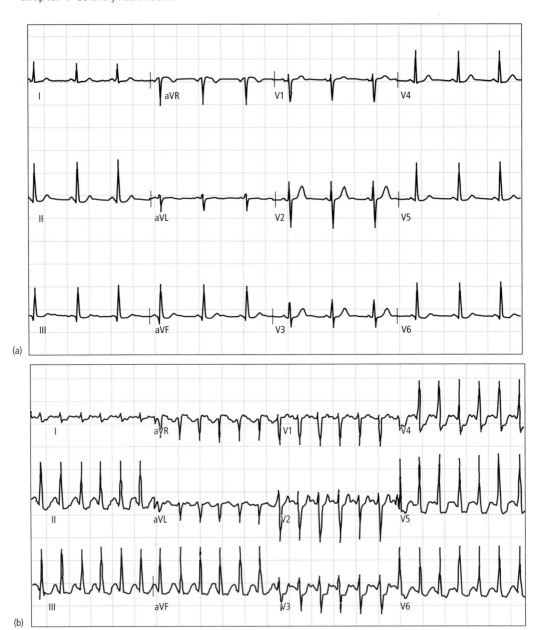

Fig. 6.4 (a) 12-lead ECG (rest). (b) 12-lead ECG (exercise) showing inferolateral ST segment depression.

shortening of the PR interval and repolarization of the atria. Rate-dependent aberrancy is an unreliable indicator of ischaemia. Some patients exhibit ST segment elevation, 'pseudonormalization' of inverted T waves or an increase in R wave amplitude, all of which may be provoked by ischaemia. Reasons for terminating an exercise test are listed in Box 6.8. A number of other conditions may give rise to repolarization changes on exercise (Box 6.9).

Radionuclide scintigraphy

Radionuclide imaging is not usually necessary in the routine investigation of patients with angina, but it may be useful in certain subgroups (Box 6.10). The patient is exercised using a standard protocol and the radionuclide (e.g. ^{201}Tl or ^{99m}Tc-sestamibi) is injected into a peripheral vein, and is taken up by perfused myocardium. The patient is then scanned using a gamma camera, and a series of tomographic (single photon emission computed tomography (SPECT)) images recorded in a variety of planes. These images are then compared with a second series of resting images recorded from similar angles (Fig. 6.5). Thus, areas of reversible ischaemia and/or infarction can be demonstrated and localized. Attention to technical detail and careful interpretation of the images, taking care not to

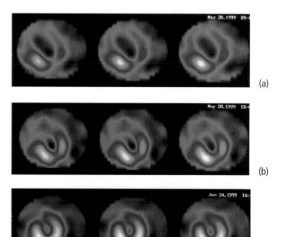

Fig. 6.5 Radionuclide scintigraphy using thallium with adenosine as a stress agent: (a) rest; (b) redistribution; and (c) re-injection traces.

over-report, are important if 'false positives' are to be avoided. Pharmacological stress using a variety of agents may be helpful in the patient who is unable to exercise (e.g. adenosine, arbutamine, dobutamine and dipyridamole).

Stress echocardiography

See Chapter 4.

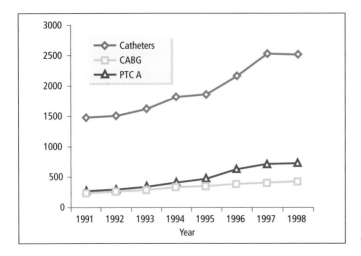

Stress magnetic resonance imaging

See Chapter 4.

Coronary arteriography

(see also Chapter 4)

Coronary arteriography is currently the only method of accurately delineating the coronary anatomy. The majority of clinical trials depend on a demonstration of the coronary anatomy to determine prognosis, and arteriography is a necessary prerequisite to CABG or percutaneous coronary intervention (PCI). It was estimated that 3418 procedures/million population were undertaken in the UK in 2005. Comparative data are available from 2003 when approximately 2 million catheter procedures where undertaken in Europe, a 5% increase on the previous year. Individual countries ranged from 100 to 5000 procedures/million population (Fig. 6.6).

Coronary arteriography, although an invasive investigation, is a low-risk procedure with a morbidity of 0.7% and a mortality of 0.07% in elective patients. Complications are higher in unstable patients, those with additional aortic valve disease, and in the setting of acute myocardial infarction or cardiogenic shock. Coronary arteriography is most commonly performed using a percutaneous femoral approach (the Judkins technique), in which preformed catheters are advanced retrogradely into

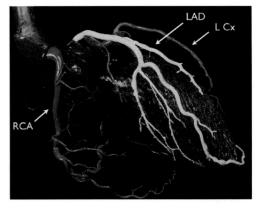

Fig. 6.7 Coronary anatomy (RCA, right coronary artery; LAD, left anterior descending; L Cx, left circumflex).

the left ventricle and each of the two coronary arteries in turn. An alternative, which is becoming more popular, is the radial artery approach. The brachial route accessed by either a cutdown (using the modified Sones technique) or percutaneously is used less frequently than formerly.

Coronary anatomy varies from patient to patient. There are two coronary arteries, the left and right (Fig. 6.7). The first segment of the left coronary artery, the left main stem, is the common trunk that divides into the anterior branch, the left anterior descending (LAD) and the posterior branch (the left circumflex). The RCA does not usually have major branches, but supplies the AV nodal artery and the posterior descending artery in about 90% of cases (right dominant anatomy). In the remaining 10% of patients, the posterior descending artery arises from the left circumflex (left dominant anatomy). The term 'three vessel disease' refers to involvement of all three major branches (i.e. the LAD, the left circumflex and the RCA). Coronary arteriography is usually combined with left ventriculography to assess ventricular systolic function and abnormalities of wall motion. Indications for invasive assessment will differ from one centre to another, but there is a general consensus that coronary arteriography is indicated in some groups of patients (Box 6.11).

The association between vascular calcification and vascular disease is well recognized, and coronary artery calcification (CAC) can be identified by electron beam computed tomography (EBCT). Although there is much commercial interest in EBCT, CAC screening was not recommended as a non-invasive screening test for risk prediction in asymptomatic patients by an ACC/AHA expert consensus document on EBCT in 2000 or an ACC/AHA guideline on stable angina in 2003.

The 'open access' chest pain clinic

Many centres offer open access clinics for the assessment of the patient with chest pain. The patient is seen by a dedicated team (who may include a cardiologist or physician, a technician and a nurse practitioner), who will take a clinical history, provide a treadmill exercise test, screen for risk factors and advise regarding risk factor modification. The general practitioner is then notified of suggested treatment options and the need for further investigation.

Medical management

General measures

Smoking

Epidemiological evidence suggests that the risk of subsequent myocardial infarction in patients suffering from angina is reduced by stopping smoking (see page 80).

Diet and weight reduction

The evidence that weight reduction *per se* favourably affects coronary risk is lacking, but there is a clear inter-relationship between obesity, systemic hypertension and abnormalities of lipids. Given that many patients who quit smoking put on weight, they should be advised that the cardiac risk of being an ex-smoker and overweight are significantly less than being a thin smoker.

Exercise and lifestyle

Regular physical exercise reduces the risk of CHD, and is likely to be associated with a healthier life-

---

Box 6.11 Indications for coronary arteriography

- Symptoms of coronary artery disease despite adequate medical therapy
- Determination of prognosis in a patient with known coronary artery disease
- Stable chest pain with marked ischaemic changes on an exercise test
- Widespread reversible ischaemia on a myocardial perfusion scan
- Patients with chest pain in whom the aetiology is unclear
- Acute coronary syndromes (ACS) (particularly with elevated troponin T or I)
- Following NSTEMI
- Following STEMI to determine revascularization strategy and future prognosis
- Survivors of near-miss sudden death
- Patients with sustained or recurrent ventricular arrhythmias (e.g. ventricular tachycardia)
- Recurrent symptoms following coronary intervention (PCI or CABG)
- In patients undergoing surgery for valvular heart disease
- Prior to surgical correction of infarct-related ventricular septal defect or papillary muscle rupture
- In patients with heart failure where the aetiology is unclear
- To determine the cause of chest pain in hypertrophic cardiomyopathy

style. Exercise may have a cardioprotective effect as well as being of therapeutic use following acute myocardial infarction.

Specific therapy (see Box 6.12)

Aspirin

All patients with angina should receive aspirin unless there is a specific contraindication. A variety of doses has been used in the available trials, but a small dose of 75 mg daily has been shown to be adequate and is only rarely associated with gastro-intestinal side-effects. Aspirin reduces platelet adhesiveness and prolongs the bleeding time. Clopidogrel, although expensive, is a more potent platelet agent, which is suitable for patients intolerant or allergic to aspirin. This drug is widely used in the treatment of acute coronary syndromes (ACS) and PCI (see pages 84 and 101).

Nitrates

The actions of nitrates are complex and include a reduction in preload due to pooling of blood in venous capacitance vessels, reduced afterload and a fall in systemic BP, direct epicardial coronary dilatation, increased coronary perfusion pressure and redistribution of myocardial blood flow. Nitrates may also enhance coronary collateral flow.

A number of nitrate preparations are available, including sublingual, buccal, oral, transcutaneous and intravenous formulations (Table 6.2). Sublingual nitrates remain one of the most effective and convenient forms of drug treatment for an acute attack of angina. The metered aerosol spray has the advantage of a 3-year shelf-life, whereas glyceryl trinitrate tablets have a shelf-life of only 2 months, which can be prolonged to 6 months by refrigeration. An advantage of the tablet preparation is that the partially dissolved tablet can be removed from the mouth once the attack has been relieved, thereby reducing

---

Box 6.12 Medical treatment of acute coronary syndrome (ACS)

- Aspirin
- Clopidogrel
- β-Blockade
- ± Calcium antagonist
- Nicorandil
- Lipid-lowering therapy
- Nitrates
- Heparin (LMWH)
- ± ACE inhibitor (in patients with impaired LV function)

Table 6.2 Nitrate preparations.

Drug name	Trade name	Route	Dose
Glyceryl trinitrate	Cor-nitro, Glytrin, Nitrolingual, Nitromin, Generic	Sublingual	0.3–0.6 mg (prn)
	Sustac	Oral	2.6–30 mg daily (bd or tds)
	Susard	Buccal SR	2–6 mg daily (tds)
	Deponit, Minitran, Nitro-Dur, Transiderm-Nitro	Patch	5–20 mg daily (om)
	Percutol	Ointment	1/2–2 inches (tds or qds)
	Nitrocine, Nitronal	IV infusion	
Isosorbide dinitrate	Cedocard, Isoket, Sorbid SA	Oral	40–160 mg daily (bd)
	Isordil	Oral, sublingual	40–120 mg daily (bd or tds)
	Isocard	Dermal spray	30–120 mg daily (om or bd)
	Isoket	IV Infusion	
Isosorbide mononitrate	Elantan, Imdur, Isib, Ismo, Isodur XL, MCR-50, Monit, Mono-Cedocard, Monomax	Oral	20–120 mg (bd or tds)

om, every morning; bd, twice daily; tds, three times daily; qds, four times daily; prn, as required.

the side-effects of headache, flushing and postural dizziness; side-effects can be minimized by taking the drug whilst sitting. Many patients are given inadequate instruction on nitrate use, which can and should be administered both prophylactically and for the relief of an angina attack once it occurs; used in this way, the beneficial effects may last up to 1 h. Administration of sublingual nitrates may be a useful diagnostic test for the differentiation between angina and other causes of chest pain. Peak levels of the drug occur within 2 min with a plasma half-life of 7 min: 75% of patients obtain symptomatic relief within 3 min and a further 15% within 15 min.

Long-acting mononitrates have largely replaced dinitrates because of the virtually complete bioavailability without the disadvantage of extensive first-pass hepatic metabolism. Tolerance to long-acting nitrates, which is an ill-understood phenomenon, is common if there is not a nitrate-free period of at least 8 h in every 24 h.

β-Blockade

β-Blocking drugs remain the mainstay of drug treatment for angina, although in the last few years calcium antagonists have made a significant impact and are now used as monotherapy in a num-

ber of patients. β-Blocking drugs are competitive inhibitors of catecholamine binding at β-receptor sites. They reduce MVO_2 by two routes: (i) a direct myocardial action reduces LV systolic pressure, and the rate of pressure rise ($\delta p/\delta t$) (i.e. contractility); and (ii) the 'double product' (heart rate × systolic BP) is reduced in response to exercise. β-Blocking drugs are effective in reducing frequency and severity of attacks of angina and also improve prognosis by reducing the incidence of major cardiac events.

Choosing the appropriate β-blocking preparation depends on a number of factors, including the dosing regimen, cardioselectivity and the side-effect profile. Side-effects sufficient to cause withdrawal of the drug occur in 5–10% of patients. β-Blockers are contraindicated in patients with severe airflow obstruction, high-grade atrioventricular block or severe peripheral vascular disease.

Many of the secondary characteristics of β-blocking drugs (e.g. partial agonist activity, membrane-stabilizing activity and local anaesthetic action) have little practical clinical importance. Low lipid solubility may be beneficial, as a failure to cross the blood–brain barrier reduces the likelihood of central nervous system side-effects. Commonly used preparations are listed in Table 6.3.

Table 6.3 β-Blocking drugs.

Drug name	Trade name	Selectivity	Secondary properties	Lipid solubility	Dose
Acebutolol	Sectral	+	ISA, MSA	Low	400–1200 mg daily (om or bd)
Atenolol	Tenormin	+	–	Low	25–100 mg daily (om or bd)
Bisoprolol	Emcor, Monocor	+	–	Moderate	10–20 mg (om)
Labetalol	Trandate	–	–	Low	200–2400 mg daily (bd, tds, or qds)
Metoprolol	Betaloc, Lopresor	+	–	Moderate	50–300 mg daily (bd or tds)
Nadolol	Corguard	–	–	Low	40–160 mg daily (om)
Oxprenolol	Trasicor	–	ISA	Moderate	80–320 mg daily (bd or tds)
Pindolol	Visken	–	ISA, MSA	Moderate	2.5–15 mg daily (om, bd, or tds)
Propranolol	Beta-Prograne, Inderal	–	MSA	High	80–240 mg daily (bd or tds)
Timolol	Betim	–	–	Low	20–60 mg daily (bd)

om, every morning; bd, twice daily; tds, three times daily; qds, four times daily; ISA, intrinsic sympathomimetic activity; MSA, membrane-stabilizing activity.

Calcium antagonists

These are a heterogeneous group of drugs that inhibit the slow current channel by which calcium ions enter the cell to initiate smooth muscle contraction and intracardiac conduction. Thus, the administration of calcium channel blockers relaxes smooth muscle, reduces afterload and has a direct effect on coronary vasomotor tone, thereby reducing coronary artery spasm. Calcium antagonists have little effect on venous capacitance vessels. All calcium antagonists are negatively inotropic, which may in clinical practice be masked by the vasodilator effect. There has been concern raised over the possible excess in cardiac mortality when hypertensive patients or those with CHD are treated with nifedipine. As a result of a number of studies, it is clear that nifedipine should be avoided as monotherapy without concomitant β-blockade. Diltiazem is well tolerated and probably the best first-generation calcium antagonist used in the treatment of angina. The properties of the calcium antagonists are very different (Table 6.4).

Other drugs

Nicorandil offers a useful alternative in the treatment of angina, usually in combination with other drugs. This potassium channel blocker relaxes smooth muscle as well as providing direct vasodilatation of the coronary arteries. Side-effects are similar to those seen with oral nitrates.

In the absence of impaired ventricular function, **angiotensin-converting enzyme (ACE) inhibitors** have no role in the treatment of angina. ACE inhibitors have been shown to reduce the long-term risk of developing unstable angina or sudden death in patients with left ventricular dysfunction.

Hormone replacement therapy (HRT) has no role in the primary or secondary prevention of cardiovascular disease in women.

'Stepped' drug therapy in the management of stable angina

All patients should be treated with aspirin 75 mg daily. For very occasional episodes of angina, sublingual nitrates may be adequate. Most patients require treatment with a cardioselective β-blocker, or, alternatively, a calcium antagonist. In 10–20% of patients, additional drugs will be needed in the form of long-acting oral nitrates, or, alternatively, a calcium antagonist can be added to the β-blocker; resistant patients may require 'triple therapy' (β-blocker + calcium antagonist + nitrate) or 'quadruple therapy' ('triple therapy' + nicorandil). The threshold for proceeding to invasive investigation (i.e. coronary arteriography) has reduced in recent years such that the majority of patients requiring multiple drug therapy for symptomatic angina should be investigated invasively unless there are specific contraindications.

Table 6.4 Calcium antagonists.

Drug name	Trade name	Dose
Amlodipine	Istin	5–10 mg (om)
Diltiazem	Adizem, Angitil, Dilzem, Slozem, Tildiem, Viazem XL	60–120 mg (tds)
Felodipine	Plendil	5–10 mg (om)
Nicardipine	Cardene	20–40 mg (tds)
Nifedipine	Adalat, Adipine, Angiopine, Cardilate, Coracten, Fortipine LA, Tensipine	5–20 mg (bd or tds)
Nisoldipine	Syscor	10–40 mg (om)
Verapamil	Cordilox, Securon, Univer	80–120 mg (tds)

om, every morning; bd, twice daily; tds, three times daily.

Lipid-lowering therapy

An elevation in blood cholesterol is an important risk factor for CHD, but should be considered in the context of other risk factors such as smoking, raised BP and a lack of exercise. A significant number of patients will respond to a low-fat diet and weight reduction alone, but up to 40% will require additional lipid-lowering therapy; this is particularly true of patients with a family history of CHD. Patients who have undergone revascularization procedures should be treated aggressively as there is clear evidence that long-term graft function following CABG and the rate of restenosis following PCI can be improved with lipid-lowering therapy.

The European Guidelines categorize cardiovascular risk based on levels of LDL-cholesterol. Target LDL-cholesterol levels should be <2.5 mmol/L for individuals with established CVD, <3.0 mmol/L for asymptomatic patients with multiple risk factors, or with a markedly raised single risk factor, type II diabetes mellitus or type I diabetes mellitus with microalbuminuria; close relatives of patients with early onset CVD should also be treated if the LDL-cholesterol level is >3.0 mmol/L. In patients with established CHD or diabetes, the target total cholesterol should be <4.5 mmol/L, with a goal of <5.0 mmol/L for the general population. There is evidence that high levels of HDL-cholesterol (>1.6 mmol/L) are protective.

The Sheffield Table for primary prevention of CHD integrates the serum cholesterol in relation to other recognized risk factors that confer a 3% risk of CHD per year and should be treated with statins (Fig. 6.8). Increasing trial evidence has demonstrated the efficacy of statin therapy in both primary and secondary prevention as part of an integrated approach to reducing cardiovascular risk. Dietary modification, weight reduction, regular exercise, blood pressure control and lipid-lowering therapy are required in many at risk patients. If the target levels of LDL-cholesterol or total cholesterol are not achieved with a combination of diet and a statin, combined therapy with the addition of a fibrate and/or a cholesterol absorption inhibitor (e.g. ezetimibe) is indicated.

Classification of hyperlipidaemia and a simple treatment algorithm are shown in Table 6.5, and the expected changes in lipids and lipoproteins in Table 6.6.

In 2004, the cost of prescriptions for lipid-lowering drugs, including statins, was £769 million, an increase of £154 million since 2003. Lipid-lowering drugs now cost the NHS more than any other class of drug (overtaking ulcer-healing drugs in 2001).

Medical management of acute coronary syndromes (ACS) (see Box 6.12)

In view of the early cardiac risk, patients with ACS should be admitted to hospital, preferably to a Coronary Care Unit (CCU) environment, and treated with bed rest, aspirin, clopidogrel, heparin and intravenous nitrates as well as additional oral anti-anginal medication (including β-blockade), with a view to early invasive investigation and revascularization. Low molecular weight heparin is easier to administer than unfractionated heparin and does not require activated partial thromboplastin time (aPTT) monitoring and dose adjustment. There is controversy over routine use and cost-effectiveness of the small molecule II/IIIa antagonists (e.g. eptifibatide and tirofiban). Emphasis should be on rapid (same hospital admission) cardiac catheterization with consideration of treatment with upstream abciximab in patients with high-risk coronary anatomy who are proceeding to PCI (Fig. 6.9). If the patient is stabilized in hospital and sent home without revascularization, there is a high chance of recurrent symptoms or a major cardiac event.

Coronary revascularization

Coronary artery bypass grafting

CABG was first performed in the early 1960s and is now one of the most common surgical procedures undertaken: in the UK, 22 700 CABG procedures were performed in 2005. Reversed saphenous vein has been the graft conduit of choice for many years, but the superior patency rates of arterial conduits (e.g. internal mammary artery)

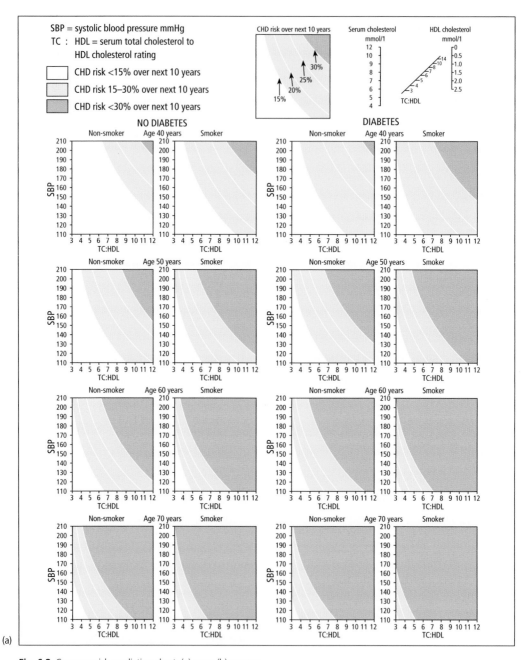

Fig. 6.8 Coronary risk prediction chart: (a) men; (b) women.

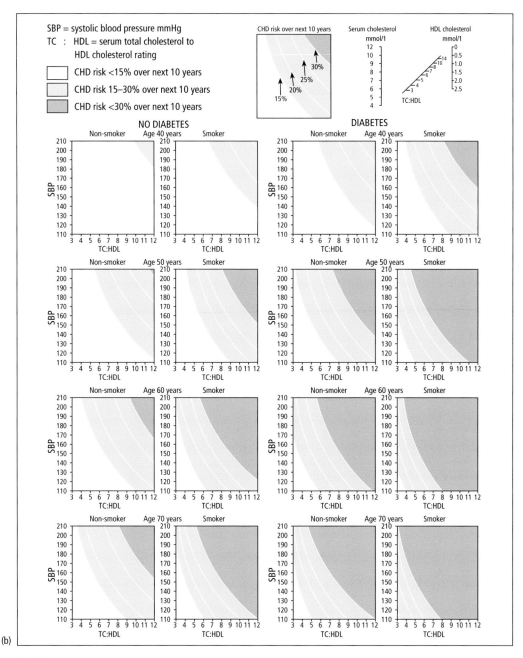

(b)

Fig. 6.8 *Continued*

Table 6.5 Classification of primary lipid disorders.

Lipoprotein (Frederickson) type	Molecular disorder	Genetic transmission	Estimated incidence	Cholesterol	Triglycerides	Clinical features
I	LPL, ApoC-II	Autosomal recessive	Rare	+++	+++	Eruptive xanthomas, hepato-splenomegaly, pancreatitis
IIa	LDL, ApoB-100	Autosomal dominant	1:500	++	Normal	Tendon xanthomas, premature atherosclerosis
IIb	Unknown	Autosomal dominant	1:200	+	+	Premature atherosclerosis
III	Apo-E	Autosomal recessive	Rare	++	+	Palmar and premature tuberoeuptive xanthomas atherosclerosis
IV	Unknown	Autosomal dominant	1:500	+	++	Usually none, or premature atherosclerosis
V	Unknown	Autosomal dominant	1:500	+++	+++	Eruptive xanthomas, premature atherosclerosis

Table 6.6 Expected changes in blood lipids with drug treatment.

	Lipids (% change)		Lipoproteins (% change)	
Drug	Cholesterol	Triglyceride	LDL	HDL
Statins	↓20–33%	↓10–30%	↓25–45%	↑2–15%
Fibrates	↓10–20%	↓30–50%	↓20–25%	↑10–25%
Nicotinic acid	↓15–30%	↓20–60%	↓5–40%	↑10–20%
Probucol	↓5–15%	↓0–5%	↓8–15%	↑10–25%
Fish oils	↓↑	↓10–60%	↓↑	↑5–10%

have resulted in most patients receiving at least one arterial graft. Early perioperative mortality for elective CABG is 1–3%. Risk factors for death include:

- poor myocardial function;
- recent myocardial infarction;
- haemodynamic instability;
- older age;
- female gender;
- diabetes mellitus;
- diffuse small vessel disease;
- environmental and institutional factors, including the choice of surgeon.

Early complications include perioperative myocardial infarction, bleeding, stroke, wound infection and atrial arrhythmias. Following successful surgery, 75–90% of patients are free from angina. Vein grafts occlude at the rate of 2–5% per annum, whereas the patency of a left internal mammary artery graft to the LAD is >90–95% at 10 years (Fig. 6.10).

In groups of patients with high-risk coronary anatomy, CABG has been shown to improve prognosis as well as symptoms: these include patients with a left main stem stenosis, triple-vessel disease, two-vessel disease including a proximal stenosis of

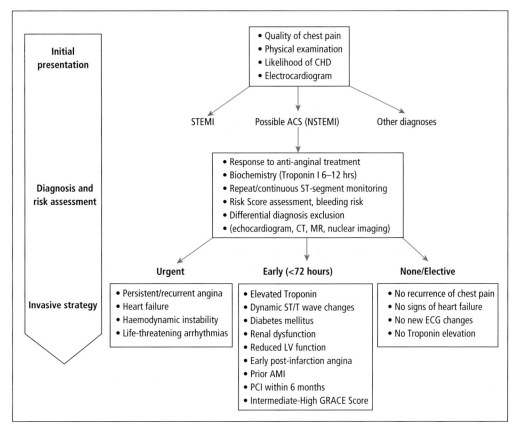

Fig. 6.9 Identification and management of acute coronary syndrome (NSTEMI). Adapted from Eur. Heart J 2007; 28:1598–1660.

the LAD and two-vessel disease with impaired ventricular function. Increasingly, patients undergoing surgical revascularization are being treated with off-pump and/or minimally invasive techniques, and complete arterial revascularization may lead to an improvement in long-term graft patency which should be translated into a more favourable long-term outcome.

Percutaneous coronary intervention (PCI)

Coronary balloon angioplasty was first performed by Andreas Gruentzig in 1977, and by 1990 the number of angioplasty procedures worldwide exceeded the number of CABG operations. In experienced centres, early mortality is approximately

1% depending on case-mix, and the rate of major complications (death, myocardial infarction and emergency CABG) is usually between 3 and 5%. Initially, simple balloon angioplasty was used to treat single, proximal, short, discrete, non-calcified lesions in large (>3 mm diameter) arteries. The procedure was carried out in centres with on-site surgical facilities because of the risk of abrupt vessel closure which followed successful dilatation in approximately 5% of patients. Abrupt vessel closure occurring as a result of arterial dissection and/or thrombus formation may result in the need for emergency CABG, acute myocardial infarction or sudden death. The major late problem associated with balloon angioplasty was restenosis, which was apparent clinically in 15–20% of patients who develop recurrent angina, or angiographically

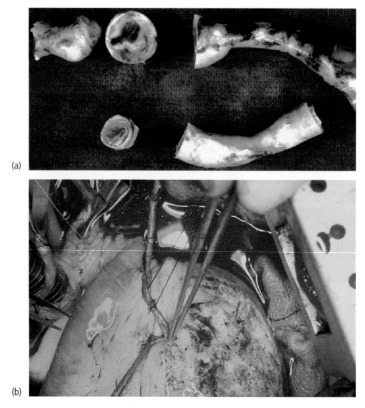

(a)

(b)

Fig. 6.10 (a) Diffuse graft atherosclerosis in an old vein graft. (b) Left internal mammary artery graft.

defined as >50% diameter restenosis in the target vessel. Restenosis occurs as a result of the migration of fibroblasts and connective tissue into the area of barotrauma resulting from balloon dilatation and intimal disruption. Restenosis appears to be more common in certain subsets of patients, including those with:

- proximal LAD lesions;
- vein graft disease;
- long lesions;
- small vessels;
- diabetes;
- restenotic lesions;
- patients who continue to smoke;
- patients with untreated hypercholesterolaemia.

No drug therapy has been shown to reduce the incidence of restenosis effectively following balloon angioplasty.

The first human implants of intracoronary stents were undertaken in 1986. The development of the stent was a landmark in interventional cardiology because the advent of intracoronary stainless steel 'scaffolding' reduced the incidence of abrupt vessel closure, acute myocardial infarction, sudden death and the need for emergency CABG (Fig. 6.11). It subsequently became clear from the BENESTENT and STRESS trials that stenting compared with simple balloon angioplasty reduced but did not abolish the incidence of late restenosis. The next important development was the introduction of drug-eluting stents which became available in Europe in 2002. The inflammation and subsequent restenosis caused by the stent itself could be reduced if the device was coated with a drug to reduce smooth cell proliferation and migration, platelet activation and extracellular matrix production. Two drugs demonstrated early efficacy;

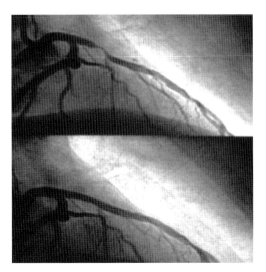

Fig. 6.11 Severe proximal stenosis (left anterior descending), before and after stent insertion.

sirolimus (rapamycin), that had been successfully used as an immunosuppressive agent, and paclitaxel, which was effective as an anti-cancer drug. The efficacy of the CYPHER stent loaded with sirolimus was demonstrated in the SIRIUS trial, and the TAXUS stent loaded with paclitaxel was extensively investigated in the TAXUS series of trials (TAXUS I–VI). Both drugs reduced angiographic restenosis compared with bare metal stents, typically from 30 to 10%, and reduced the need for ischaemia-driven target lesion revascularization from 16 to 6%, although there is no beneficial effect on all-cause mortality. By 2005, >3 million patients had been treated with >5 million drug-eluting stents worldwide; in the USA, >90% of patients undergoing percutaneous intervention received a drug-eluting stent.

The advent of stents has increased the applicability of percutaneous intervention to other patient subsets including those with multivessel disease, long lesions and vein grafts. Antiplatelet therapy in patients treated with drug-eluting stents includes pre-treatment with aspirin and clopidogrel, peri-procedural heparin, post-procedural clopidogrel for 12 months, and low-dose aspirin is continued indefinitely. With current antiplatelet regimens, early stent thrombosis occurs in approximately 0.5% of patients. High-risk subgroups (e.g. diabetics, patients with small vessels, and those undergoing multivessel intervention) may be treated with a IIb/IIIa antagonist (e.g. abciximab), which has been shown to reduce the risk of subsequent cardiac events. There has been recent concern related to the occurrence of late stent thrombosis which may occur many months or years after apparently successful stent implantation. Late stent thrombosis frequently results in acute myocardial infarction or death. It seems likely that that these events relate to incomplete endothelialization caused by the drug coating. The role of prolonged dual antiplatelet therapy, modified drug dosing and the application of bioerodable polymers are being extensively investigated in an attempt to reduce this infrequent, but often catastrophic complication.

PCI is effective in reducing or abolishing attacks of angina in selected patients with lesions amenable to balloon dilatation and stent implantation. At present, there is little evidence that PCI improves life expectancy when compared with medical therapy, and it is probably similar to CABG in terms of morbidity and mortality when similar patient groups are compared. Early trials comparing PCI and CABG prior to the advent of stents demonstrated a high redo rate in the PCI group, with significant numbers of patients with recurrent symptoms crossing to the surgical arm. Currently, there are a number of trials comparing the use of drug-eluting stents vs. CABG in multivessel and left main stem disease. Until the results of these trials are available, PCI tends to be reserved for patients at the 'simple' end of the spectrum with one or two lesions, and patients with three-vessel disease are treated with CABG. In many ways, the two revascularization techniques should be viewed as complementary rather than in competition. A comparison of the two techniques is shown in Table 6.7. In the UK, the number of PCIs continues to increase at a rate of 10–20% per annum (to >70 000 procedures in 2005), whereas the number of patients treated with CABG has been falling in recent years. The ratio of PCI:CABG procedures undertaken in the UK is 3.1:1 and increasing.

Table 6.7 Comparison between percutaneous coronary intervention and coronary artery bypass grafting.

Percutaneous coronary intervention (PCI)	Coronary artery bypass grafting (CABG)
Indications	
Discrete single vessel disease	Diffuse multivessel disease
Multivessel disease	Small calibre vessels
Complex disease (e.g. bifurcations)	Long lesions
Chronic total occlusions	Chronic total occlusions
Left main stem disease (±)	Left main stem disease
Primary PCI (STEMI)	Additional valve surgery
Rescue PCI (STEMI)	
Salvage PCI (cardiogenic shock)	
Advantages	
Short hospital stay	More complete revascularization
Major surgery avoided	Good symptomatic relief
Fewer cerebral events	Improved prognosis
Less periprocedural infarcts	
Disadvantages	
Less complete revascularization	Longer hospital stay
Symptom recurrence	Increased initial costs
More subsequent procedures	Periprocedural complications

Natural history

It is clear from the literature that the prognosis of the patient with stable angina has improved with the passage of time. Patients can now be more easily divided into high- and low-risk subsets on clinical history, treadmill exercise testing and coronary arteriography. Furthermore, aggressive risk factor modification coupled with effective drug therapy and successful methods of revascularization has reduced risk and improved prognosis. Prognosis in individual patients is difficult to estimate, but varies from an annual mortality of 1–2% for single vessel disease, 3.5–7.5% for three vessel disease to 10–13% for left main stem disease.

Acute myocardial infarction

Epidemiology

The true incidence of acute myocardial infarction is unknown, but CHD caused approximately 105 000 deaths in the UK in 2004. The incidence and mortality of acute myocardial infarction are improving with time as a result of efforts targeted at primary prevention, risk factor reduction, patient awareness, paramedic ambulance personnel, CCUs, drug therapy (e.g. aspirin, β-blockade, ACE inhibitors, statins), thrombolysis, primary PCI, rehabilitation, post-infarct risk stratification and revascularization (PCI, CABG).

Pathophysiology

An acute myocardial infarct occurs when myocardial ischaemia, usually occurring as a result of atherosclerotic coronary artery disease, is sufficient to result in irreversible necrosis of cardiac muscle.

Coronary thrombosis

Angiographic and post-mortem studies of patients very early after the onset of symptoms demonstrate a high (>85%) incidence of occlusive thrombus in the culprit artery (Fig. 6.12). The thrombus is a mixture of white (platelet-rich) and red (fibrin/erythrocyte-rich) clot. Even without treatment, the incidence of thrombosis falls to 65% by 24h, suggesting that spontaneous thrombolysis occurs if the patient survives the acute event.

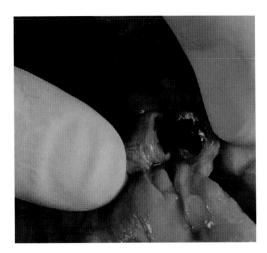

Fig. 6.12 Coronary thrombosis.

Plaque-fissure

Coronary thrombosis commonly occurs in association with a plaque-fissure (see page 83).

Coronary artery spasm

In a small minority (<5%) of patients, acute myocardial infarction occurs in the setting of normal coronary arteries. It is assumed that coronary artery spasm plays a role in some of these cases. Spasm may also be superimposed on 'fixed' atherosclerotic disease that can lead to a critical occlusion, often with added thrombus sufficient to cause infarction.

Collateral vessels

One of the major determinants of the extent of myocardial necrosis is the presence of a collateral blood supply to the area undergoing infarction. In patients suffering acute myocardial infarction, following a long history of chronic stable angina, collateral vessels may be well developed such that the size of the infarct is small. In the young patient with a sudden occlusion of the LAD, the consequence is usually an extensive anterior infarct because of the paucity of collateral vessels.

Box 6.13 Symptoms in acute myocardial infarction

- Prolonged chest pain
- Anxiety, apprehension
- Sweating
- Breathlessness
- Nausea

Clinical history (see Box 6.13)

Chest pain

The majority (>80%) of patients present with chest pain. The symptoms are typical and can be compared with a prolonged attack of severe angina. Whereas a typical attack of angina lasts 5–10 min, the chest pain of myocardial infarction usually lasts at least 30 min. The pain or tightness is oppressive and may be associated with sweating or fear. Although the pain may radiate to the arm(s) or jaw, occasionally the symptoms may be mainly arising from the epigastrium, which can cause diagnostic difficulty. In the elderly and diabetics, pain may be slight or absent.

An acute infarct often occurs after extremes of exertion or emotion, rarely at the peak of exercise. Up to 50% of patients are awoken from sleep by chest pain, and approximately one-third of patients continue with their activities despite the presence of chest pain. On direct questioning, many patients admit to vague symptoms in the days or weeks before the event, including malaise, fatigue or non-specific chest pain.

Breathlessness

Breathlessness may be due to a sudden rise in left ventricular end-diastolic pressure, indicative of incipient ventricular failure, and may occasionally occur as the sole manifestation of myocardial infarction. Anxiety may result in hyperventilation. In silent infarction, breathlessness is indicative of significant left ventricular dysfunction.

Gastrointestinal symptoms

An increase in vagal activity results in nausea and vomiting, and is said to be more common in inferior infarction. Diaphragmatic stimulation in inferior infarction may also cause hiccoughs.

Other symptoms

These include palpitation, dizziness or syncope from ventricular arrhythmias, and symptoms from arterial embolism (e.g. stroke, limb ischaemia).

Physical examination

General appearance

The patient appears pale, sweaty and apprehensive due to sympathetic overactivity. There may be obvious respiratory distress with tachypnoea and breathlessness. A moderate fever of usually less than 38 °C occurs 12–24 h after the infarct and may be useful in diagnosis if cardiac enzyme estimations are not yet available.

Pulse and BP

A sinus tachycardia (100–120/min) occurs in one-third of patients; with adequate analgesia, the pulse usually slows unless there is impending cardiogenic shock. A slow heart rate may indicate a sinus bradycardia or heart block complicating the infarct. A moderate increase in BP is attributable to catecholamine release. Hypotension occurs as a result of vagal overactivity, dehydration, right ventricular infarction, or may be indicative of cardiogenic shock.

Examination of the heart

Palpation of the precordium may reveal an area of dyskinesia, particularly in patients who have sustained an extensive anterior infarct. An S4 is common, but may be transient. More severe left ventricular dysfunction is accompanied by an S3, and/or reversed splitting of the S2. Late systolic murmurs of mild MR come and go depending on ventricular loading conditions. Pericardial friction rubs are rarely heard until the second or third day, or much later (up to 6 weeks) as a feature of Dressler syndrome (see page 107).

Examination of the lungs

End-inspiratory crackles may be evident, even in the absence of radiographic pulmonary oedema. Frank pulmonary oedema is seen as a complication of extensive, usually anterior, infarction.

Other features

Clinical evidence of hyperlipidaemia, peripheral vascular disease, diabetes and hypertensive retinopathy may all be present.

Investigations (see Box 6.14)

Markers of myocardial damage

Following death of myocardial tissue, the cytoplasmic constituents of myocardial cells are released into the circulation. Creatine phosphokinase (CPK) is detectable 6–8 h after acute infarction peaking at 24 h and returning to normal after another 24 h. An isoenzyme (CPK-MB) is specific for heart muscle, but can also be released in myocarditis, cardiac trauma and following direct current (DC) countershock.

An elevation of one or more serum markers defines the presence of an acute myocardial infarct according to the 2000 ACS criteria (see page 84). The troponins (T and I) are regulatory proteins located within the myocyte contractile apparatus and are sensitive markers of myocardial cell injury; they can conveniently be measured by a bedside test kit. The sensitivity of troponin elevation is relatively low for at least the first 4–6 h following the onset of symptoms, and some patients do not show an elevation in troponin until 12 h. Troponin positivity allows stratification for risk in patients pre-

---

Box 6.14 Investigations in acute myocardial infarction

- FBC, ESR, CRP
- Resting ECG
- Cardiac enzymes (including troponin I or T)
- Echocardiography
- Exercise testing
- ± Coronary arteriography

senting with ACS. Troponin elevation may also be seen in patients with heart failure, left ventricular hypertrophy, chronic kidney disease and diabetes. It is important therefore that an elevated troponin value should be assessed in the context of the clinical history and the ECG.

Aspartate aminotransferase (AAT), a non-specific enzyme commonly run as part of a biochemical screen, can be detected as early as 12h, peaks at 36h and returns to normal by 4 days. Hepatic congestion, primary liver disease and pulmonary embolism may all be associated with an elevation in AAT. Like CPK, AAT is also found in skeletal muscle. An increase in the non-specific enzyme lactate dehydrogenase (LDH) occurs late in myocardial infarction: elevated levels are detectable at 24h, peaking at 3–6 days with an increase which may remain detectable for 2 weeks. Its isoenzyme LDH_1 is more specific but its clinical use has been superseded by measurement of the troponins.

Serial estimates of a panel of cardiac enzymes are measured daily for the first 3 days: a significant elevation is defined as twice the upper limit of the laboratory normal. Time–activity curves of the various enzymes are shown in Fig. 6.13.

Other blood tests

Non-specific changes in routine blood tests include an elevated white cell count after 48h, typically 10 000–15 000, predominantly polymorphs, and an elevated erythrocyte sedimentation rate (ESR) and C-reactive protein (CRP) peaking at day 4 with a second peak as a feature of Dressler syndrome. Mild hyperglycaemia as a result of carbohydrate intolerance may persist for some weeks. Catecholamine release, recumbency and a change in diet alter estimates of lipid levels, which should therefore be deferred for 4–6 weeks.

Electrocardiography

The combination of a typical history in association with elevated cardiac enzymes is more reliable than the ECG in the diagnosis of acute myocardial infarction. The ECG has a positive predictive accuracy of approximately 80%; thus a normal ECG does not exclude infarction. Serial ECGs are valuable in documenting the evolution of electrical disturbances. ECG changes evolve in a well-defined order (Fig. 6.14).

In ST segment elevation myocardial infarction (STEMI), incomplete repolarization of damaged myocardium causes ST segment elevation ('current of injury') overlaying the affected region. In patients seen very early after infarction, tall, symmetrical T waves may be apparent which invert as the ST segments rise. Reciprocal ST segment depression is seen in the leads opposite the infarct. The ST segments return to the isoelectric line within a few days depending on the magnitude of the infarct, followed by T wave inversion, which may remain indefinitely. Subsequently, pathologi-

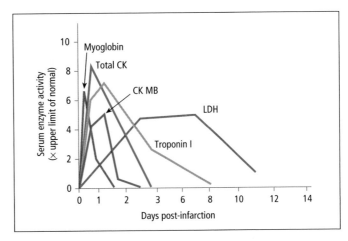

Fig. 6.13 Time–activity curves for a panel of cardiac enzymes.

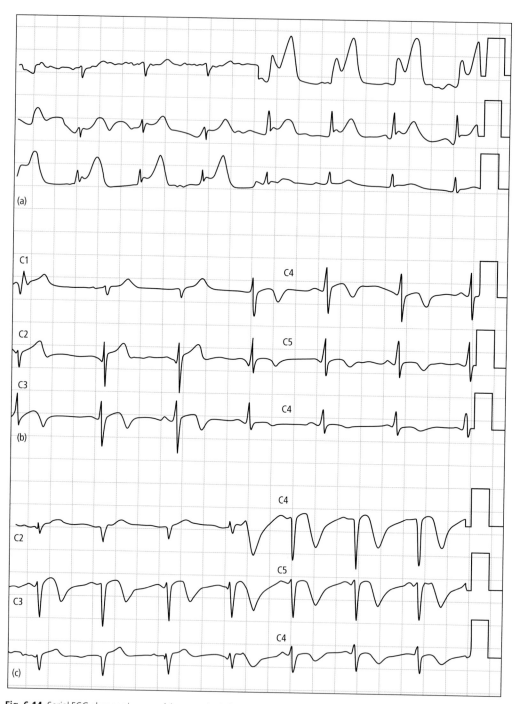

Fig. 6.14 Serial ECG changes in an evolving anterior infarct (a–c).

cal Q waves develop, defined as any Q wave in leads V_1–V_3, or a Q wave with a duration $\geq$30 ms in leads I, II, AVL, AVF or V_4–V_6: the Q wave must be present in any two contiguous leads and have a depth $\geq$1 mm. Q waves are not specific as they may be seen in cardiomyopathy and ventricular hypertrophy. In one-third of patients, Q waves resolve within 18 months of the acute event. A proportion of the 20% of patients who have a documented infarct by clinical and enzyme criteria have the infarct in an area that is electrically silent to the surface 12-lead ECG.

Non-ST segment elevation myocardial infarction (NSTEMI) is characterized by ST segment depression and/or T wave inversion, without ST segment elevation or the development of Q waves. The pattern of ST segment depression is variable (horizontal, upsloping or downsloping), and usually overlies the area of ischaemic myocardium, but may be more generalized. Pathological ST segment depression is defined by ST segment depression of $\geq$1 mm, 80 ms after the J point. ECG changes of STEMI and NSTEMI may be indistinguishable at the time of initial evaluation.

The relationship between the ECG and the pathological severity of infarction is unreliable, thus a patient with Q waves may have sustained a transmural or a subendocardial infarct. The same is true for the patient with ST segment depression or fixed T wave inversion (NSTEMI), which is not specific for subendocardial infarction. Although subendocardial infarction is less likely to result in cardiogenic shock or myocardial rupture, minor degrees of infarction may result in sudden death from ventricular arrhythmias or be the harbinger of a later transmural infarct (the so-called 'stuttering' infarct). The prognosis of a non-Q wave infarct is less favourable than that of Q-wave infarction.

Echocardiography

Following myocardial infarction, regional wall motion abnormalities, reduced fractional shortening and ejection fraction, mural thrombus, pericardial fluid and abnormalities of valve function can all be detected by cross-sectional echocardiography (see Chapter 4).

Radionuclide scintigraphy

Infarct-avid myocardial scintigraphy with a radionuclide with a short half-life (^{99m}Tc-pyrophosphate) can be used to make a semi-quantitative assessment of infarct size, but this is not used as a routine investigation (see Chapter 4).

MRI scanning

See Chapter 4.

Coronary arteriography

Urgent (same hospital admission) coronary arteriography is required in all patients with troponin-positive ACS, and is often combined with PCI if technically feasible, so-called 'angioplasty query proceed'. Patients undergoing primary PCI for STEMI are often taken directly to the cardiac catheterization laboratory by the ambulance paramedics (see General measures below).

Differential diagnosis

Aortic dissection

Retrosternal pain radiates through to the back, with clinical evidence of reduced or absent pulses and/or aortic regurgitation. Diagnosis is confirmed by computed tomographic (CT)/magnetic resonance scanning or transoesophageal echocardiography (see Chapter 4).

Acute pericarditis

- Chest pain is relieved by sitting forward.
- Previous viral infection, fever, systemic upset, friction rub and typical ECG (see Chapter 3).

Acute pulmonary embolism

- Marked breathlessness with little or no chest pain.
- Pleuritic pain and haemoptysis may accompany peripheral emboli.
- Elevated venous pressure, right-sided S3, pleural rub.

- Arterial hypoxaemia, typical ECG, oligaemic chest radiograph.
- Confirm with V/Q scan, spiral CT, pulmonary arteriography (see Chapter 16).

Chest wall pain

- Differentiated on the clinical history.
- Superficial, localized pain, often transient, may be provoked by activity or changes in posture. Responds to minor analgesics or NSAIDs. Similar symptoms from costo-chondritis (Tietze syndrome) localized to the costo-chondral junction (often the second).

Gastrointestinal disorders

Disorders of the upper gastrointestinal tract (oesophageal reflux, spasm, hiatus hernia, peptic ulceration or acute pancreatitis) may all cause diagnostic difficulty in occasional patients.
- ST/T wave changes and a response to nitrates may occur with oesophageal spasm, pancreatitis and cholecystitis.
- A careful clinical history and investigation of the gastrointestinal tract will help clarify the diagnosis.

Treatment (see Box 6.15)

General measures

Once admitted to hospital, the patient should be transferred rapidly to the CCU. If paramedic ECG telemetry is available in the ambulance, it may be possible to bring the patient directly to the CCU,

---

> ### Box 6.15 Treatment in acute myocardial infarction (NSTEMI and STEMI)
>
> - Analgesia (opiate)
> - Aspirin
> - Clopidogrel
> - Heparin (LMWH)
> - Thrombolysis
> - β-Blockade
> - ± Diuretics
> - ACE inhibitor
> - Oxygen

---

rather than endure the inevitable delays associated with the Accident and Emergency Department. The patient with a STEMI should be treated with either thrombolysis (pre-hospital or hospital) or primary PCI, depending on local resource availability (see pages 111 and 112). In some hospitals, thrombolysis is administered in the Accident and Emergency Department; in others, the patient is admitted to the CCU first. Either way, there should be the shortest possible delay before the patient is monitored for disturbances of heart rhythm, and a venous cannula inserted for vascular access. Rather than undergo a formal admission procedure, it is preferable for the patient to be admitted to the CCU inappropriately and then moved to another ward if it transpires that the diagnosis was incorrect. Central venous cannulation and arterial access is not required in uncomplicated patients (Killip I).

Routine blood tests should include haematology and a biochemical screen including a panel of cardiac enzymes. A portable (AP) chest radiograph is taken together with daily ECGs. Uncomplicated patients usually remain in hospital for 48 h for an STEMI treated with primary PCI, or 5 days if treated with a thrombolytic.

Analgesia

Adequate analgesia and if necessary light sedation are important, as a comfortable, relaxed patient is less likely to suffer from arrhythmias, and a reduction in endogenous catecholamines will reduce the chance of subendocardial ischaemia. Small doses of intravenous opiates (diamorphine 2.5–5.0 mg or morphine sulphate 5–10 mg) are effective analgesics with additional vasodilating properties, which may be particularly useful in the patient suffering from pulmonary oedema. Because of the side-effects of nausea and vomiting, prophylactic anti-emetics (prochlorperazine 10 mg, metoclopramide 10 mg or cyclizine 50 mg) should also be administered. The initial pain usually settles within 24 h in Killip I patients. Recurrent pain after a few days may be indicative of pericarditis, or, later still, Dressler syndrome, both of which are best treated with NSAIDs.

Anxious patients may benefit from a short-acting benzodiazepine (e.g. lorazepam 0.5–1.0 mg). Bed rest is only necessary as long as the patient is in pain, or there is evidence of arrhythmia or haemodynamic disturbance.

Oxygen

There is little evidence that oxygen supplements are necessary in the uncomplicated infarct, although many patients will experience psychological benefit from oxygen which is widely prescribed. Nasal cannulae delivering 2–4 L/min of humidified oxygen are convenient, although oxygen delivery is variable. In patients with pulmonary oedema, transcutaneous oxygen monitoring is helpful, and arterial blood gas estimates usually unnecessary.

Antiplatelet therapy

All patients with ACS should be commenced on dual antiplatelet therapy with aspirin and clopidogrel as soon as possible after presentation to hospital (or, if possible, in the ambulance on the way to hospital). The benefit of the early administration of aspirin 300 mg in STEMI has been documented in a number of clinical trials (e.g. ISIS-2). Long-term treatment with aspirin following myocardial infarction also reduces all-cause mortality, including reinfarction and non-fatal stroke. The beneficial effect of aspirin and clopidogrel is especially marked in NSTEMI; the minimum effective and best tolerated dose of aspirin is 75 mg daily, which should be continued indefinitely. Patients are usually loaded with clopidogrel 600 mg (previously 300 mg), and continued on clopidogrel 75 mg daily thereafter. Evidence suggests that clopidogrel should be continued for 3 months following STEMI and 12 months after a NSTEMI. Patients treated with drug-eluting stents usually continue dual antiplatelet therapy for a minimum of 12 months (see page 103).

Anticoagulation

Heparin reduces the risk of systemic and pulmonary embolism and has also been shown to facilitate the resolution of apical thrombus demonstrated on echocardiography. Most of the data favourable to the routine use of heparin preceded the thrombolytic era. Heparin can be administered by either the subcutaneous or the intravenous route; low molecular weight heparin (LMWH) is convenient to administer as it does not require routine monitoring. Formal anticoagulation with heparin followed by warfarin should be reserved for patients with extensive myocardial infarction, cardiogenic shock, left ventricular aneurysm or sustained atrial arrhythmias. In the GUSTO-I trial, clinical outcome in patients treated with heparin following myocardial infarction was clearly related to the level of anticoagulation: the optimal range for the aPTT was 50–70 s; more aggressive anticoagulation was associated with an increased risk of bleeding.

Reperfusion therapy

Thrombolysis

Early mortality and long-term outcome following acute myocardial infarction relates to early and complete reperfusion as judged by normal (TIMI-3) flow in the target artery. The rapid intravenous administration of a thrombolytic agent has been shown to improve prognosis in a number of clinical trials (e.g. ISIS-3, GISSI-2, GUSTO-I). Arterial patency at 90 min following infusion appears to be the main determinant of long-term outcome: a patent vessel favourably improves survival, ventricular function and the incidence of late sudden death. A number of thrombolytic agents are effective (Table 6.8), and although accelerated tissue plasminogen activator (t-PA) is superior to streptokinase, the routine use of t-PA is prohibitive. Most patients are now treated with tenectplase because of the ease of administration.

All patients presenting within 12 h of the onset of symptoms from an STEMI should be considered for reperfusion therapy, either thrombolysis or primary PCI. Thrombolytic therapy was, until recently, the mainstay of treatment for STEMI, although it was clear that a number of patients did not receive a lytic because of contraindications (Box 6.16). Even when thrombolysis is administered promptly, normal (TIMI 3) flow in the culprit

Table 6.8 Fibrinolytic agents for use in acute myocardial infarction.

Drug name	Trade name	Dose
Alteplase	Actilyse	100 mg IV over 90 min (symptoms <6 h) or over 3 h (symptoms 6–12 h)
Anistreplase	Eminase	30 units IV over 4–5 min (symptoms <6 h)
Reteplase	Rapilysin	2 × 10 units IV over <2 min, 30 min apart (symptoms <12 h)
Streptokinase	Kabikinase	1.5 million units IV over 1 h
Streptokinase	Streptase	1.5 million units IV over 1 h

Box 6.16 Contraindications to thrombolysis

Absolute
- Previous haemorrhagic stroke (at any time)
- Other strokes or cerebrovascular events (within 1 year)
- Intracranial neoplasm
- Active internal bleeding
- Suspected aortic dissection

Relative
- Severe or uncontrolled systemic hypertension (BP >180/110 mmHg)
- History of previous cerebrovascular event
- Current use of anticoagulants
- Known bleeding diathesis
- Recent major trauma, including head injury (within 4 weeks)
- Recent major surgery (within 4 weeks)
- Prolonged cardiopulmonary resuscitation
- Non-compressible vascular punctures (especially arterial)
- Recent internal bleeding (within 4 weeks)
- Prior administration (within 2 years) or allergic reaction to streptokinase or anistreplase
- Active peptic ulceration
- Pregnancy
- Delay in presentation (>12 h from symptom onset)

---

artery is only restored in 60% of patients. The decision as to whether to offer the patient thrombolysis or primary PCI depends on a number of factors, including time to presentation, distance from the cardiac centre and the availability of local resources, infrastructure and expertise. Patients who present within 3 h of the onset of chest pain are on the steep part of the survival vs. time-to-reperfusion curve and in many centres would be best treated with thrombolysis for maximum efficacy, particularly if they presented within 60 min.

Following thrombolytic treatment, it is important to emphasize that the clinical (bedside) assessment of reperfusion is unreliable. Normalization of the ST segment is not a surrogate for arterial patency, although this combined with the resolution of chest pain and a 'reperfusion' arrhythmia (e.g. accelerated idioventricular rhythm) is highly suggestive of a restoration of arterial patency.

Primary percutanous coronary intervention (PPCI)

A number of clinical trials have demonstrated superior TIMI-3 (i.e. normal) flow in patients undergoing primary angioplasty, with or without stenting, following myocardial infarction, when compared with a variety of thrombolytic agents. Vessel patency, myocardial salvage, reinfarction, mortality and the incidence of cerebral haemorrhage are all superior following PPCI, providing the delay between drug administration with a thrombolytic and balloon inflation time is less than 90 min. For every 10 min delay to PCI there is a 1% reduction in absolute mortality difference between the two techniques. There is no doubt that a strategy of primary intervention requires a huge resource, including a dedicated and experienced team, 24-hour catheter laboratory availability and a mechanism for rapid access to allow the shortest possible elapse from the onset of chest pain to restoration of arterial patency. Patients presenting very early after the onset of symptoms are best treated with a thrombolytic (see above). It is likely that a mixed and pragmatic reperfusion strategy will be applicable to most health care systems. In the UK in 2006 it was estimated that 30% of PCI centres could offer daytime PPCI, and 14% offered 24/7 PPCI: in 2005, 7% of all PCI procedures were PPCI.

β-Blockade

β-Blocking drugs reduce heart rate, systemic BP and cardiac output. Cardiac work and peak δp/δt are lowered, thus there is a significant reduction in MVO_2. In numerous clinical trials, β-blockers have been shown to reduce all-cause mortality, including sudden death and non-fatal reinfarction. The absolute benefit is most marked in the elderly, and those with a previous myocardial infarct, diabetes mellitus, left ventricular dysfunction and electrical instability. β-Blockade is well tolerated in the majority of patients. Despite the widespread use of other drugs post-infarction (e.g. aspirin, ACE inhibitors), there is evidence that β-blockers offer an additional benefit over the other drugs. The majority of the benefit is seen in the first year following infarction, but late sudden death is reduced by β-blockade, suggesting that the drug should be continued in the long term. A once-daily selective β-blocking agent (e.g. atenolol 25–50 mg daily) is commonly prescribed.

Nitrates

Most of the data relating to the beneficial effects of nitrates are derived from the pre-thrombolysis era. Nitrates are commonly used for the relief of chest pain and are particularly effective when combined with heparin in the management of the patient with unstable or post-infarction angina. They are effective venous and arteriolar dilators and may therefore be used to control systemic hypertension, or to offload the myocardium in the patient with cardiogenic shock. If nitrates are used in the post-infarct patient, the intravenous route is preferable in doses sufficient to reduce systolic BP to 100 mmHg.

ACE inhibitors

A variety of ACE inhibitors have been studied following acute myocardial infarction using a variety of dosing regimens, in either unselected patients (e.g. CONSENSUS II, GISSI-3, ISIS-4) or selected high-risk patients (e.g. SAVE, AIRE). In general, the trials show a significant reduction in all-cause mortality, including late sudden death and reinfarction. Secondary end-points also show a significant reduction in the incidence of heart failure and the need for early revascularization.

ACE inhibitors should be started early (within 24 h) and are most beneficial in the elderly, and in patients with clinical evidence of heart failure or left ventricular dysfunction on echocardiography. ACE inhibitors are well tolerated, with side-effects (e.g. systemic hypotension, cardiogenic shock, renal dysfunction) occurring in only a small minority of patients. The benefit of ACE inhibitors appears to occur in addition to the benefit seen with the concomitant use of β-blockers.

Calcium channel blockade

The calcium antagonists are a heterogeneous group of drugs with differing clinical properties. The short-acting dihydropyridines (e.g. nifedipine) have no role in treating the post-infarction patient, except possibly in combination with β-blockade. Used alone, a number of trials have shown that nifedipine and similar agents may actually increase mortality compared with placebo. Diltiazem may have a role in patients with non-Q wave myocardial infarction, and verapamil in patients in whom β-blockers may be contraindicated. Both drugs are usually well tolerated, although side-effects of heart failure, hypotension or symptomatic heart block may occasionally be seen.

Diabetes

Because of the adverse prognosis in diabetic patients with cardiac disease, tight control of risk factors is important, particularly following myocardial infarction. Patients with type II diabetes usually controlled on oral hypoglycaemics should be switched to a modified GIK (glucose–insulin–potassium) regimen during the early phase after an infarct, and insulin should be continued for 3 months thereafter according to the DIGAMI study.

Diuretics

See Chapter 9.

Other vasodilators

See Chapter 9.

Inotropic support

See Chapter 9.

Anti-arrhythmic agents

See Chapter 13.

Magnesium

See Chapter 13.

Mechanical support

See Chapter 9.

DC cardioversion

See Chapter 13.

Endocardial pacing

See Chapter 13.

Complications

Arrhythmias

See Chapter 13.

Cardiogenic shock

See Chapter 9.

Acute mitral regurgitation

Mild MR following myocardial infarction is heard in up to 50% of patients and occurs as a result of abnormal papillary muscle geometry, malaligned mitral cusps or annular dilatation. Typically, a late systolic murmur comes and goes depending on loading conditions.

Severe MR as a result of papillary muscle rupture is rare (Fig. 6.15), occurring in <1% of all infarcts. It is seen more frequently complicating inferior infarcts because the posteromedial papillary muscle has only a single blood supply and is therefore more susceptible to ischaemic insult. Typically, the patient appears in acute pulmonary oedema (Fig.

6.16) or cardiogenic shock within the first 10 days after an infarct; sudden death may also occur. A pansystolic murmur, which may be inconspicuous and cannot be differentiated on clinical grounds from an infarct-related ventricular septal defect (VSD), may be present. Cross-sectional echocardiography is diagnostic, with a flail leaflet prolapsing into the left atrium in association with detachment of all or part of the subvalve apparatus. Without surgical intervention (mitral repair or replacement), >75% of patients are dead within 24 h. Surgical mortality should be in the order of 10% depending on the condition of the patient.

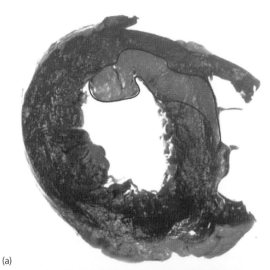

(a)

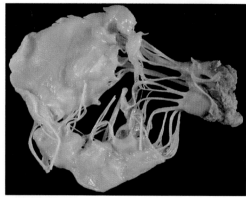

(b)

Fig. 6.15 (a) Transmural infarction involving a papillary muscle. (b) Papillary muscle rupture.

Ventricular septal defect

Acquired VSD occurs in 1–3% of cases of acute myocardial infarction (Fig. 6.17). VSD complicating anterior infarction is more common than those involving inferior infarcts, although the latter have a worse surgical mortality. Necrotic muscle results in a 1–2 cm defect in the muscular septum, often in association with a left ventricular aneurysm. Most patients with an acute VSD have had a sizeable infarct, whereas patients with acute MR have often sustained only a small infarct involving the papillary muscle. Diagnosis is confirmed on cross-sectional imaging, with Doppler flow clearly visible from the left to right ventricle. Cardiac catheterization is usually required to document the coronary anatomy and/or to insert an intra-aortic balloon. Operative mortality is in the region of 20–30% in experienced centres, and right ventricular function appears to be a major determinant of late survival. Immediate resuscitation and urgent surgical referral reduce the chance of multisystem failure occurring as a consequence of low cardiac output.

Free-wall rupture

Up to 15% of patients dying suddenly following myocardial infarction die from free-wall rupture (Fig. 6.18). This complication appears to have reduced in frequency since the routine use of β-blockade. Cardiac rupture is more common in the elderly, in females and following extensive transmural infarction. A small minority of patients survives the acute event as a result of a sealed defect or pseudoaneurysm formation. Diagnosis is usually evident on echocardiography, and the treatment is surgical.

Systemic thromboembolism

Even in the presence of mural thrombus on echocardiography, systemic thromboembolism is rare, occurring in <5% of patients overall. Systemic emboli usually pass to the cerebral circulation.

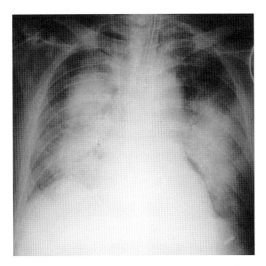

Fig. 6.16 Chest radiograph demonstrating acute pulmonary oedema in a patient with papillary muscle rupture (note the small heart).

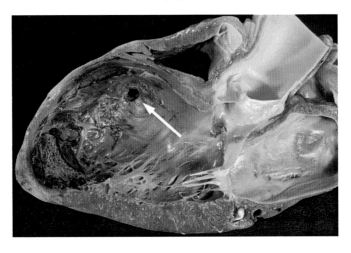

Fig. 6.17 Anterior myocardial infarct complicated by an acute VSD.

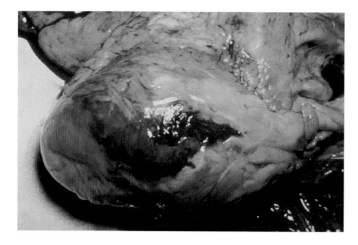

Fig. 6.18 Left ventricular free-wall rupture.

Formal anticoagulation (heparin followed by warfarin) should be reserved for patients with poor ventricular function (ejection fraction <40%), left ventricular aneurysm or atrial arrhythmias (especially AF).

Pulmonary embolism

As a result of the liberal use of heparin and thrombolytics, coupled with rapid mobilization, the incidence of pulmonary embolism has fallen. Pulmonary embolism if it occurs should be treated in the routine manner (see Chapter 16).

Pericarditis and the post-myocardial infarction syndrome

Early pericarditis (within 1 week of infarction) is characterized by typical pericardial pain (see Chapter 12) and an audible friction rub in association with ST/T wave changes. It is more common following extensive transmural infarction, but seems to be occurring less frequently since the advent of thrombolytic therapy, now reported in 6–7% of patients. Symptoms respond rapidly to NSAIDs in the majority of patients.

Post-myocardial infarction (Dressler) syndrome consists of pleuro-pericarditis occurring 2–6 weeks after myocardial infarction, in association with a fever-elevated ESR, CRP and white cell count. The condition appears to have an immune basis, and

may occur without preceding (early) pericarditis. A minority of patients have a pericardial effusion, and occasional cases of pericardial tamponade or constriction have been reported. The syndrome is indistinguishable from post-cardiotomy syndrome following cardiopulmonary bypass procedures. Symptoms usually respond rapidly to NSAIDs, but some patients require a short course of oral steroids.

Left ventricular aneurysm

Transmural apical infarction is particularly prone to aneurysm formation. Early infarct expansion may be associated with myocardial thinning, dilatation and fibrosis, such that a discrete bulge occurs, within which there is paradoxical movement (i.e. systolic expansion), thereby detracting from overall ventricular function. Symptoms of recurrent chest pain, breathlessness, intractable arrhythmias and systemic thromboembolism are typical. Clinical features include a dilated heart, dyskinetic or paradoxical apex, an S3 and possible MR. Chronic cases have a typical appearance on the chest radiograph, often with calcification within the wall of the aneurysm (Fig. 6.19). The diagnosis can be confirmed on cross-sectional echocardiography (which often demonstrates thrombus within the aneurysm), magnetic resonance scanning or cine-angiography.

The early use of ACE inhibitors and thrombolytics has reduced the incidence of aneurysm forma-

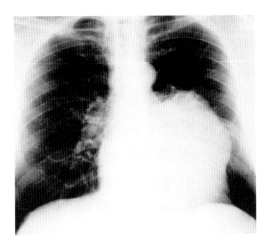

Fig. 6.19 Chest radiograph in a patient with a left ventricular aneurysm.

tion. Left ventricular aneurysm formation ± CABG has an early mortality of <5% in experienced centres.

Rehabilitation and risk factor modification

Prior to leaving hospital, patients should be counselled by a cardiac rehabilitation nurse. During their inpatient stay, the patient will be receptive to reassurance and encouragement, and the opportunity should not be missed to address the correction of risk factors. Explanations are important and lead to realistic expectations in the post-infarct recovery period. Specific advice should be given regarding diet, smoking, physical activity, sex and plans for return to work. If facilities are available, a formal rehabilitation programme and group activity should be encouraged, with emphasis on a progressive increase in dynamic (isotonic) exercise (e.g. walking, swimming and cycling).

Post-infarct investigations

Lipids

Despite the fact that only 75% of patients who have sustained a myocardial infarct will have an abnormal lipid profile, the aggressive reduction of cholesterol with a statin should be commenced in all patients (regardless of cholesterol levels) as

statins significantly reduce all-cause mortality, re-infarction, ventricular dysfunction (heart failure), hospital readmission, stroke and the need for subsequent revascularization. Reduction in cholesterol using statins is at least as effective as aspirin and β-blockade in reducing mortality following myocardial infarction. The aim should be to reduce LDL-cholesterol to <2.6 mmol/L and total cholesterol to <4.5 mmol/L. In combined hyperlipidaemia, or where cholesterol levels are resistant, fibrates should be added to a statin and/or a cholesterol absorption inhibitor (e.g. ezetimibe).

Coronary arteriography and revascularization

The published literature supports an early invasive strategy for patients presenting with ACS, particularly in patients presenting with ST segment depression and an elevated troponin (e.g. FRISC II, ISAR-COOL and RITA 3). Thus, the majority of patients presenting with ACS will have undergone diagnostic coronary arteriography ± PCI before hospital discharge.

Functional testing and risk stratification

In patients who have not undergone early coronary arteriography, post-infarct exercise testing offers a simple non-invasive method to identify the presence of inducible ischaemia and thus to be able to stratify patients for risk and the need for coronary arteriography at a later date. Most of the studies of post-infarct exercise testing relate to the pre-thrombolytic era. As most of the studies show a very low (1–2% at 1 year) mortality in patients receiving thrombolysis, the value of routine exercise testing has recently been questioned, particularly in relation to 'false-positive' responders. Nevertheless, a pre-discharge or 6-week post-infarct exercise test does provide useful information, and can determine the need for further investigation (Box 6.17).

Natural history and prognosis

Early 30-day and late mortality following myocardial infarction is related to the territory and extent of

---

Box 6.17 Exercise testing following myocardial infarction

Poor prognostic features:
- Exercise-induced chest pain (angina)
- ST segment depression
- Abnormal blood pressure response
- Flat heart rate response (chronotropic incompetence)
- Exercise-induced ventricular arrhythmias

Box 6.18 Factors associated with a poor prognosis following myocardial infarction

- Increasing age
- Female gender
- Extensive infarction (determined by cardiac enzymes or widespread ECG changes)
- Mechanical complications of myocardial infarction (e.g. VSD, free-wall rupture, acute mitral regurgitation
- Anterior infarction
- Inferior infarction with right ventricular involvement
- Diabetes mellitus
- Previous angina or myocardial infarction
- Impaired ventricular function (S3, pulmonary oedema)
- Failure to perfuse with thrombolysis or PCI
- Anterior infarction associated with atrioventricular block
- Recurrent infarction/ischaemia whilst still an inpatient
- Electrical instability (e.g. secondary VT/VF)
- Depressed heart rate variability
- Abnormal late potentials

---

the ECG changes. Limited inferior infarcts have a 30-day and 12-month mortality of 4.5 and 6.7%, respectively, whereas anterior infarcts with widespread ST segment elevation and bundle branch block have mortalities of 19.6 and 25.6%, respectively. Additional information can be gained from classification according to the haemodynamic (Killip) class:

- the majority of patients (85%) have no evidence of heart failure (Killip I);
- an S3 and bibasal crackles define Killip II (10%);
- frank pulmonary oedema (Killip III) and cardiogenic shock (Killip IV) together account for only 5% of patients.

The major determinants of prognosis after myocardial infarction are age, systolic BP, heart rate, infarct location and Killip class. Factors associated with a poor prognosis are listed in Box 6.18.

Further reading

Bertrand ME, Simoons ML, Fox KAA, Wallentin LC, Hamm CW, McFadden E, De Feyter PJ, Specchia G, Ruzyllo W. Management of acute coronary syndromes in patients presenting without persistent ST-segment elevation myocardial. The Task Force on the Management of Acute Coronary Syndromes of the European Society of Cardiology. *European Heart Journal* 2002; 23: 1809–1840.

British Cardiovascular Interventional Society Website. www.bcis.org.uk

British Heart Foundation Statistics Website. www.heartstats.org

The Joint European Society of Cardiology/American College of Cardiology Committee. Myocardial Infarction Redefined — A Consensus Document of The Joint European Society of Cardiology American College of Cardiology Committee for the Redefinition of Myocardial Infarction. *Journal of the American College of Cardiology* 2000; 36: 959–969.

Van de Werf F, Ardissino D, Betriu A, Cokkinos DV, Falk E, Fox KA, Julian D, Lengyel M, Neumann FJ, Ruzyllo W, Thygesen C, Underwood SR, Vahanian A, Verheugt FW, Wijns W.; Task Force on the Management of Acute Myocardial Infarction of the European Society of Cardiology. Management of acute myocardial infarction in patients presenting with ST-segment elevation. The Task Force on the Management of Acute Myocardial Infarction of the European Society of Cardiology. *European Heart Journal* 2003; 24: 28–66.

Chapter 7

Thrombosis in cardiovascular disease

Introduction

The formation of blood clot (coagulation) is a complex and dynamic process that involves interaction between endothelium, platelets, white blood cells and a wide range of clotting factors and mediators. Counteracting systems inhibit coagulation and can break down forming or even established thrombus. In normal individuals this balance between clotting and anticoagulant/fibrinolytic mechanisms is sophisticated. However, iatrogenic manipulation of this balance is often required for patients with cardiovascular disease, and an understanding of thrombotic and antithrombotic mechanisms is therefore important.

Components of clot formation

The endothelium

The endothelium is a layer of cells that line the luminal side of blood vessels. It was previously thought that these cells simply represented an inert barrier between blood and vessel wall. In fact, carrier mechanisms in endothelial cell membranes specifically transport the vasoactive substances **serotonin, adenosine and adenine nucleotides**, and **angiotensin-converting enzyme** (ACE) on the outer cell surface inactivates the vasodilator **bradykinin**. The cells themselves also synthesize vasoactive substances and **platelet-activating fac-**

tors **(PAFs)**. Thus, the endothelium plays a crucial role in the setting of blood vessel tone and response to vessel injury:

- *Nitric oxide*: this small molecule is constantly produced by healthy endothelium, but in variable quantity. It is a potent vasodilator and inhibits platelet aggregation.
- *Prostacyclin*: this prostaglandin is a vasodilator that inhibits platelets.
- *Endothelin-1 and thromboxane*: are both potent vasoconstrictors that are procoagulant.

Furthermore, damage to the vessel wall exposes subendothelial and endothelial **collagen** fibres which promotes adhesion of platelets to the site of injury, a process mediated by **von Willebrand factor** which forms links between some of the platelet surface glycoprotein receptors (Ib, V and IX) and the collagen fibrils. Platelets then become activated and release the contents of their granules into the plasma, which in turn sets off further procoagulant responses (see below).

Platelets

Plaque inflammation, erosion, disruption or injury are central pathophysiological mechanisms in acute coronary syndromes (including ST segment elevation myocardial infarction (STEMI) and non-ST segment elevation myocardial infarction (NSTEMI)) and in angioplasty/stenting. Circulating platelets are attracted to subendothelial connective tissue at sites of vessel injury, adhere together, are activated by the exposed collagen (and later by thrombin and norepinephrine), and express other platelet receptors (particularly the glycoprotein IIb/IIIa receptor (GP IIb/IIIa)). They also release the contents of their granules into the plasma; these include several mediators (calcium, adenosine diphosphate (ADP), serotonin and thromboxane A$_2$) which induce further platelet aggregation and activation. It is the platelet membrane GP IIb/IIIa receptor that links with plasma fibrinogen to produce a platelet aggregate. The process leading to platelet plug formation is sometimes described as 'primary haemostasis'.

Secondary haemostasis: the coagulation cascade

The process of forming a clot (thrombus), rather than just an aggregate of platelets, is dependent upon the coagulation cascade, and the mechanics of its formation are dynamic and complex. **Thrombin** converts **fibrinogen** to **fibrin**, and also activates several other clotting factors in the cascade (Fig. 7.1) that amplify the process of coagulation and, more specifically, its own production. Fibrin

strands consolidate clot and trap circulating red and white cells.

The end point of thrombin, fibrinogen and fibrin production can be achieved by two pathways of the coagulation cascade. Both involve a series of reactions that chemically convert an inactive component to an active component which then in turn catalyses the next conversion in the series. These 'coagulation factors' are mostly enzymes (factor V and VIII are glycoproteins) and are labelled by Roman numerals, with an 'a' added to distinguish the active part.

The most important pathway for the initiation of coagulation is the **'tissue factor'** (previously termed 'extrinsic') pathway. This pathway is initiated by the release of **tissue factor** from damaged endothelium which then forms a complex with **factor VIIa** and this complex then trips the cascade. The system has several positive feedback loops, particularly centred around thrombin, which, for example, stimulates the generation of more VIIa, Va and VIIIa. The second coagulation cascade pathway is known as the **'contact activation'** (previously termed 'intrinsic') pathway. This pathway is initiated by exposure of collagen that leads to complex formation with **high molecular**

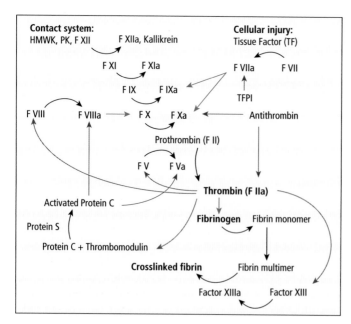

Fig. 7.1 The coagulation cascade. HMWK, high molecular weight kininogen; PK, prekallikrein; TFPI, tissue factor pathway inhibitor. Black arrow, conversion/activation of factor; red arrows, action of inhibitors; blue arrows, reactions catalysed by activated factor; grey arrow, various functions of thrombin.

weight kininogen, **prekallikrein** and **factor XII**; the generated activated factors then trip this cascade. The clotting cascades are dependent upon cofactors such as **calcium and phospholipid**. **Vitamin K** is also an essential cofactor for the liver enzyme responsible for the production of factors II, VII, IX and X, protein S and protein C. Those with low levels of vitamin K, or who have liver disease (e.g. cirrhotics), therefore often have a bleeding tendency. Warfarin inhibits this vitamin K-dependent mechanism.

Inhibitors of coagulation

The body has a natural ability to counterbalance clot formation through the presence of natural inhibitors (anticoagulants), with deficiencies in these inhibitors being associated with prothrombotic clinical conditions. **Protein C** is a protease enzyme that is activated by thrombin and, together with its co-enzyme, **protein S**, acts to degrade factors Va and VIIIa. **Antithrombin** breaks down thrombin and factor Xa and IIa; its activity is enhanced by the presence of heparins which increase its binding affinity for these factors.

Fibrinolysis (Fig 7.2)

Naturally occurring fibrinolysis is a dynamic, balanced process that results in the breakdown of established clot. **Tissue-type plasminogen activator (t-PA)** and **urokinase-type plasminogen activator** work by converting **plasminogen** to **plasmin**, which breaks up fibrin to produce **fibrin degradation products (FDPs)**. There are also naturally occurring inhibitors of this fibrinolytic pathway **(plasminogen activator inhibitors-1 and -2)**, excessive levels of which can produce a thrombotic tendency and have been reported in venous thromboembolism, sepsis, obesity and acute coronary syndromes.

Antithrombotic drugs

Heparin

Unfractionated heparin (UFH) refers to a family of mucopolysaccharide chains. It accelerates the action of naturally occurring antithrombin III and, at high doses, heparin cofactor II. In plasma, approximately 20 times more UFH is needed to inactivate fibrin-bound thrombin than to inactivate free thrombin. This explains why more heparin is needed to prevent the extension of venous thrombosis than to prevent formation of the initial thrombus. Heparin is not absorbed through the gastrointestinal mucosa, and cannot therefore be administered orally. When in the bloodstream after parenteral administration, heparin binds to endothelial cells, mononuclear macrophages and numerous plasma proteins. Elevated levels of these proteins explain the variable individual doses of heparin required to produce the same antithrombotic effect, and the 'heparin resistance' seen in patients with inflammatory and malignant diseases.

The pharmacokinetics of UFH are complicated, and the dose (usually 24000–36000 IU/24 h) needs to be monitored regularly, most commonly by the **activated partial thromboplastin time (aPTT)**, to ensure adequate levels of anticoagulation. Bleeding is the most common side-effect and is higher when UFH is given by intermittent (14%) rather

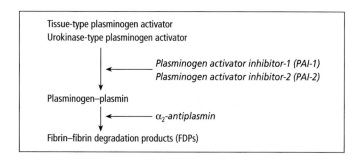

Fig. 7.2 Fibrinolytic pathway.

than continuous infusion (7%), or subcutaneously (4%). **Heparin-induced thrombocytopaenia (HIT)** occurs in 2.4% of patients receiving therapeutic doses.

Some of the limitations of unfractionated heparin can be overcome with **low molecular weight heparins (LMWHs;** including **enoxaparin, dalteparin** and **fondaparinax)**, which have the advantages of less protein binding, reduced plasma clearance, less effect on platelets and fewer bleeding complications. Their long half-life and predictable anticoagulant response to weight-adjusted doses allow once- or twice-daily subcutaneous administration without routine laboratory monitoring. The usual dose of enoxaparin for prophylaxis against deep venous thrombosis (DVT) is 20–40 mg per day, and for more complete anticoagulation (treatment for DVT, unstable angina) is 0.75–1.0 mg/kg/12 h.

Oral anticoagulants

Warfarin and related coumarin agents inhibit hepatic production of vitamin K-dependent clotting factors (II, VII, IX, X) and of proteins C and S. The intensity of the effect of warfarin differs between patients and varies in the same individual over time. Its action is affected by many drugs, foods and intercurrent illnesses such as hepatic failure, heart failure and hyperthyroidism. The laboratory test used to monitor its effect is the **prothrombin time**, now standardized into the **international normalized ratio (INR)**. At the start of warfarin treatment, the prothrombin time is prolonged but the 'contact pathway' for coagulation may still be temporarily unaffected. This is the reason why, in switching from heparin to warfarin, heparin is often continued for at least 24 h after an adequate INR has been achieved. The usual maintenance dose of warfarin is between 1 and 12 mg once daily. Bleeding is the most common side-effect and is influenced by other factors, particularly age, hypertension and malignant disease. On average, the overall annual bleeding risk is 6%, with major and fatal episodes being 2 and 0.8%, respectively. A rare complication is coumarin-induced skin necrosis, the aetiology of which is unknown and which oc-

> ### Box 7.1 Reducing platelet activity
>
> - Inhibition of prostaglandin synthase (aspirin, sulfinpyrazone, flurbiprofen, indobufen)
> - Inhibition of thromboxane synthase (aspirin)
> - Blockade of endoperoxide-thromboxane receptors
> - Inhibition of the activation pathway or glycoprotein IIb/IIIa (ticlopidine, clopidogrel)

curs on the third to eighth day after starting. Coumarin drugs readily cross the placenta and may be teratogenic, particularly during the first trimester of pregnancy.

Antiplatelet agents (see Box 7.1)

Aspirin is an inhibitor of the cyclooxygenase enzyme that is responsible for the generation of prostaglandins (such as prostacyclin) and thromboxane. It is a potent inhibitor of platelet aggregation. It is prescribed in almost all patients with coronary disease and continued for life (75–150 mg per day). Aspirin can cause upper gastrointestinal irritation which sometimes leads to bleeding.

Clopidogrel is a thienopyridine derivative. It inhibits ADP-induced platelet activation and aggregation. The maintenance dose is 75 mg once per day; where its early full effect is required (PCI or acute coronary syndromes), a loading dose of 300–600 mg is given. Clopidogrel may be given alone to reduce the risk of cardiovascular events in high-risk patients but more commonly is used for patients with acute coronary syndromes and/or coronary stenting, in combination with aspirin (see Chapter 6). The actions of aspirin and clopidogrel are by distinct mechanisms so the combination is at least additive. Clopidogrel has largely rendered its predecessor ticlopidine, obsolete. A new antiplatelet drug, **prasugrel**, is similar in action to clopidogrel but more potent and is undergoing clinical trials.

Glycoprotein IIb/IIIa inhibitors

Exposure of GP IIb/IIIa receptors at the platelet surface is the end-point of all pathways leading to platelet aggregation. The monoclonal antibody recombinant **abciximab** (ReoPro) was the first specific IIb/IIIa receptor inhibitor and is given intravenously. It can reduce the incidence of myocardial infarction following complex or high-risk angioplasty/stenting procedures. Synthetic IIb/IIIa inhibitors **(tirofiban, eptifibatide)** are reversible receptor antagonists and have shorter durations of action than abciximab. Both these agents can reduce cardiovascular events in patients with NSTEMI syndromes.

Specific thrombin inhibitors

Recombinant **hirudin** is obtained from *Escherichia coli* and yeast. Unlike heparin which requires endogenous cofactors (antithrombin III, heparin cofactor II), does not penetrate the thrombus and does not reduce platelet deposition, hirudin is active against thrombin without cofactors, penetrates the thrombus, neutralizes thrombin bound to fibrin and reduces platelet deposition and thrombus growth. **Hirulog** is the synthetic analogue of hirudin. Neither has an antidote, but the half-life is short (around 2 h). These agents have been used in some trials but infrequently in clinical practice.

Thrombolytic drugs (see Chapter 6)

STEMI occurs as a result of clot formation at the site of an inflamed atheromatous plaque, occlusion of the coronary artery, downstream ischaemia and then infarction. The combination of aspirin with thrombolysis has been shown to restore antegrade blood flow in >50% of STEMI patients.

Streptokinase is a non-enzyme protein produced by several strains of haemolytic streptococci and indirectly activates the conversion of plasminogen to plasmin. Most people have circulating antibodies to streptokinase, due to previous streptococcal exposure, so a sufficient dose must be infused to overcome this resistance. Antibody titres rise rapidly a few days after streptokinase administration, so further doses are considerably less effective and produce an allergic response if given within 4–6 months. It lacks specificity, has a long half-life and is less effective than some of the newer agents.

Anisoylated plasminogen–streptokinase activator complex (APSAC) was developed to create a more predictable thrombolytic effect. It requires deacylation *in vivo* before being effective in converting plasminogen to plasmin. Antibodies to streptokinase also cross-react with APSAC.

Urokinase, a trypsin-like serine protease, can be isolated from human urine or cultured human embryonic kidney cells. It has been used as an alternative to streptokinase in the USA but rarely used in the UK. Recombinant prourokinase was later produced.

Recombinant tissue-type plasminogen activator (rt-PA) is a serine protease which is converted to plasmin by hydrolysis *in vivo*. The presence of fibrin enhances the efficiency of plasminogen activation by rt-PA. The high affinity of rt-PA for plasminogen in the presence of fibrin thus allows its activation at the site of the fibrin clot, without plasminogen activation in the plasma, making it more clot-specific. rt-PA is a commonly used thrombolytic and is now being superseded by similar agents that are even easier to administer, such as **reteplase** and **tenecteplase**.

Specific cardiovascular conditions

Risk reduction

Any intervention, such as drug therapy, to reduce risk in those known to have cardiovascular disease is termed '**secondary prevention**'; intervention in those who may be at risk but who are not yet known to be affected is termed '**primary prevention**'. Of all the risk factors for cardiovascular events (lipids, smoking, hypertension, family history, etc.), the most important for the prediction of future events is the presence of pre-existing disease. Any strategy for risk reduction will reduce the **absolute** number of future events much more in those at highest than those at lowest risk. For instance, take 100 individuals with a risk of a future 'event' over the next year of 10% (group A), and another 100 with a risk of 2% (group B). An intervention which reduces **relative** risk by 50% will decrease the **absolute** number of events from 10 to five in group A, and from two to one in group B.

Thus, although the **relative** risk reduction is the same (50%), the **absolute** reduction in number of events is quite different (5 vs. 1). Health economists place great importance on the magnitude of absolute number of events avoided, because this markedly affects their assessment of cost–benefit. Aspirin is of proven benefit as secondary prevention for patients with vascular disease (see below), but its benefit in primary prevention is still debated. Any absolute risk reduction is much smaller than with secondary prevention though the risk of side effects is the same.

NSTEMI (see Chapter 6)

Aspirin (75–150 mg daily) unequivocally reduces cardiovascular event rates, particularly myocardial infarction, in these patients, and trials (such as CURE) have shown benefit from **clopidogrel** (75 mg daily) given in addition. Combined antiplatelet therapy is now standard. **Heparin** also reduces event rates in these patients, with LMWH being more effective and easier to administer (no blood monitoring) than UFH. Thrombolytic agents have not been found to be beneficial in this group of patients.

Acute STEMI (see Chapter 6)

Thrombolysis reduces mortality in patients with STEMI if given within 12 h of symptom onset. Aspirin also reduces mortality in its own right, and should be given in addition. Recent data from trials (COMMIT, CLARITY) suggest early benefit from clopidogrel in STEMI.

Coronary bypass grafting

(see Chapter 6)

The original Mayo Clinic trial on saphenous vein coronary grafts showed aspirin and dipyridamole to reduce the early graft occlusion rate from 10 to 2%. Aspirin (75–300 mg) is usually prescribed indefinitely. Dipyridamole is no longer routinely used.

Coronary angioplasty and stenting (PCI)

(see Chapter 8)

Aspirin (75 mg daily) and **clopidogrel** (preloading dose 600 mg, then 75 mg daily) have been shown to reduce both peri-procedural and long-term events (MI) after PCI. **Unfractionated heparin** is also commonly given during the procedure (70 U/kg). **Abciximab** has strong evidence to support its use in high-risk or complex PCI, and there are some data to support the use of tirofiban and eptifibatide. The combination of aspirin (for life) and clopidogrel (the duration depends on the type of stent) minimizes the risk of subsequent stent thrombosis; drug-eluting stents require clopidogrel to be given for at least 1 year.

Valve disease

Native valves

Atrial thrombus occurs mainly in patients with mitral valve disease and may embolize and cause stroke. Imaging thrombus in this area is unreliable with transthoracic echocardiography (TTE), but transoesophageal echocardiography (TOE) has higher sensitivity because it gives excellent images of the left atrium (LA) and atrial appendage (see Chapter 3). From autopsy studies in non-anticoagulated patients with rheumatic heart disease, about 50% of patients with atrial fibrillation (AF) have atrial thrombus compared with 15% of those in sinus rhythm. Up to 75% of clinically significant embolic episodes from LA thrombus involve the cerebral circulation. The risk of emboli increases with age and previous episodes of embolization. In the absence of AF, pure mitral regurgitation (MR) has a low incidence of embolic episodes. Mitral valve prolapse and aortic valve disease have a very low incidence.

Patients in AF with mitral stenosis (MS) are at highest risk and should be anticoagulated to an INR of 2.5–3.5. Patients with mixed MS and MR or severe pure MR should be maintained at an INR of 2.0–3.0. Those with mitral valve prolapse and a history of a transient cerebral event (transient ischaemic attack (TIA)) should be treated with aspirin, but those who have had a stroke, in the absence of an alternative cause, should be considered for anticoagulation (INR 2.0–3.0). Anticoagulation is not required for aortic valve disease or infective endocarditis, unless AF is present.

Prosthetic heart valves

The risk of thromboembolism varies depending on the type of valve (bioprosthetic or mechanical), the particular design (e.g. Starr Edwards, St Jude, Carbomedics, etc.), the position (mitral or aortic) into which it is inserted and the presence of other factors (AF, LV dysfunction, previous emboli, etc.). Overall, the risk of thrombus formation on prosthetic valves has decreased as their design has improved, and hence the degree of anticoagulation required has tended to be lowered. A balance has always to be struck between optimum protection from thrombus development and minimizing bleeding complications. The most important thing to stress to patients requiring anticoagulation is the need to maintain adequate and consistent anticoagulation.

General agreement exists that all mechanical prostheses should be anticoagulated, with the risk of emboli being higher for valves in the mitral than the aortic position. An INR of 2.5–3.5 is sufficient for those with no other embolic risk factors, but an INR of 3.0–4.5 should be achieved for those at higher risk. Several trials have suggested an even lower rate of embolism and death when antiplatelet agents (usually aspirin) are combined with warfarin, but this additional benefit may have been due to a reduction in the rate of myocardial infarction in these patients. Patients who require anticoagulation, but also have coronary disease, are often treated with a combination of warfarin and low-dose (75 mg) aspirin. In the absence of other risk factors, bioprostheses (xenografts) do not require long-term anticoagulation, although some advocate anticoagulation (INR 2.0–3.0) for 3 months after surgery, a time when the risk of thrombus forming on the bioprosthesis is highest.

Patients with prosthetic valves should not have their anticoagulants stopped unless absolutely necessary. When patients undergo non-cardiac surgery, and anticoagulation is felt to be hazardous, warfarin can be stopped 3–4 days before the proposed surgery and UFH substituted to maintain an aPTT ratio of 2.0–2.5 times normal. The heparin can then be stopped 4–6 h preoperatively, allowing near normal coagulation for the operative period, and restarted as soon as haemostasis is felt to be satisfactory. Patients with a prosthetic valve who are anticoagulated and have a stroke should have an urgent computed tomographic (CT) or magnetic resonance imaging (MRI) scan of the head; if the stroke is embolic and only of moderate size, anticoagulation can be continued, unless temporarily contraindicated by severe systemic hypertension, and the later addition of an antiplatelet agent should be considered. If the stroke is haemorrhagic or due to a large embolic infarct, anticoagulation should be omitted acutely and a management plan discussed.

Non-valvular atrial fibrillation

The lack of uniform contraction in the left atrium, and particularly its appendage, during AF increases the risk of clot formation, and AF carries a substantially increased risk of embolic stroke even in the absence of valvular disease. In a study of over 27 000 men and women (Frost *et al.*, 2000), AF increased the stroke rate 2.4 times for men and 3.0 times for women when compared with the general population. The incidence of stroke increases with age, the stroke rate (% per patient per year) in the above study being:

50–59 years	1.3%
60–69 years	2.2%
70–79 years	4.2%
80–89 years	5.1%

The absolute risk of emboli in non-valvular AF depends crucially on the presence of risk factors, being positively correlated with:
• increasing age (as above);
• presence of systemic hypertension;
• diabetes;

- previous stroke;
- cerebral TIA;
- recent heart failure;
- other structural heart disease.

Echocardiographic predictors of increased risk include LA enlargement, the presence of spontaneous contrast formation (sluggish blood flow) and impaired LV function. TOE provides the best images of the LA. It has recently been established that the risk of thromboembolic complication is also elevated in patients with paroxysmal AF, as well as in those in whom the AF is persistent, particularly when an attack lasts >48–72h.

All these factors need to be taken into account when considering whether a patient should be recommended for anticoagulation with warfarin. In general, patients under 65 years who are in AF, without additional risk factors, should be advised to take daily aspirin (300mg), and those with additional risk factors should be anticoagulated (INR 2.0–3.0). Each patient needs to be considered individually, and their thrombotic vs. bleeding risk assessed.

Cardioversion

Systemic embolization is a complication of electrical or pharmacological cardioversion of AF to the mechanically more efficient sinus rhythm. In the absence of a contraindication, it is generally accepted that all patients who have been in AF for longer than 48h should be anticoagulated (INR 2.5–3.0) for at least 3 weeks before, and at least 3 weeks after, successful cardioversion. Few data are available for patients with AF of less than 48h, but most would anticoagulate with heparin. Increasingly, TOE is undertaken in this situation to help determine whether intracardiac thrombus is present.

Ventricular thrombus

Before the era of aggressive therapy for acute myocardial infarction (thrombolytics, PCI), left ventricular thrombus probably occurred in up to 30%

of anterior myocardial infarcts and 5% of those with inferior infarcts. In modern practice, the risk of ventricular thrombus has declined. Factors that predict the development of thrombus include poor ejection fraction, size of infarct and the presence of AF. When ventricular thrombus does occur, it generally does so in the first 7 days after infarction. About 75–90% will be detectable on TTE. Meta-analysis of a number of trials suggests that anticoagulation reduces the risk of emboli. Randomized trial data are lacking, so decisions regarding anticoagulation are usually made on an individual patient basis, taking account of perceived risk. In the first 3 months after infarction, left ventricular aneurysms have a 10% risk of embolization and oral anticoagulation is advisable for this period. Chronic left ventricular aneurysms carry a surprisingly low risk of embolization and do not routinely require long-term anticoagulation. Patients with aneurysms and global severe left ventricular dysfunction, mobile thrombus in the left ventricle or those with previous emboli should be anticoagulated long term (INR 2.0–3.0).

Dilated cardiomyopathy

In dilated (idiopathic) cardiomyopathy, autopsy studies show a high risk of mural thrombi (50% in LV, 25% in RV, 20% in RA and 8% in LA). Patients not receiving anticoagulants have an overall risk of around 18% of an embolic episode (14% if in sinus rhythm and 33% if in AF). The risk increases with the severity of LV dysfunction. Anticoagulation (INR 2.0–3.0) should be considered for all patients who are significantly affected by this condition; it is hard to give clear guidance because of lack of good trial data, though all in AF should be anticoagulated. For some reason, the risk of emboli is much lower in ischaemic cardiomyopathy, and anticoagulation is indicated only for those in AF, those with previous embolism and those with poor ejection fraction together with LV thrombus visible on echocardiography.

Further reading

Frost L, Engholm G, Johnsen S, Møller H, Husted S. Incident of stroke after discharge from the hospital with a diagnosis of atrial fibrillation. *American Journal of Medicine* 2000; 108: 36–40.

Fuster V, Topol EJ, Nabel EG, eds. *Atherothombosis and Coronary Artery Disease*, 2nd edition. Philadelphia, Lippincott Williams & Wilkins, 2005.

Chapter 8

The myocardium

Introduction

Myocardial structure and function

The myocardium of the left (LV) and right (RV) ventricles can generate a cardiac output of 5–20 L/min depending on physiological conditions, and contraction is dependent on the highly specialized cardiac cell, the myocyte. Myocytes are connected by intercalated discs, membranes that facilitate electrical and chemical transmission between cells. Each myocyte contains between 100 and 150 thin myofibrils, with each myofibril made up of multiple sarcomeres, the basic unit of contractile myocardial function (Fig. 8.1). The thin, actin filaments are anchored to the Z-line, and are composed of actin molecules with the proteins tropomyosin and troponin. The thick myosin filaments interdigitate with the actin filaments and the myosin 'heads' interact with the actin filaments dependent on the concentration of intracellular calcium. The majority of myocardial fibres are oriented circumferentially around the LV, but there are also fibres oriented in a longitudinal direction, many being found in the subendocardial region of the myocardium. During systole, fibre shortening results in LV contraction both circumferentially and longitudinally, and thereby reduces the short and long axis diameters of the LV, respectively.

Contraction and relaxation

Electrical stimulation of the myocyte causes influx of calcium through calcium channels in the T-tubules. These are invaginations of the cell membrane related to individual sarcomeres, and influx of calcium causes further intracellular calcium release from the sarcoplasmic reticulum. The increase in intracellular calcium causes the myosin heads to move along the actin molecules, causing reduction in sarcomere length and thereby resulting in myocardial contraction, with conversion of ATP to ADP providing the required energy. Increasing concentrations of intracellular calcium then activate calcium/ATPase pumps, returning calcium to the sarcoplasmic reticulum, and also activate sodium-dependent calcium exchange channels which remove calcium into the extracellular space. This reduction in intracellular calcium results in myocardial relaxation. Myocytes are also rich in mitochondria, and energy release from metabolic pathways regenerates ATP from ADP and phosphate.

Myocardial oxygen usage

Determinants of myocardial oxygen consumption (MVO_2) are important as they are major factors in the development of myocardial ischaemia, particularly where myocardial oxygen delivery may be

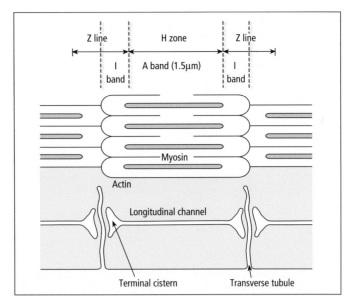

Fig. 8.1 Schematic diagram of a sarcomere element of the myofibril within a cardiac myocyte.

reduced, as occurs in significant coronary artery disease. The four major determinants of MVO$_2$ are:

1 heart rate;
2 preload;
3 afterload; and
4 contractility.

Preload and the Frank–Starling relationship

Preload is the load on the ventricle before systolic contraction and reflects ventricular end-diastolic volume. An increase in preload occurs as a consequence of increasing end-diastolic volume, resulting in augmented ventricular contraction and increased stroke volume. This relationship between preload and augmentation of stroke volume is known as Starling's Law (Fig. 8.2). Increasing preload stretches the individual sarcomeres and augments contraction by optimizing sarcomere length and increasing sensitivity to calcium. Beyond this optimal point, additional stretching causes ventricular stroke volume to fall.

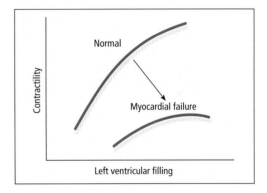

Fig. 8.2 Frank–Starling curve demonstrating the relationship between left ventricular filling and contractility.

Afterload

Afterload is the load, or wall stress, experienced by the ventricle when it contracts during ventricular ejection, and occurs after the onset of systolic contraction. Major determinants of LV afterload are the peripheral arterial vascular resistance (a major determinant of BP; see Chapter 5) and arterial wall compliance. In most clinical circumstances, alteration in BP is a useful indicator of changes in afterload. However, LV myocardial wall stress, and hence afterload, can also be increased by aortic stenosis (AS), a condition where aortic impedance (or resistance) to ejection is increased but arterial BP may be normal or even low. Wall stress increases with LV dilatation (Law of Laplace) and is reduced by LV hypertrophy. The same principles apply to RV function.

Contractility

Contractility, or the inotropic state of the myocardium, is the force of myocardial contraction independent of any other haemodynamic factors such as heart rate, preload or afterload. It is well recognized that contractility can be increased with adrenergic stimulation, calcium or other positively inotropic agents such as digoxin or dobutamine, whereas agents such as β-blockers and calcium channel blockers are negatively inotropic agents and reduce contractility. Because measurement of contractility should be independent of other haemodynamic factors, it is almost impossible to measure in the clinical setting, but the concept is important, particularly as decreased contractility is often the principal abnormality causing heart failure in primary myocardial disease.

Myocardial hypertrophy and dilatation

The LV myocardium responds to pressure overload and volume overload in different ways.

Pressure overload: as occurs in conditions such as arterial hypertension or AS, results in ventricular hypertrophy without any overall change in LV dimension. This so-called 'concentric hypertrophy' results in a reduced cavity size as the ventricular muscle thickens. Myocardial hypertrophy occurs as a result of increasing thickness of individual cardiac myocytes due to increasing numbers of myofibrils, rather than an increase in myocyte numbers. This hypertrophy compensates for the increased aortic pressure or impedance and maintains a normal overall wall stress.

Volume overload: as occurs in conditions such as aortic or mitral regurgitation, causes an increase in preload and results in LV dilatation. This is due to myocyte elongation resulting from longitudinal sarcomere proliferation in the myofibrils. The increase in LV internal dimension increases wall stress and there is compensatory myocyte hypertrophy, though in a pure volume overload situation this hypertrophy is minimal, sufficient only to normalize wall stress from dilatation.

Myocarditis

Acute myocarditis is relatively uncommon, and the diagnosis is often a presumptive one based on clinical symptoms and signs, though strictly speaking it is a histological diagnosis based on the presence of myocyte necrosis and inflammatory infiltration. The natural history of acute myocarditis is highly variable. In many patients, the condition is mild and self-limiting, and the patient may be asymptomatic. However, in some patients, a severe myocarditis may cause profound cardiac failure and death. If the patient survives even a severe acute episode, recovery is highly variable. Some will develop chronic inflammation and heart failure, whereas in others the inflammatory process may resolve, leaving many patients with varying degrees of dilated cardiomyopathy. The aetiology of myocarditis is often unknown and labelled as 'idiopathic', though there are many recognized infective and non-infective causes. Almost any infection (bacterial, viral, fungal, protozoal, etc.) can cause acute myocarditis, though viral infections, particularly Coxsackie, are common in Europe and the USA, whereas trypanosomiasis (Chagas' disease) is common in South America. Acute myocarditis can also occur as a manifestation of HIV infection either directly or as a result of opportunistic infection. See Box 8.1 for non-infective causes of myocarditis.

Clinical features

The presentation of myocarditis is highly variable and may be recognized only because of associated pericarditis (see Chapter 12) as part of a myopericarditis, with chest pain, concave upwards ST elevation and a troponin rise; many patients will also describe a prodromal flu-like illness. The patient may complain of generalized tiredness and

Box 8.1 Non-infective causes of myocarditis
Autoimmune disorders
• Rheumatoid arthritis
• Systemic lupus erythematosus
• Polymyositis
• Systemic sclerosis
• Thyrotoxicosis
• Sarcoidosis
• Diabetes mellitus
Hypersensitivity reactions
• Heavy metals
• Drugs (particularly anthracyclines, cyclophosphamide, fluorouracil)
• Radiation
• Electricity
• Transplant rejection

lethargy or occasionally palpitation as a result of ventricular arrhythmias or atrial fibrillation (AF). Dyspnoea is usually an indication of more serious myocardial dysfunction or a significant pericardial effusion. In severe cases, the presentation may be that of acute pulmonary oedema and severe haemodynamic compromise requiring circulatory support.

Management

Although the diagnosis is primarily histological, myocardial biopsy is rarely performed in mild cases and may not be performed even in severe myocarditis as there is no evidence that anti-inflammatory agents (steroids or immunosuppressive therapy) influence the prognosis. Hence, at present, the biopsy result will often not influence patient management although it may allow a firm diagnosis to be made. Management is largely supportive, with circulatory support and treatment of heart failure in severe cases. If significant pericardial effusion or tamponade is present, pericardial drainage is indicated and, from an analysis of the drained fluid, may help in determining aetiology. In mild cases, NSAIDs are often prescribed for pericardial pain. Steroids and immunosuppressive agents have been used in more severe cases, though their value is unproven.

Cardiomyopathies (See Box 8.2, p. 136)

Dilated cardiomyopathy

Dilated cardiomyopathy is characterized by ventricular dilatation and symptoms and signs of ventricular failure. The term is generally applied to cases of dilated and poorly functioning left ventricles where the aetiology is uncertain ('idiopathic'), thereby excluding ventricular dysfunction secondary to ischaemic or valvular heart disease, or hypertension. A similar clinical picture may occur with chronic ischaemia where severe LV dysfunction results, with or without symptomatic angina, but this is more usually termed 'ischaemic cardiomyopathy'. Some cases of dilated cardiomyopathy may have an autoimmune aetiology, progression from viral myocarditis to dilated cardiomyopathy can occur in up to 10% of patients, and dilated cardiomyopathy can result from non-infective external agents such as alcohol. It can also occur rarely in post-partum women. A genetic predisposition to the development of dilated cardiomyopathy has been recognized in 30–50% of cases where, unlike hypertrophic cardiomyopathy, there is variable gene penetrance and expression. Autosomal dominant, recessive, X-linked and other mutations, such as mitrochondial mutations, have all been associated with dilated cardiomyopathy. The diagnosis of familial dilated cardiomyopathy is generally reserved for situations where abnormalities in LV function can be found in at least two first- or second-degree relatives.

Clinical features

The clinical features are those associated with LV or RV dysfunction. Tiredness, lethargy and dyspnoea are common, and occasionally the patient may present with frank pulmonary oedema. Palpitation due to atrial or ventricular arrhythmias may occur, particularly AF which is common. Systemic or pulmonary embolization may occur secondary to atrial or ventricular thrombus formation, particularly if AF is present. Right heart failure may predominate, with a raised jugular venous pressure (JVP), ascites and peripheral oedema, particularly if there is significant tricuspid regurgitation as a result of RV dilatation, usually manifesting late in the condition. On examination, the LV apex may be displaced and a LV or RV third heart sound may be present. There may be clinical evidence of pulmonary oedema and functional mitral and/or tricuspid regurgitation. Pulsus alternans may be noted.

Investigations

The electrocardiogram (ECG) may show atrial or ventricular arrhythmias, non-specific ST/T wave changes, and poor 'r' wave progression across the anterior chest leads, which is common and occurs as a result of ventricular dilatation. The chest radiograph will often show pulmonary venous congestion or pulmonary oedema. Echocardiography usually demonstrates dilatation of both LV and RV, with globally poor ventricular function, often with associated atrial distension and atrioventricular (AV) valve regurgitation. The global nature of the ventricular dysfunction is important as the presence of regional dysfunction would favour ischaemic heart disease as the underlying aetiology. Sluggish blood flow in the dilated, poorly contracting LV may result in the development of thrombus, particularly in the apex of the ventricle, often visualized by two-dimensional echocardiography. Exercise testing with assessment of oxygen consumption by respiratory gas analysis can provide an objective assessment of functional capacity, as well as demonstrating underlying ECG abnormalities that may reflect myocardial ischaemia. Cardiac catheterization allows measurement of pulmonary artery pressure and pulmonary capillary wedge pressure, and LV end-diastolic pressure, all of which tend to rise with increasing severity of the condition. LV angiography further characterizes the nature and extent of LV dysfunction, and the severity of functional mitral regurgitation. Coronary arteriography excludes ischaemic heart disease as an underlying aetiology. Myocardial biopsy can occasionally be helpful, particularly in myocardial infiltration (see below).

Management

The management of dilated cardiomyopathy is largely based on the management of heart failure (see Chapter 9).

Diuretics, digoxin, angiotensin-converting enzyme (ACE) inhibitors and long-acting nitrates. All of these have a role, with the ACE inhibitors being of particular importance because of their beneficial effects on mortality.

β-*Blockers.* Metoprolol, bisoprolol and carvedilol, for example, have also been shown to be effective in some patients, though the mechanism remains unclear and may be diverse. Anti-arrhythmic drugs are restricted because many of them have negative inotropic effects and may exacerbate heart failure.

Amiodarone. This is commonly prescribed for both atrial and ventricular arrhythmias as it is both effective and generally well tolerated, being relatively free from negative inotropy. Aggressive, life-threatening ventricular arrhythmias may require insertion of an internal defibrillator.

Anticoagulation. Generally recommended in patients with dilated cardiomyopathy especially when associated with atrial arrhythmias or in the presence of ventricular thrombus. However, even in patients without evidence of thrombus and who remain in sinus rhythm, many would still advise anticoagulation if there is severe LV dysfunction and/or atrial dilatation.

Cardiac transplantation. Reserved for younger patients with severe functional incapacity or deteriorating heart failure. Difficulty in obtaining sufficient donor organs led to the development of alternative surgical techniques, ventricular reduction surgery, but these have not been proven to provide benefits in morbidity and mortality.

Stem cell implantation. This remains experimental, but the transformation of injected stem cells into functioning myocardium holds promise for the treatment of dilated cardiomyopathy.

Hypertrophic cardiomyopathy

Hypertrophic cardiomyopathy (HCM) is characterized by unexplained, usually patchy, hypertrophy of the LV and occasionally RV myocardium. It occurs in the absence of secondary causes of ventricular hypertrophy such as AS or systemic hypertension, and is often localized to the upper portion of the interventricular septum (IVS) and anterior free wall of the LV. If the RV is involved, it is almost always in association with LV disease. Histologically, there is hypertrophy associated with myocardial cell disarray as well as disruption of the myofibrillar components within the hypertrophied myocytes. There is usually a variable degree of associated fibrosis.

HCM is inherited as an autosomal dominant disorder with causative genetic mutations of the sacromere proteins, many of which have been isolated, including the β-cardiac myosin heavy chain on chromosome 14 and the cardiac troponin T gene on chromosome 1. Hence, there is often a family history of the condition, in addition to cases due to spontaneous mutation. Late onset in the elderly is also well recognized, associated with mutation of myosin-binding protein C.

Clinical features

Symptoms include dyspnoea, chest pain, palpitation, dizziness or syncope. Occasionally sudden death may be the first presentation. Clinical signs of HCM can be minimal. An ejection systolic murmur at the left sternal edge is most commonly heard. The pulse is usually normal, though a 'jerky' rapidly rising pulse is described. The apex beat may be rather sustained as a function of ventricular hypertrophy.

Investigations

Transthoracic **echocardiography** (TTE) is the main diagnostic investigation (Fig. 8.3) most commonly demonstrating asymmetric septal hypertrophy of the LV, although isolated apical or posterior wall hypertrophy may also occur. Doppler ultrasound can assess the severity of LV outflow tract obstruction, the most significant obstruction usually occurring in late systole after most of the left ventricular ejection has already occurred. Systolic anterior motion of the mitral valve occurs so that the tips of the mitral leaflets may appose the interventricular septal, and mitral regurgitation of varying degree is commonplace. In families with known HCM, the diagnosis may be made at a screening echocardiographic examination and, in some cases, may be identified incidentally in patients undergoing echocardiography for other reasons. Where the diagnosis is uncertain on conventional TTE, transoesophageal echocardiography (TOE) or magnetic resonance imaging (MRI) provide useful alternatives for diagnostic confirmation.

The **ECG** can show a variety of abnormalities — the QRS complexes may be broad and bizarre, there may be voltage criteria for LV hypertrophy, widespread ST–T changes, interventricular conduction defects and AF, although the

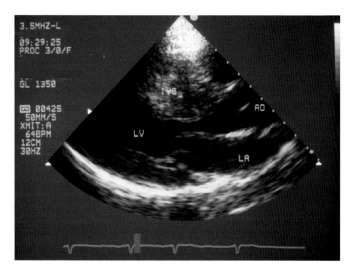

Fig. 8.3 Two-dimensional echocardiogram from a patient with hypertrophic cardiomyopathy. Note the grossly thickened interventricular septum (IVS) in comparison with the normal left ventricular posterior wall.

ECG is normal in 5 to 25% of patients. In patients with confirmed HCM, **ambulatory ECG** (Holter) monitoring is important as the presence of significant ventricular arrhythmias can occur in up to 25% of adults and may be asymptomatic. The presence of significant ventricular arrhythmias is associated with increased mortality.

Cardiac catheterization may be necessary, particularly in patients with chest pain, in order to determine whether there is co-existing coronary artery disease. LV angiography often demonstrates cavity obliteration during systole. Measurement of the gradient across the left ventricular outflow tract can be performed, confirming the severity of outflow tract obstruction.

Management

Management is aimed at symptomatic relief, treatment of potentially life-threatening arrhythmias and assessment of risk. Symptoms may be due to poor myocardial relaxation, hyperdynamic systolic function with significant LV outflow tract obstruction, arrhythmias, particularly AF, or the presence of significant mitral regurgitation. Due to the presence of severe and extensive ventricular hypertrophy, ischaemic symptoms can occur even in the absence of coronary artery disease.

β-Blockers and calcium channel blockers, particularly verapamil, have been used to promote myocardial relaxation and reduce ventricular outflow tract obstruction. Where outflow tract obstruction is the predominant feature, surgical myomectomy or percutaneously delivered septal alcohol ablation may be beneficial. Mitral valve replacement may be necessary if MR is severe. Dual-chamber cardiac pacing has also been recommended in some patients; alteration in the timing of atrial and ventricular electrical activation may augment ventricular filling and reduce outflow tract obstruction.

Increased risk of sudden death can be predicted by a family history of sudden death, the presence of ventricular arrhythmias, a hypotensive response to exercise, a history of syncope and a septal thickness greater than 3 cm. Patients with high risk of sudden death should be considered for prophylactic treatment with an implantable defibrillator.

Restrictive cardiomyopathy

Restrictive cardiomyopathy is the most uncommon type of cardiomyopathy outside certain geographical regions, such as Africa, where **endomyocardial fibrosis** is more prevalent. The presentation of restrictive cardiomyopathy is often similar to, if not identical with, that of constrictive pericarditis (see Chapter 12). Differentiation of the two conditions is important as constrictive pericarditis can be successfully treated by surgery whereas the management of restrictive cardiomyopathy is largely supportive. There are a number of other causes of restrictive cardiomyopathy that occasionally occur in adults:

1 amyloid;
2 sarcoid; and
3 haemochromatosis.

Clinical features

These result from diastolic dysfunction with restricted ventricular relaxation. Systolic contraction is usually well maintained until late in the natural history of the disease when ventricular dilatation and dysfunction develops. Dyspnoea and exercise intolerance predominate, and clinical signs are mainly those of RV dysfunction, such as a raised JVP with its further increase on inspiration (Kussmaul's sign), peripheral oedema, hepatomegaly and ascites. There may be a third and/or fourth heart sound present. Pulmonary oedema is rarely present until late in the disease process.

Investigations

ECG and chest radiograph findings are nonspecific, although the presence of pericardial calcification strongly favours the diagnosis of constrictive pericarditis rather than restrictive cardiomyopathy. On echocardiography, the myocardium is usually thickened, with abnormal left ventricular filling on Doppler ultrasound. In amyloidosis, myocardial deposition produces a characteristic 'ground-glass' textured appearance to the thickened myocardium. The ventricles are not usually dilated until end-stage disease, but there is early biatrial dilatation which may become considerable ('giant atria'). Useful information may be obtained on cardiac MRI scanning.

Cardiac catheterization demonstrates raised right atrial pressure with a prominent 'a' wave and rapid 'x' and 'y' descents. Left and right ventricular filling pressures are abnormal with an initial rapid fall in pressure at the onset of diastole, followed by a rapid rise in diastolic pressure in both ventricles to a raised plateau throughout the rest of diastole, the so-called 'dip-and-plateau' or 'square root' appearance (see Fig. 12.2). A similar pattern is also seen in constrictive pericarditis, although in constriction ventricular diastolic pressures are closely similar, whereas they are often quite different in restriction. In practice, it is often impossible to distinguish the two based on their haemodynamics. Myocardial biopsy is an important diagnostic part of cardiac catheterization. The presence of amyloid, sarcoidosis or haemochromatosis can usually be identified from either right or left ventricular biopsy material.

Management

This is generally supportive, with treatment of fluid retention and arrhythmias. Calcium channel blockers may improve ventricular relaxation. The clinical course is usually that of progressive deterioration, although its onset and rapidity are variable. In haemochromatosis, repeated venesection and the use of chelating agents may be beneficial. If investigations fail to exclude pericardial constriction, then it may be appropriate to consider exploratory thoracotomy, because patients with constriction may respond very well to pericardiectomy and such a treatable condition should not be missed. In restriction, cardiac transplantation should be considered for those most severely affected.

Miscellaneous

Acromegaly

The cardiac effects of acromegaly are ill under-

stood. A cardiomyopathy characterized by dilatation of all four chambers occurs late in the disease and appears to be related to elevated levels of growth hormone, which, when corrected, result in some improvement in the cardiac dysfunction. Disproportionate cardiac enlargement, compared with other organs, occurs in 75% of affected patients. Histology demonstrates an increase in both collagen and fibrous connective tissue which results in poor contractility. Systemic hypertension is present in 30% of acromegalics, and this may result in LV hypertrophy. Other cardiac manifestations of acromegaly include conduction disturbance, arrhythmias, hyperlipidaemia (in the presence of diabetes mellitus, which complicates 15–20% of cases) and atherosclerotic coronary disease. Treatment is directed towards suppression of the increased growth hormone secretion by surgical removal or irradiation of the pituitary adenoma, together with conventional treatment for any heart failure.

Hypothyroidism

Hypothyroidism may be associated with a cardiomyopathy characterized by dilatation of all four cardiac chambers with an increase in interstitial fibrosis and swelling of the myofibrils on histology. The consequent reduction in systolic function causes breathlessness and fluid retention. Pericardial effusions are common, occurring in approximately 30% of patients. There appears to be little correlation between the severity of the biochemical derangement and the severity of any cardiomyopathy or the size of an effusion. Electrocardiographic features include a sinus bradycardia, low voltages, conduction abnormalities and nonspecific repolarization changes. Cardiac arrhythmias (including ventricular tachycardia) have also been described. Untreated hypothyroidism is associated with an elevated cholesterol which may predispose to premature coronary artery disease. Treatment involves the cautious administration of thyroid replacement using L-thyroxine (T4), initially at a dose of 25 μg, increasing progressively after a few weeks until the level of thyroid-stimulating hormone returns to normal.

Box 8.2 Cardiomyopathies

Dilated cardiomyopathy
- Hereditary
- Secondary
  - Coronary artery disease
  - Myocarditis
  - Autoimmune disorders
  - Cardiotoxins (see causes of myocarditis)
  - Post-partum
Hypertrophic cardiomyopathy
Restrictive cardiomyopathy
Hereditary neuromyopathic
Miscellaneous

Connective tissue diseases

A number of connective tissue diseases including rheumatoid arthritis and systemic lupus erythematosus can affect the myocardium, resulting in ventricular dysfunction, though they more commonly cause pericarditis and pericardial effusion. Systemic sclerosis frequently causes myocardial fibrosis as seen at autopsy (80%), but this is not usually sufficient to cause symptomatic ventricular dysfunction. Cardiomyopathy can occur with either a restrictive or a dilated pattern.

Hereditary neuromyopathic conditions

Erb's limb girdle dystrophy

This is an autosomal recessive condition which is most commonly expressed during the second and third decades of life. Progressive weakness of the limb girdle musculature is the major clinical feature. Cardiac involvement is usually limited to abnormalities of sinus node and AV node function, and the conduction system.

Facioscapulohumeral dystrophy

This is a rare autosomal dominant condition with marked weakness of the facial, arm and shoulder musculature, and is usually evident at the end of the first decade of life. Atrial standstill is a rare cardiac manifestation.

Duchenne muscular dystrophy

This is an X-linked recessive disorder. It has an early onset and is rapidly progressive, with skeletal muscle weakness and dystrophy. A late onset and less rapidly progressive form (Becker dystrophy) is also seen. Cardiac muscle may be affected by dystrophic fibrosis and fatty infiltration, giving rise to the clinical features associated with a cardiomyopathy. All cardiac structures may be affected, including abnormalities of the specialized conduction system, coronary arteries and the papillary musculature, in addition to the myocardium. Arrhythmias, valvular disease, and systolic and diastolic ventricular dysfunction may all be apparent.

Dystrophia myotonica

This condition is inherited as an autosomal dominant trait and is one of the more common neuromuscular disorders. Weakness of the flexor muscles of the neck and sternocleidomastoid muscles is an early clinical manifestation. Cardiac abnormalities include disease of the specialized His–Purkinje conduction system, and a dilated cardiomyopathy.

Friedreich's ataxia

This spinocerebellar degenerative disease is inherited as an autosomal recessive trait and has a spectrum of neurological involvement, which are classified by their clinical manifestations. Cardiac involvement is common and often the cause of death. Some develop regional ventricular dysfunction, some more global hypokinesia, and others develop a hypertrophic form of cardiomyopathy.

Chapter 9

Heart failure

Introduction

Heart failure is a clinical syndrome and is the final common pathway for a variety of diseases which affect the heart. Overall cardiovascular mortality rates have declined in industrial countries over the last few decades, but the prevalence of heart failure is increasing. More patients now survive myocardial infarction, but many will subsequently develop heart failure in later life, with its consequent disability. Heart failure has a worse prognosis than most cancers; 40% of patients die within the first year of diagnosis. However, there is a variety of proven medical, surgical and device therapies, which can improve both symptoms and prognosis.

Definition

When few cardiac investigations were available, the definitions of heart failure tended to be pathophysiological, with later definitions placing an increased emphasis on heart failure being a clinical diagnosis (see Box 9.1). Most recent definitions have required supportive evidence from cardiac investigations, most commonly echocardiography, with left ventricular (LV) dysfunction usually defined as ejection fractions of <30–45%. Whilst no universally accepted definition for chronic heart failure (CHF) exists, it is recognized clinically by a constellation of signs and symptoms produced by

> **Box 9.1 Definitions of heart failure**
>
> 'A pathophysiological state in which the heart fails to maintain an adequate circulation for the needs of the body despite a satisfactory filling pressure'. (Paul Wood, 1958)
>
> 'A pathophysiological state in which an abnormality of cardiac function is responsible for the failure of the heart to pump blood at a rate commensurate with the requirements of the metabolizing tissues'. (Eugene Braunwald, 1980)
>
> 'A syndrome in which cardiac dysfunction is associated with reduced exercise tolerance, a high incidence of ventricular arrhythmias and shortened life expectancy'. (Jay Cohn, 1988)
>
> 'The presence of heart failure symptoms (at rest or during exercise), together with objective evidence of cardiac dysfunction (preferably by echocardiography). In cases of doubt a response to treatment is required'. (European Society of Cardiology, 2005)

complex circulatory and neurohumeral responses to cardiac dysfunction. In cases of doubt, a response to treatment directed towards heart failure is required.

Epidemiology

- CHF affects 1–2% of the adult population in economically developed countries (similar numbers have asymptomatic LV dysfunction).
- CHF prevalence increases with age (6–10% of people over 65 years affected).

- Lifetime risk of developing CHF is approximately 1 in 5 for a person aged 40 years.
- CHF is the most common cause of admission to hospital in those >65 years.
- CHF accounts for 5% of all medical admissions in the UK, with a bed occupancy rate of 10% reflecting the prolonged admissions typical of this syndrome.
- 1–2% of health care budgets are spent on CHF management in industrialized countries (annual cost estimated at ~1.9% of the total NHS budget in 2000; 70% of this being hospital costs).

Aetiology

Heart failure is a clinical state and not a diagnosis; the cause should always be sought (Box 9.2). It

---

Box 9.2 Causes of heart failure

Coronary artery disease
- Myocardial infarction
- Ischaemia

Hypertension

Cardiomyopathy
- Dilated
- Hypertrophic
- Restrictive

Valvular and congenital heart disease
- Mitral and/or aortic valve disease
- Atrial and/or ventricular septal defect

Arrhythmias
- Tachycardias
- Bradycardia

Alcohol

Drugs
- Cardiodepressants
- Chemotherapeutic agents

High output failure
- Anaemia
- Thyrotoxicosis
- Arteriovenous fistula

Pericardial disease
- Constrictive pericarditis
- Pericardial effusion

Right heart failure
- Pulmonary hypertension
- Pulmonary embolism
- Tricuspid incompetence

---

usually arises as a consequence of an abnormality in cardiac structure, function, rhythm or conduction. In economically developed countries heart failure is most commonly due to failure of myocardial contractility, as may occur with myocardial infarction, longstanding hypertension (see Chapter 5) or a cardiomyopathy (see Chapter 8). However, under certain conditions, even myocardium with good contractility may be unable to maintain sufficient forward blood flow to meet the body's metabolic needs. Such conditions include mechanical problems such as severe valvular regurgitation and, more rarely, arteriovenous fistulae, thiamine deficiency (beriberi) and severe anaemia. These high cardiac output states may themselves cause heart failure but, when less severe, may precipitate heart failure in those with underlying cardiac disease.

The prevalence of aetiological factors will depend on the population being studied, coronary heart disease (see Chapter 6) and hypertension being the most common causes in Western societies, whereas valvular heart disease and nutritional deficiencies may be more important in developing countries. Independent risk factors for the development of heart failure are similar to those for coronary artery disease (raised cholesterol, hypertension, smoking, diabetes and obesity), but there is also a strong association between the presence of LV hypertrophy (LVH) on the resting electrocardiogram (ECG) and the development of heart failure. The prevalence of aetiological factors has changed with time: cohort data from the Framingham Study, which was started in the 1940s, identified a history of hypertension in >75% of patients with heart failure, whereas more recent studies suggest much lower prevalences (10–50%), perhaps due to the better treatment of hypertension. Effective treatment of hypertension may therefore reduce the incidence of heart failure by as much as 50%.

Excess **alcohol** and some **drugs** such as chemotherapeutic agents (e.g. doxorubicin) can be cardiotoxic. Other drugs may reduce myocardial contractility (negative inotropism), such as some calcium antagonists and the acute use of β-blockers (see later for their place in the management of CHF).

Arrhythmias reduce cardiac efficiency, as occurs when atrial contraction is lost (atrial fibrillation, AF) or dissociated from ventricular contraction (heart block). Tachycardias (ventricular or atrial) reduce ventricular filling time, increase myocardial workload and oxygen demand leading to myocardial ischaemia, and, when prolonged, may cause ventricular dilatation and worsening ventricular function. Arrhythmias are common consequences of heart failure itself, whatever the aetiology, with AF reported in up to 20–30% of cases of heart failure at first presentation. Arrhythmias are a common cause of patients with stable heart failure symptoms becoming symptomatic with worsening heart failure. Ventricular arrhythmias are a common cause of sudden cardiac death in this condition.

Pathophysiology

When a primary disturbance of myocardial contractility exists or an excessive haemodynamic burden is placed on a normal ventricle, the heart depends on a number of adaptive mechanisms to maintain cardiac output and blood pressure (see Box 9.3 and Fig. 9.1). Most important amongst these adaptive mechanisms are the following:

- The **Frank–Starling mechanism**, in which an increased preload helps to sustain cardiac performance.
- Activation of neurohumeral systems, especially the release of **norepinephrine** (noradrenaline), which augments myocardial contractility, and activation of the **renin–angiotensin–aldosterone system (RAAS)**, as well as other neurohormones, which act to maintain arterial pressure and perfusion of vital organs.
- **Myocardial remodelling** with or without cardiac chamber dilatation, in which the mass of contractile tissue is augmented.

These compensatory mechanisms can provide immediate haemodynamic benefits, but they do so at the expense of longer-term adverse consequences, which themselves contribute to the

> **Box 9.3 Adaptive mechanisms**
>
> - Myocardial hypertrophy
> - Neurohormonal
> - Activation of renin–angiotensin–aldosterone system
> - Activation of sympathetic nervous sytem
> - Natriuretic peptides, antidiuretic hormone (ADH) and endothelin
> - Frank–Starling mechanism

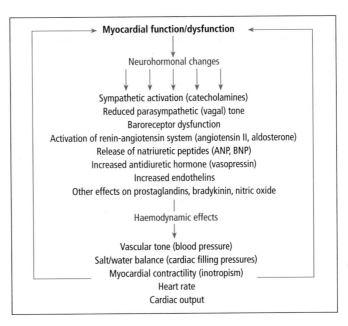

Fig 9.1 Diagram showing the relationship between myocardial function, adaptive mechanisms occurring in heart failure and the haemodynamic consequences of these interactions.

development of CHF (Fig. 9.1). For instance, **myocardial hypertrophy** increases the mass of contractile elements and improves systolic contraction, but also increases ventricular wall stiffness, impairing ventricular filling and diastolic function.

In the setting of CHF, vascular redistribution of blood occurs to allow the limited cardiac output to be most useful for survival. Thus vasoconstriction occurs earliest in areas that are not vital for **immediate** survival, such as the skin, skeletal muscle, gut and kidney. Reduced renal perfusion causes stimulation of the RAAS, resulting in increased levels of **renin, plasma angiotensin II** and **aldosterone**. Angiotensin II is a powerful vasoconstrictor of the renal efferent (and systemic) arterioles, where it stimulates the release of norepinephrine (noradrenaline) from sympathetic nerve endings, inhibits vagal tone and promotes the adrenal release of aldosterone, causing sodium and water retention and renal excretion of potassium. Impaired hepatic function in heart failure may reduce aldosterone metabolism, increasing aldosterone levels still further.

The **sympathetic nervous system** is activated in CHF via baroreceptors, resulting initially in enhanced myocardial contractility. However, prolonged activation of the RAAS, and other neurohormones, leads to increased venous (cardiac preload) and arterial (cardiac afterload) tone, increased plasma norepinephrine, progressive retention of salt and water, and oedema. Chronic sympathetic stimulation results in the down-regulation of cardiac β-receptors, attenuating the heart's usual response to stimulation, for example in response to exercise. This contributes to the exercise intolerance associated with heart failure.

Natriuretic peptides exert a wide range of effects on the heart, kidney and central nervous system.
• **Atrial natriuretic peptide** (ANP) is released from the cardiac atria in response to stretch, leading to natriuresis and vasodilatation.
• In humans, **brain natriuretic peptide** (BNP) is also released from the heart, predominantly from the ventricles, and has actions similar to

ANP. The natriuretic peptides act as physiological antagonists to the effects of angiotensin II on vascular tone, aldosterone secretion and renal sodium reabsorption.

Antidiuretic hormone (**arginine vasopressin**) levels are also increased, causing vasoconstriction and contributing to water retention and hyponatraemia.

Endothelin-1 (ET-1) is a highly potent vasoconstrictor peptide secreted by vascular endothelial cells. Plasma ET-1 concentrations are increased in relation to the symptomatic and haemodynamic severity of heart failure. ET-1 plays an important role in mediating pulmonary hypertension, promotes renal retention of sodium and works synergistically with the RAAS.

Constriction of the systemic veins and sodium and water retention increase atrial pressure and ventricular end-diastolic volume and pressure, sarcomeres lengthen and myofibril contraction is enhanced (**Frank–Starling mechanism**).

With such a complex interplay of influential factors, cardiac output in the resting state is a relatively insensitive index of cardiac function, because these compensatory mechanisms work to maintain it as the myocardium fails, but each of these compensatory mechanisms has a price. For instance, catecholamine- and angiotensin-induced vasoconstriction will increase systemic vascular resistance and tend to maintain blood pressure but increase cardiac work and myocardial oxygen consumption.

Non-cardiac abnormalities

The **vascular endothelium** plays an important role in the regulation of vascular tone, locally releasing constricting and relaxing factors. The increased peripheral vascular tone in patients with chronic heart failure is due to increased sympathetic activity, activation of the RAAS and impaired release of nitric oxide (formerly known as endothelium-derived relaxing factor). Some of the beneficial effects of exercise and certain drug treatments (angiotensin-converting enzyme (ACE) inhibitors) may be due to improvements in endothelial function.

Diastolic dysfunction

Impaired myocardial relaxation, due to increased ventricular wall stiffness and reduced compliance, results in impaired diastolic ventricular filling. Ischaemic myocardial fibrosis (coronary artery disease) and LVH (hypertension, hypertrophic cardiomyopathy) are the most common causes, but it may rarely be due to myocardial infiltration, by, for instance, amyloid. Diastolic dysfunction often coexists with systolic failure, but may occur in isolation in 20–40% of patients presenting with heart failure. The diagnosis of diastolic dysfunction is both complex and controversial, and is usually made using a variety of echocardiographic measurements. Differentiation between diastolic and systolic heart failure may make little difference to management because it remains uncertain how best to treat diastolic dysfunction.

Myocardial remodelling, hibernation and stunning

After extensive myocardial infarction, regional hypertrophy of the non-infarcted segments, with wall thinning and cavity dilatation of the infarct territory, constitutes the process of remodelling. This is most pronounced when the infarct-related coronary artery remains occluded rather than recanalized. Even after successful reperfusion, myocardial recovery may be delayed (myocardial stunning). This is in contrast to myocardial hibernation, which describes more persistent myocardial dysfunction at rest, secondary to reduced myocardial perfusion, even though cardiac myocytes remain viable and contractility may improve with revascularization. The stunned or hibernating myocardium remains responsive to inotropic stimulation, and can be assessed by stress echocardiography, radionuclide myocardial perfusion scanning, magnetic resonance imaging or positron emission tomography (PET).

Clinical presentation

This is determined by the relative contribution of three main factors:

1 cardiac damage;

2 haemodynamic overload; and

3 the secondary compensating mechanisms that arise as heart failure develops.

Initially the compensatory mechanisms may be effective at maintaining cardiac output, and the symptoms associated with heart failure may only be present on exercise. Symptoms later occur at rest as the condition worsens.

Clinical manifestations are also influenced by the rate of progression of the disease and whether compensatory mechanisms have had time to develop. For instance, the sudden development of mitral regurgitation may be tolerated poorly and cause acute heart failure (AHF), whereas the gradual development of the same amount of mitral regurgitation may be tolerated with few symptoms. In the earlier stages of heart failure, symptoms may be non-specific (malaise, lethargy, fatigue, dyspnoea, exercise intolerance) but, as the condition progresses, the clinical features may become overtly indicative of cardiac disease.

Heart failure may principally affect the left heart, right heart or both (biventricular or congestive failure), but in practice the left heart is most often affected. Isolated right heart failure may occur due to major pulmonary embolism, pulmonary hypertension or pulmonary valve disease. The ventricles share the interventricular septum, so dysfunction of either ventricle can potentially influence function of the other. Patients often present with a mixture of symptoms and signs related to both ventricles, but it simplifies matters to consider them as if they occur in isolation.

Left heart failure (see Box 9.4)

An increase in left atrial pressure raises pulmonary venous pressure and results in pulmonary congestion and eventually alveolar oedema, causing breathlessness, coughing and occasionally haemoptysis. Dyspnoea will initially be present on exercise, but as LV failure progresses may occur at rest, causing orthopnoea and paroxysmal nocturnal dyspnoea (PND).

Examination will often be normal but, as heart failure progresses, the following may be observed.

Box 9.4 Clinical features of left heart failure

Symptoms
- Reduced exercise capacity
- Dyspnoea (wheeze, orthopnoea, PND)
- Cough (haemoptysis)
- Lethargy and fatigue
- Reduced appetite and weight loss

Signs
- Cool skin
- Blood pressure (high, low or normal)
- Pulse (normal or low volume, alternans, tachycardia, arrhythmias)
- Displaced apex
- Third sound, summation gallop
- Functional mitral regurgitation
- Pulmonary crepitations
- (± Pleural effusion)

Box 9.5 Clinical features of right heart failure

Symptoms
- Ankle swelling
- Dyspnoea (but not orthopnoea or PND)
- Reduced exercise capacity
- Chest pain

Signs
- Pulse (tachycardia arrhythmias)
- Raised JVP (±tricuspid regurgitation)
- Oedema
- Hepatomegaly and ascites
- Parasternal heave
- RV S3 or S4
- (Pleural effusion)

- The **skin** may be cool and pale reflecting peripheral vasoconstriction.
- The **blood pressure** may be high in the case of hypertensive heart disease, normal, or low as cardiac dysfunction worsens.
- The **pulse** may be low volume and the rhythm may be normal, or irregular due to ectopics or AF. **Pulsus alternans** may be noted.

Resting sinus **tachycardia** usually reflects severe heart failure and sympathetic activation. The jugular venous pressure (JVP) is normal in isolated left heart failure. On palpation, the **apex** may be displaced laterally (LV dilatation), the beat sustained (LV hypertrophy) or dyskinetic (LV aneurysm). On **auscultation**, there may be a left ventricular third sound (S3), summation gallop, and the murmur of mitral regurgitation secondary to dilatation of the mitral valve ring. Other murmurs may suggest intrinsic valvular heart disease. The pulmonary second heart sound may be accentuated as pulmonary arterial pressure increases secondary to pulmonary venous hypertension. Pulmonary **crackles** (crepitations) arise due to alveolar oedema, and oedema of the bronchial wall may cause wheezing.

Right heart failure (see Box 9.5)

Symptoms may be minimal, especially if diuretics have already been given, but when present include fatigue, dyspnoea (but not orthopnoea or PND), ankle swelling and reduced exercise capacity. As right ventricular (RV) pressure rises or the RV becomes more dilated, chest pain is common. On examination, the **pulse** may show similar abnormalities to left heart failure, the **jugular venous pressure** is often elevated, unless reversed by diuretic treatment, and may show large systolic waves of tricuspid regurgitation. Peripheral **oedema**, **hepatomegaly and ascites** may be present. On palpation there may be a left parasternal heave suggesting RV hypertrophy and/or dilatation, and on auscultation a right ventricular S3 or S4. A pleural effusion may be present with right or left heart failure. Most commonly, the right heart fails secondary to left heart disease, but myocarditis and dilated cardiomyopathy may affect each chamber equally. When the right heart fails sufficiently, the symptoms and signs of left heart failure may diminish because of the inability of the right heart to maintain an output sufficient to keep left-sided filling pressures elevated.

The reduction in cardiac output and reduction in perfusion to organs such as the brain, kidneys and skeletal muscle, whether caused by severe left or right heart failure, results in general symptoms such as mental confusion, tiredness, fatigue and reduced exercise tolerance. The New York Heart Association (NYHA) has classified functional limitation (see Box 9.6).

Box 9.6 Functional classification of heart failure (NYHA)

- Class I: no limitation in physical activity
- Class II: slight limitation of exercise (fatigue, dyspnoea)
- Class III: marked limitation of activity (comfortable at rest but slight exertion causes symptoms)
- Class IV: symptoms even at rest

Prognosis

The 1-year mortality in patients with heart failure is high and correlates with its severity. Framingham data, collected before the widespread use of vasodilator treatment for heart failure, indicated an average 1-year mortality of 30% when all patients with heart failure are grouped together, and >60% for those in NYHA class IV. However, as medical and device treatment for heart failure advances, the prognosis of heart failure improves, such that now a patient with stable NYHA class II/III heart failure aged 60, on optimal medical therapy, has an annual mortality of <10%. Death occurs typically due either to progressive cardiac failure or to sudden death, which is predominantly due to arrhythmias (ventricular tachycardia or ventricular fibrillation; less commonly bradyarrhythmias). Patients who are well (NYHA class I/II) are more likely to die of sudden death, whereas patients with advanced heart failure (NYHA class IV) are more likely to die a progressive heart failure death.

Predicting the prognosis of a patient with heart failure is particularly challenging due to these differing modes of death. Many indices have now been shown independently to predict a poor outcome in heart failure, but practically three separate measures seem to allow a degree of risk stratification:

- an assessment of **LV function** (e.g. LV ejection fraction (LVEF));
- an assessment of symptoms or **exercise tolerance** (NYHA class, 6 min walk time, oxygen consumption (VO_2 max));
- an assessment of **neurohormonal** activation (simple measures such as hyponatraemia or

elevations in norepinephrine, BNP and ET-1 are associated with a poor prognosis).

Predicting arrhythmic death is difficult, but is potentially important as implantable cardioverter defibrillators (ICDs) provide an effective therapy. As yet we have no reliable risk stratification, though patients with very low ejection fractions and prolonged QRS duration appear to be at greatest risk.

Investigations

- **Electrocardiography** shows some abnormality in almost all heart failure patients. Indeed a normal ECG virtually precludes the diagnosis of heart failure. Common abnormalities include Q waves, ST/T wave changes, LV hypertrophy, conduction disturbance, axis change and arrhythmias such as AF.
- **Chest radiography** will often show cardiomegaly (cardiothoracic ratio (CTR) >50%), especially when heart failure is chronic. A normal heart size does not exclude the diagnosis, and may be seen when left ventricular failure is acute, such as occurs with myocardial infarction, acute valvular regurgitation or post-infarct ventricular septal defect (VSD). Cardiomegaly may be due to left or right ventricular dilatation, LVH or occasionally a pericardial effusion. The degree of cardiomegaly correlates poorly with left ventricular function.

Normally, lung perfusion favours the bases, but with pulmonary venous congestion (LV failure) upper lobe diversion occurs and, as pulmonary venous pressure rises above 20 mmHg, interstitial oedema develops causing septal lines especially at the bases (known as Kerley B lines). As pressures rise above 25 mmHg, hilar oedema develops in a butterfly or bat's wing distribution, and perivascular oedema produces haziness of the vessels. Engorgement of the superior vena cava (SVC) and azygos veins may be visible. When heart failure causes pleural effusions they are usually bilateral, but if unilateral tend more commonly to occur on the right. Interestingly, this is because patients with advanced heart failure and high filling pressures tend to find it uncomfortable sleeping on their left side and so usually sleep on their right side; thus the dependent oedema collects on the right side. Unilateral left-sided effusions should make one think of other causes such as malignancy.

- **Blood tests** are recommended to exclude anaemia and assess renal function before treatment is started. Thyroid dysfunction (both hyper- and hypothyroidism) may cause heart failure, so tests of thyroid function should also be requested. BNP can now be measured in many centres. Whilst a high BNP level is not specific for heart failure, a low BNP can be helpful in excluding the possible diagnosis of heart failure. **Echocardiography** should be undertaken in all patients in whom there is justifiable clinical suspicion of heart failure. Cardiac cavity dimensions, wall thickness, ventricular function (systolic and diastolic) and wall motion abnormalities can be assessed, and valvular heart disease can be excluded. Mitral regurgitation found in the presence of left ventricular dysfunction is often due to left ventricular enlargement causing mitral ring (annular) dilatation. **Stress echo**, which involves the administration of dobutamine to increase contractility and heart rate, can assess the presence of ischaemia and/or viability of the myocardium.
- **Exercise testing** is often undertaken to assess the presence of myocardial ischaemia and in some cases to measure maximum oxygen consumption (VO_2 max). This is the level beyond which oxygen consumption does not rise any further despite increasing levels of exertion. It represents the limit of aerobic exercise tolerance and is often considerably reduced in heart failure. It is often used as a guide in assessing the need for cardiac transplantation.
- **Ambulatory ECG** monitoring should be undertaken if arrhythmias are suspected.
- **Radionuclide imaging** provides another method of assessing ventricular function and is useful when adequate echocardiographic images are difficult to obtain. Measurements of LVEF are more accurate than with echo, and so these techniques are often used in clinical research. Myocardial perfusion scanning may also be helpful in assessing the functional significance of coronary artery disease and determining whether the myocardium is viable or infarcted.

- **Cardiac magnetic resonance imaging** is becoming increasingly important in patients with heart failure. The quality of imaging allows very accurate measurements of structure and LV function. It is useful in the diagnosis of restrictive cardiomyopathies and can demonstrate evidence of pericardial constriction. Increasingly, use of the non-ionic contrast agent gadolinium has allowed demonstration of areas of completed myocardial infarction and, importantly, the presence of viable myocardium.
- **Cardiac catheterization** should be undertaken when there is a history of angina and revascularization may be required. It can be argued that almost all patients with heart failure should undergo angiography to determine the presence or absence of coronary artery disease as this may alter management (need for aspirin, statins, revascularization). Right heart catheterization with direct measurement of right atrial pressure, pulmonary artery pressure and pulmonary artery capillary wedge pressure allows assessment of the haemodynamic impact of heart failure. These measurements can guide medical therapy, with alteration in diuretic and vasodilator therapy as required. In rare cases, myocardial biopsy is performed (e.g. restrictive cardiomyopathy). When cardiac catheterization is indicated, contrast ventriculography is usually undertaken and provides another measure of LV function.

Management

General and lifestyle factors

- **Physical activity** should be tailored to the level of symptoms. Judicious exercise training reduces sympathetic tone, encourages weight reduction and improves symptoms, the sense of well-being and exercise tolerance in stable, compensated heart failure. Exercise, however, has not been shown to alter outcome in patients with heart failure.
- **Sodium and fluid** restriction is widely advocated in heart failure management, but interestingly without strong supporting evidence; patients

who are oedematous certainly benefit, particularly those with low serum sodium. Hyponatraemia in heart failure reflects sodium and particularly water retention, not sodium depletion.

- **Smoking** tends to reduce cardiac output, and increases heart rate and both systemic and pulmonary vascular resistance; it should be strongly discouraged.
- Although moderate **alcohol** consumption has not been shown to be harmful, alcohol alters fluid balance, is negatively inotropic and may worsen hypertension and precipitate arrhythmias (particularly AF). Its consumption should therefore be kept to a minimum or avoided altogether, especially when thought to be the cause of a cardiomyopathy.

Treatment of underlying causes

The common underlying causes (coronary artery disease, hypertension, cardiomyopathy) should be optimally treated (see Chapters 4, 5 and 8). For patients with coronary artery disease, revascularization (coronary artery bypass graft (CABG) or percutaneous transluminal coronary angioplasty (PTCA)) may improve cardiac function by reducing ischaemia, and prolong survival. Surgery may also be of benefit when significant valve disease (usually aortic or mitral) is present. Attention should be paid to any factors which may have precipitated or exacerbated heart failure (e.g. infection, alterations in drug therapy, worsening angina, electrolyte disturbance).

Drug therapy (see Table 9.1)

Diuretics

Diuretics are used for relief of dyspnoea and signs of sodium and water retention. They are needed in virtually all patients with symptomatic heart failure, but are usually not required for patients with

Table 9.1 Evidence-based pharmacological treatment of heart failure.

Drug	Major trials and year	Starting dose (mg)	Target total daily dose (mg)	Doses per day	Mean trial total daily dose (mg)
ACE inhibitors					
Captopril	SAVE 1992	6.25	150	3	121
Enalapril	CONSENSUS 1987	2.5	20–40	2	16.6
Lisinopril	ATLAS 1999	2.5–5.0	20–35	1	
Ramipril	AIRE 1993	2.5	10	1 or 2	8.7
Trandalopril	TRACE 1995	1.0	4	1	3
β-Blockers					
Bisoprolol	CIBIS II 1999	1.25	10	1	6.2
Carvedilol	COPERNICUS 2001	3.125	50–100	2	37
Metoprolol XL	MERIT-HF 1999	12.5 or 25	200	1	159
Nebivolol	SENIORS 2005	1.25	10	1	7.7
ARBs					
Candesartan	CHARM 2003	4	32	1	24
Losartan	ELITE I/II 1997/2000	12.5	50	1	
Valsartan	Val-HeFT 2001	40	320	2	254
Aldosterone antagonists					
Eplerenone	EPHESUS 2003	25	50	1	43
Spironolactone	RALES 1999	25	50	1	26
Hydralazine + ISDN					
Hydralazine	V-HeFT 1986	37.5	225	3	143
ISDN	A-HeFT 2004	20	120	3	60

asymptomatic LV dysfunction. Their accepted use pre-dates evidence-based trials. They are best used flexibly and in the minimum dose to maintain 'dry weight' and to avoid electrolyte disturbance (hypokalaemia and hyponatraemia), hyperuricaemia (gout) and renal dysfunction.

Loop diuretics (furosemide 40–240 mg daily, bumetanide 1–5 mg daily) increase renal sodium and water excretion by their effect on the ascending limb of the loop of Henle, but their effect when given orally may diminish in chronic severe heart failure due to impaired gut absorption. They can also be given intravenously. Torasemide (10–80 mg daily) is a newer oral loop diuretic that has more reliable gut absorption. These agents cause significant potassium loss and may cause hyperuricaemia. The starting dose for furosemide is typically 20–40 mg daily, but for refractory heart failure doses as high as 240 mg in divided doses are not exceptional.

Thiazide diuretics (bendroflumethiazide 2.5–10 mg daily, hydrochlorothiazide 25–50 mg daily, indapamide 2.5 mg once daily, xipamide 20–80 mg daily and metolazone 2.5–10 mg daily) inhibit salt reabsorption in the distal tubule and promote calcium reabsorption. They are less effective at salt and water removal in heart failure than the loop diuretics and are largely ineffective when the glomerular filtration rate (GFR) falls below around 30% (common in the elderly). The combined use of loop and thiazide diuretics is synergistic and is very useful to treat fluid overload in refractory heart failure. The thiazides have a direct vasodilatory effect on peripheral arterioles, and may cause carbohydrate intolerance, a slight rise in cholesterol and triglycerides, and hyperuricaemia.

Potassium-sparing diuretics fall into two groups: (i) the aldosterone antagonists (spironolactone and eplerenone; see page 147); and (ii) inhibitors of sodium conductance in the collecting duct (amiloride 5–20 mg daily and triamterene 100–250 mg daily in divided doses) which diminish renal potassium and hydrogen ion secretion. These agents are generally used to offset the potassium- and magnesium-losing effects of the loop diuretics. Magnesium deficiency probably occurs more often than is appreciated because, being principally an intracellular ion, blood levels are maintained at the expense of intracellular depletion. Deficiency may increase the risk of arrhythmias and cause muscle weakness and fatigue. Supplements are best given intravenously because gut absorption is poor.

Osmotic diuretics (e.g. mannitol 50–200 g infusion over 24 h) are able to maintain urine flow at a low GFR and may be used in acute severe heart failure, as may occur in the early stages following cardiac bypass surgery. They are filtered by the glomerulus but are not reabsorbed or metabolized by the kidney.

ACE inhibitors

ACE inhibitors are both veno- and arterial dilators but work particularly on the arteriolar bed. They cause a decrease in angiotensin II and a rise in renin. They interfere with the breakdown of the vasodilator bradykinin and decrease circulating catecholamines (angiotensin II promotes the release and inhibits the reuptake of norepinephrine in the sympathetic nervous system), thus activating additional vasodilator mechanisms. ACE inhibitors improve symptoms, reduce hospital admissions for heart failure and reduce mortality (overall 24% decrease in mortality in clinical trials). As such they are recommended for all patients with left ventricular systolic dysfunction.

The main causes of intolerance are cough, symptomatic hypotension and renal dysfunction. Rarely angioedema can occur. They tend to increase serum potassium, so caution is required when used with potassium-sparing diuretics. Renal impairment is not a contraindication to the use of ACE inhibitors; indeed patients with high serum creatinine have a poor outlook and potentially have much to gain from this therapy as ACE inhibitors delay the progression of renal failure. ACE inhibitors are, however, contraindicated in patients with bilateral renal artery stenosis because they can cause anuria. Hypotensive patients and those with pre-existing renal impairment require particularly close monitoring of renal function.

ACE inhibitors should be started at low dose and then gradually increased to the maximum tolerated. The ATLAS trial showed improved outcome with high rather than low doses of lisinopril; interestingly, high dose lisinopril had the most benefit in milder heart failure, emphasizing the need to increase doses of ACE inhibitors even when patients are relatively asymptomatic.

Angiotensin receptor blockers

Angiotensin receptor blockers (ARBs) (e.g. candesartan, irbesartan, losartan, valsartan) prevent binding of angiotensin II to its type I receptor and are similar to ACE inhibitors in terms of haemodynamic effects. Tolerability is better than with ACE inhibitors, with a lower incidence of cough. In the trial CHARM-Alternative (for patients intolerant of an ACE inhibitor), candesartan was well tolerated and resulted in a 13% reduction in mortality compared with placebo. As this mortality reduction is less than that typically seen with ACE inhibitors, this suggests that ACE inhibitors should still be the first-line therapy, with ARBs reserved for patients intolerant of ACE inhibitors. Candesartan led to angioedema in only three of 39 patients who had previously developed angioedema with ACE inhibitors.

ARBs can be given together with ACE inhibitors; angiotensin II levels remain high despite ACE inhibitors, and combination therapy leads to further neurohormonal suppression and greater reverse remodelling of the left ventricle. The combination of an ACE inhibitor and candesartan was studied in the trial CHARM-Added; there was a 15% reduction in combined cardiovascular death/hospitalization for heart failure, but no overall mortality benefit. Importantly there was a high incidence of renal impairment when patients were taking spironolactone (11 vs. 4% with placebo). It remains to be seen whether an ARB or spironolactone is the better add-on therapy for patients already taking an ACE inhibitor and a β-blocker.

β-Blockers

β-Adrenoreceptor blockers used to be avoided in heart failure because of their negatively inotropic action. However, it has now been proven that β-blockers (bisoprolol, carvedilol, metoprolol succinate and nebivolol), when started at low doses in stable heart failure, improve symptoms, LV function and survival (CIBIS II, COPERNICUS, MERIT-HF and SENIORS trials, respectively, Table 9.1). β-Blockers reduce sympathetic activation in heart failure, work to block the adverse effects of norepinephrine and epinephrine (adrenaline), and reduce renin secretion. They may improve cardiac function by reducing heart rate, resulting in lower myocardial energy expenditure, prolonged diastolic filling and increased effective myocardial blood flow due to prolonged coronary (diastolic) perfusion time. β-Blockers may also reduce mortality by reducing the frequency of supraventricular and ventricular arrhythmias.

β-Blockers should only be started when the patient is stable, and gradually up-titrated over weeks and months. Patients may feel worse when β-blockers are first started, and indeed may need increased diuretic doses for a few days, with the symptomatic benefit becoming noticeable after approximately 3 months. β-Blockers can be safely started in all classes of heart failure (including NYHA IV) provided the patient is stable with no signs of fluid overload. Overall mortality is reduced by about a third with a β-blocker. It should also be remembered that stopping a β-blocker can be harmful, both when the patient is stable and importantly when in decompensated heart failure. When patients are admitted with AHF, the β-blocker should be continued unless the patient is unacceptably bradycardic or hypotensive.

Aldosterone antagonists

Aldosterone antagonists were initially used as diuretic agents for the treatment of heart failure. It has now been recognized that aldosterone has a number of adverse effects in heart failure: it promotes vascular and myocardial fibrosis, potassium and magnesium depletion, sympathetic activation and baroreceptor dysfunction. The RALES mortality trial showed that low-dose **spironolactone** (12.5–50 mg daily), when used with an ACE inhibitor, loop diuretics and digoxin in NHYA class III/IV heart failure, reduced mortality and heart failure admissions by approximately a third. At these low doses, spironolactone did not have an appreciable diuretic effect. The RALES trial was conducted before the use of β-blockers was standard therapy, but similar efficacy was seen in the 11% of patients taking β-blockers. Whether spironolactone is of benefit in milder heart failure remains unknown. The main adverse effects seen with spironolactone were renal dysfunction, and antiandrogenic side-effects such as breast pain and gynaecomastia in men.

Eplerenone, which selectively blocks the mineralocorticoid receptor (and not the glucocorticoid, progesterone and androgen receptors), was used in the EPHESUS trial, which involved over 6000 patients with reduced ejection fraction post-myocardial infarction. Eplerenone (25–50 mg daily) resulted in a 15% reduction in mortality, and lower heart failure admissions, during a mean follow-up of 16 months. Seventy-five per cent of these patients were taking β-blockers. Eplerenone was well tolerated, with no increased risk of gynaecomastia. Whilst hyperkalaemia was more common with epleronone, hypokalaemia was less common, perhaps contributing to the reduction in sudden cardiac death seen with eplerenone.

Digoxin

In 1785 William Withering described the use of an extract of foxglove (*Digitalis purpurea*). Experimentally, glycosides such as digoxin increase the velocity of myocardial contraction, and digoxin has traditionally been thought of as a positive inotrope, though it also has autonomic, neurohumoral and diuretic actions. Digoxin is a potent inhibitor of the cellular sodium pump (Na-K ATPase) activity, which results in increased Na–Ca exchange and a rise in intracellular calcium. The effect of this is to increase the availability of calcium ions to the myocardial contractile element at the time of excitation–contraction coupling. The main electrophysiological effect of clinical importance is slowing of conduction through the AV node, thus digoxin is frequently used to control ventricular rate in AF.

Early studies suggested an increased risk of worsening heart failure on withdrawal of digoxin. Digoxin, however, had no effect on mortality in the DIG trial, but did reduce hospitalizations for heart failure and had modest symptomatic benefit. Subsequent reports from this trial have suggested that there was an increase in death in women treated with digoxin and better outcome with low serum digoxin levels (<0.5 ng/mL). Thus the primary indication for digoxin in heart failure is for patients with persisting symptoms or signs, despite use of the standard pharmacological agents described above, or for rate control in addition to a β-blocker, for those in poorly controlled AF.

Contraindications to the use of digoxin include bradycardia, second- and third-degree heart block, Wolff–Parkinson–White syndrome, hypertrophic cardiomyopathy (increased LV outflow tract obstruction) and amyloid heart disease (digoxin accumulates in the myocardium). Magnesium or potassium depletion increases the risk of digoxin-induced arrhythmias. Digoxin toxicity causes anorexia, nausea, headache, fatigue, malaise, confusion and various visual disturbances including changes in colour vision; patients are at risk of life-threatening ventricular arrhythmias. Toxicity is most likely in the setting of renal impairment, and with co-existent administration of drugs such as amiodarone and verapamil which increase digoxin levels.

Other drug therapy

Nitrates (glyceryl trinitrate (IV), isosorbide dinitrate (ISDN) 30–120 mg in divided doses) or mononitrate (20–120 mg in divided doses)) work principally as venodilators in usual therapeutic doses. Nitrate tolerance tends to occur with prolonged use, and so intermittent therapy is preferred. Their use is mainly for heart failure patients with angina or those intolerant of the ACE inhibitors and ARBs.

Hydralazine (usually 25–75 mg tds for use in heart failure) acts directly on arteriolar smooth muscle, but side-effects (headaches, flushing, nausea, rashes) are common with high doses and the drug may rarely cause a lupus-like syndrome. A combination of hydralazine and isosorbide dinitrate was shown to improve survival in patients with heart failure (V-HeFT I trial) prior to the landmark ACE inhibitor trials. A later trial comparing the ACE inhibitor enalapril with the combination of hydralazine and isosorbide dinitrate (V-HeFT II) showed enalapril had a greater mortality benefit but, interestingly, exercise capacity was improved to a greater extent by the nitrate–hydralazine combination. A further trial addressed the benefits of the nitrate–hydralazine combination in black patients in addition to standard therapy (A-HeFT). The trial was stopped early due to a 43% reduction in death in the nitrate–hydralazine arm when compared with placebo. Quality of life was also improved and hospitalizations for heart failure were reduced. Black patients were chosen for this trial on the basis that this subgroup seemed to respond well to this combination therapy in earlier trials and because they tend to have a lower bioavailability of nitric oxide than Caucasians, with a less active renin–angiotensin system.

Calcium antagonists (nifedipine, verapamil, diltiazem, amlodipine, felodipine) are vasodilator drugs but also tend to be negatively inotropic, may cause peripheral oedema and are not generally used in the treatment of heart failure. Trials of amlodipine (PRAISE) and felodipine (VHeFT III) suggest that their use is safe, making them potentially useful agents when hypertension or angina coexist with heart failure.

Anticoagulant and antiplatelet agents

The annual overall incidence of stroke or thromboembolism in heart failure is about 2%. Predisposing factors include immobility, low cardiac output, ventricular cavity dilatation or aneurysm, and AF. The annual risk of stroke in heart failure trials has been around 1.5% in mild/moderate heart failure and 4% when severe, compared with 0.5% in controls. However, the place of oral anticoagulation with warfarin is less clear. Patients with a history of AF or with mitral stenosis, and those with evidence of intracardiac thrombus on investigation, should be anticoagulated unless there are contraindications, aiming for an international normalized ratio (INR) of 2.5–3.0. Controversy exists as to whether aspirin may have harmful effects in heart failure. Aspirin has been shown to block some of the haemodynamic effects of ACE inhibitors in acute studies. A small randomized study compared warfarin with aspirin and with placebo in patients with CHF (WASH study); there was a significantly higher risk of heart failure in the aspirin group compared with warfarin or placebo. In a further small study of warfarin vs. aspirin vs. clopidigrel (WATCH), there was again an increased risk of heart failure hospitalization in the aspirin group compared with warfarin or clopidigrel. These studies are not conclusive, but they do suggest that in patients with non-ischaemic cardiomyopathy, aspirin should be avoided unless there are other good indications for this therapy.

Antiarrhythmic agents

With the exception of β-blockers, anti-arrhythmic agents are not of prognostic benefit in patients with CHF. If an anti-arrhythmic agent is required to maintain sinus rhythm for a patient with paroxysmal AF, or to improve the chances of successful cardioversion, amiodarone is the drug of choice. Rate control with β-blockers +/- digoxin is appropriate for persistent AF. If patients have heart failure with preserved systolic function, verapamil can also be used. The SCD-HeFT study compared ICDs with amiodarone and with placebo in patients with stable NYHA class II/III CHF. This study confirmed that amiodarone has no favourable effect on survival in CHF and should therefore be reserved for patients with symptomatic arrhythmias. Patients with ventricular arrhythmias should also be considered for insertion of an ICD.

Device therapy

Implantable cardioverter defibrillators (ICDs)

Patients with heart failure are likely to die either of progressive heart failure or sudden cardiac death, which is frequently due to an arrhythmia. ICDs offer the potential to reduce the risk of sudden death and improve outcome for selected patients with CHF. ICDs are used for secondary prevention when the patient has suffered a ventricular arrhythmia or unexplained syncope thought to be due to an arrhythmia (see Chapter 13).

Two major landmark studies have shown improved outcome with primary prevention ICDs in CHF. MADIT II demonstrated that patients with prior myocardial infarction and LVEF ≤30% benefited from ICD therapy with a 31% reduction in mortality. SCD-HeFT enrolled a population with ischaemic and non-ischaemic cardiomyopathy (NYHA class II/III) with LVEF <35%, and showed a 23% reduction in mortality with an ICD after 5 years of follow-up. The ICD seemed of particular benefit in class II heart failure in this study. Importantly, not all primary prevention ICD trials have been positive. The DINAMIT study randomized patients 6–40 days after myocardial infarction with LVEF ≤35% and impaired autonomic function (as demonstrated on a 24-hour tape) to ICD or standard medical care. Prophylactic ICD therapy did not affect overall mortality in this study as there were excess non-arrhythmic deaths in the medical treatment group. The benefit of ICD therapy depends on competing risks, the sicker the patient, and hence the greater risk of non-arrhythmic death, the less likely they are to benefit.

Cardiac resynchronization therapy (CRT)

In a number of patients with heart failure, the disease process affects not only cardiac contractility, but also affects electrical conduction leading to dyssynchronous contraction between the walls of the left ventricle (typically in patients with left bundle branch block). There may also be abnormalities in atrioventricular timing (reflected by a prolonged PR interval) and interventricular timing. This abnormal timing leads to inefficient ventricular emptying and, in many cases, mitral regurgitation. The ECG has commonly been used as a surrogate for evidence of ventricular dyssynchrony, though echo studies show that its reliability is variable. Approximately 25–30% of patients with moderate to severe heart failure have a QRS duration >120 ms. QRS prolongation is an independent predictor of prognosis in heart failure.

CRT (see also Chapter 13) aims to retime the failing heart and has been shown acutely to increase cardiac output and systolic blood pressure, to increase diastolic filling time, lower pulmonary artery wedge pressure, reduce mitral regurgitation and, importantly, to improve LV function without increasing myocardial oxygen consumption. CRT can be delivered as either a CRT pacemaker (CRT-P) or as a CRT defibrillator which, by incorporating an ICD, offers additional protection against sudden cardiac death.

Trials have now conclusively shown that CRT, with or without a defibrillator, improves exercise tolerance and quality of life, reduces hospitalizations for heart failure and reduces mortality in selected patients with CHF and a prolonged QRS. The 'CARE-HF' trial compared CRT-P with optimal medical therapy and demonstrated a 36% reduction in mortality over a mean follow-up of 29 months. Patients were entered into the study if they fulfilled the following criteria:

- optimal medical therapy for heart failure;
- LVET ≤35%;
- NYHA class III–IV;
- QRS duration ≥150 ms or QRS duration 120–149 ms and echo evidence of dyssynchrony;
- they were in sinus rhythm.

In this study, 7% of patients in the CRT group died suddenly, suggesting that additional benefit might have been gained by implanting an ICD (CRT-D). In the COMPANION trial, which compared CRT-P with CRT-D and with medical therapy, only CRT-D reduced the risk of death compared with medical therapy, though there was a strong trend to reduction in mortality with CRT-P.

Not all patients respond to this therapy; typically 70% of patients are said to improve following CRT, but some of this benefit may be a placebo response. Successful CRT depends upon appropriate patient selection, optimal lead positioning, pacemaker programming and careful follow-up with continuing optimization of medical therapy. A number of questions remain: which patients are most likely to benefit from CRT; should patients receive CRT-P or CRT-D; and is CRT-D cost-effective when compared with CRT-P? Traditionally, CRT has been reserved for patients in sinus rhythm; however, similar benefits seem to apply in patients with AF with a well-controlled ventricular response rate. Further studies should help clarify these issues.

Surgical management of heart failure

Surgical management is indicated for heart failure secondary to intrinsic valve disease, e.g. aortic and mitral stenosis, and aortic and mitral regurgitation, even in the presence of LV dysfunction. In patients with angina, revascularization usually improves ischaemic symptoms and may reduce the risk of sudden death for patients with low ejection fractions. Patients without angina, but who have evidence of inducible ischaemia or viability on imaging, may also benefit from surgery, but this has yet to be proven in a randomized outcome trial. Patients with CHF often develop mitral regurgitation due to annular dilatation, which occurs as a result of LV dilatation, and may benefit from mitral valve repair.

Increased left ventricular volume is associated with worse outcome in CHF; in an attempt to overcome this, there is now considerable interest in surgical ventricular restoration (SVR), which involves remodelling the left ventricle to eliminate or exclude areas of infarction, thus reducing left ventricular volumes and wall stress. The STICH trial is an ongoing randomized comparison of medical therapy vs. CABG in patient with heart failure and LVEF <35%. Patients undergoing CABG are further randomized to CABG alone or to CABG + SVR. This trial may have a major impact on determining the frequency with which heart failure patients are put forward for revascularization in the future.

Acute heart failure

AHF is defined as the rapid onset of symptoms and signs secondary to abnormal cardiac function. The most common cause is acute myocardial infarction; others include myocarditis, acute valvular regurgitation (mitral, aortic), post-infarct VSD and intractable arrhythmias. The cardiac dysfunction can be related to systolic or diastolic dysfunction, to abnormalities in cardiac rhythm, or to preload

and afterload mismatch. The principles of managing acute, sudden-onset heart failure are similar to those of the more chronic variety. However, when the heart sustains an acute insult, the cardiovascular and neurohormonal systems have little time to adapt and initiate compensatory changes. Patients therefore tolerate AHF much less well than the same degree of cardiac impairment occurring gradually, and as such the mortality is high.

Patients present in a variety of ways:
- Acute decompensated heart failure with signs and symptoms of AHF which are mild and do not fulfil criteria for cardiogenic shock, pulmonary oedema or hypertensive crisis.
- Hypertensive AHF: signs and symptoms of heart failure are accompanied by high blood pressure and relatively preserved left ventricular function with a chest X-ray showing pulmonary oedema.
- Pulmonary oedema accompanied by severe respiratory distress, with orthopnoea and pulmonary crackles with hypoxia.
- Cardiogenic shock: cardiogenic shock is defined as evidence of tissue hypoperfusion induced by heart failure after correction of preload. Cardiogenic shock is usually characterized by systolic BP <90 mmHg and low urine output (<0.5 ml/kg/h) with a pulse rate >60 bpm with or without evidence of organ congestion.
- High output failure, characterized by high cardiac output, usually with a high heart rate, warm peripheries, pulmonary congestion and often low blood pressure.
- Right heart failure: low output syndrome with increased jugular venous pressure and hypotension.

Management

AHF should be assessed and treated urgently. Attention should be paid to any factors which may have precipitated or exacerbated heart failure (e.g. infection, alterations in drug therapy, worsening angina, electrolyte disturbance). The underlying aetiology should be identified and managed. Atrial or ventricular arrhythmias should be treated. The patient should ideally be managed in a high dependency or intensive care area, with continuous ECG monitoring, frequent blood pressure monitoring and measurement of arterial oxygen saturation using pulse oximetry. A urinary catheter is frequently used to monitor hourly urine volumes.

Patients require adequate levels of oxygenation aiming for an arterial oxygen saturations of 95–98%. There is no evidence that hyperoxia is helpful, and indeed it may be harmful (it may reduce cardiac output and coronary blood flow, and increase systemic vascular resistance). If adequate oxygenation is not achieved with supplemental oxygen, non-invasive ventilation can be helpful and reduce the need for tracheal intubation and mechanical ventilation. Ventilation may, however, sometimes be required to relieve respiratory distress and to reverse hypercapnia and hypoxaemia.

Medical therapy

- **Morphine** induces venodilatation and mild arterial dilatation and may help reduce the heart rate as anxiety and breathlessness are reduced.
- **Vasodilators** are indicated as first-line therapy if hypoperfusion is associated with an adequate blood pressure and signs of congestion, to reduce afterload and preload. **Nitrates** relieve pulmonary congestion without increasing myocardial oxygen demand. At low doses they induce venodilation, but as the dose is increased they cause the arteries to dilate, including coronary arteries. Dose titration to achieve the highest tolerable dose of intravenous nitrate, together with low-dose furosemide, is superior to high-dose furosemide alone. Indeed, in one randomised study IV nitrate alone was superior to IV furosemide alone. **Sodium nitroprusside** (SNP) is an alternative, very short-acting vasodilator which is useful in severe heart failure. It is also a mixed vasodilator and is particularly useful for patients with increased afterload, for example in hypertensive heart failure. Hydrocyanic acid is released, which can cause cyanide poisoning when SNP is used for more than 2–3 days.
- **Diuretics** are usually given intravenously. As well as being a diuretic, furosemide exerts a vasodilating effect when given intravenously, though

higher doses can cause vasoconstriction. Use of a furosemide infusion after the bolus dose can be very effective in achieving a sustained diuresis.
- There is no evidence to support the introduction of **ACE inhibitors or β-blockers** in the acute management of AHF. They should be introduced once stabilized. However, if the patient is taking these agents already, they should be continued.
- **Inotropic agents** (see below) are indicated in the presence of tissue hypoperfusion (hypotension, decreased urine output) refractory to volume replacement (if appropriate), diuretics and vasodilators at optimal doses. Their use, however, is potentially harmful as they increase myocardial oxygen demand and they have repeatedly been shown to be associated with adverse outcome in longer-term clinical trials. They may, however, be life-saving when patients do not respond to standard measures.

Inotropic therapy

Dopamine is an endogenous catecholamine and the immediate precursor of norepinephrine. Its effects are dose-dependent and involve dopaminergic, β-adrenergic and α-adrenergic receptors. At low dose (<2 μg/kg/min IV) it acts on peripheral dopaminergic receptors causing vasodilatation in the renal, splanchnic and coronary beds. At this dose, dopamine may improve renal blood flow and GFR, and work synergistically with diuretics. At higher doses (>2 μg/kg/min IV) it stimulates β-adrenergic receptors which increases myocardial contractility. At high doses (>5 μg/kg/min IV) it acts on α-adrenergic receptors leading to an increase in vascular resistance.

Dobutamine (dose 2.5–10 mg/kg/min) acts mainly through stimulation of $β_1$ and $β_2$ receptors. It is a positive inotrope and increases cardiac output. It has chronotropic effects (increases heart rate) which may not always be beneficial. At low doses, dobutamine induces mild arterial vasodilatation which augments stroke volume by reductions in afterload. Use of dobutamine is associated with increased risk of both atrial and ventricular arrhythmias. It should be used with caution as its use has been linked to adverse outcomes in heart failure. **Phosphodiesterase inhibitors** (milrinone and enoximone) are positive inotropic agents and cause peripheral vasodilatation through inhibition of phosphodiesterase III which is responsible for breakdown of cAMP, thus raising intracellular levels of cAMP. They are used intravenously when there is peripheral hypoperfusion with preserved systolic blood pressure, but trials have consistently highlighted their pro-arrhythmic effects.

Levosimendan is a calcium-sensitizing agent which acts as an inotrope and causes vasodilatation by smooth muscle K^+ channel opening. It is currently undergoing clinical trials and appears to be associated with better outcome than dobutamine. Its haemodynamic effects are prolonged. It is not currently licensed for use in the UK.

Where patients respond poorly to inotropic therapy, a pulmonary artery flotation catheter (Swan–Ganz catheter) may be used to measure cardiac filling pressures and cardiac output directly. Systemic and pulmonary vascular resistance can be calculated. These measurements can guide the clinician to optimize treatment. Vasopressors such as epinephrine and norepinephrine may be required to maintain blood pressure in the setting of life-threatening hypotension. These agents, however, tend to increase afterload, which is already usually increased in the setting of severe heart failure and as such these agents should be used cautiously and for short periods only. Arterial blood pressure monitoring is required during infusion of these agents, usually using a radial arterial cannula.

Intra-aortic balloon counterpulsation

In severe LV dysfunction, where the natural history of the underlying condition is one of possible improvement (e.g. early following cardiac surgery or myocardial infarction, in acute myocarditis or occasionally in unstable angina), the use of aortic balloon counterpulsation may help support the circulation for a number of days or even a few weeks. It may also be used as a bridge towards cardiac transplantation while a donor organ is being sought. A long balloon is inserted percutaneously, usually via a femoral artery, and positioned to lie between the upper part of the descending thoracic aorta, just beyond the origin of the left subclavian artery and the suprarenal section of the abdominal aorta. A predetermined volume of an inert gas is used to fill the balloon, and subsequent inflation by a bedside pump is synchronized with the ECG to occur in diastole, and deflation to occur at the onset of systole. By so doing, coronary perfusion pressure is increased in diastole and left ventricular afterload is reduced in systole. With current balloons, the use of heparin is often not required. After removal of the balloon, haemostasis is achieved either by local femoral pressure or by surgical arterial repair.

Ventricular assist devices

Ventricular assist devices are mechanical pumps that partially replace the mechanical work of the ventricle. They unload the ventricle, thereby decreasing myocardial work, and pump blood into the arterial system, increasing peripheral and end-organ flow. A variety of these devices are available. Some devices require a median sternotomy and complex surgery. Others simply extract blood from the arterial system, pumping the blood again into the arterial or venous vascular system (these tend to be used for patients requiring short-term support). Left ventricular assist devices (LVADs) are used to support critically ill patients until a transplant becomes available ('bridge to transplant'), or in rare cases as a 'bridge to recovery' (e.g. myocarditis). LVADs have also been used as 'destination therapy' for patients ineligible for transplant; the REMATCH trial showed improved outcome with an LVAD compared with standard medical care in a study population of very advanced heart failure, most of whom could not be weaned from inotropic support. Median survival was 408 days in the LVAD group, compared with 150 days in the medical treatment group. Infection, bleeding, thromboembolism and device failure were common adverse events in the LVAD group, side-effects which may become less frequent as the technology improves.

Cardiac transplantation

Cardiac transplantation is indicated for patients with severe symptoms of heart failure, with no alternative form of treatment, medical, surgical or electrical (including CRT when appropriate), with a poor prognosis (life expectancy <1 year). Although no controlled trials have ever been performed, transplantation is considered to increase survival, exercise capacity, return to work and quality of life compared with conventional treatment (assuming strict selection criteria are applied). Recent results suggest that patients on triple immunosuppressive therapy have a 5-year survival of 70–80%. Besides shortage of donor hearts, the main problem with transplantation is rejection of the allograft, which is responsible for a considerable number of deaths in the first postoperative year. The long-term outcome is limited predominantly by the consequences of immunosuppression (infection, hypertension, renal failure, malignancy and by coronary artery disease developing in the transplanted heart).

Selection of appropriate patients is important to define the patients most likely to benefit from transplantation and to avoid transplanting patients likely to do well with standard therapy. Older patients (age >65 years) are less likely to be accepted for transplantation, as are patients with impaired renal function, other co-morbidities or a high pulmonary vascular resistance (PVR) measured at cardiac catheterization (as the transplanted heart's right ventricle may fail if PVR is high). Patients' risks are assessed using heart failure survival scores to identify prospective candidates. Fewer ambulant patients are now being transplanted, with organs usually going to inpatients with severe decompensated heart failure requiring inotropic support. It is important to involve the transplant centre early in the course of the admission when transplantation seems likely to be appropriate.

Palliative care

Despite optimal care, many CHF patients will die from progressive heart failure, which can be very distressing. It is important to recognize when medical therapies have failed and focus on the physical and psychological needs of the patient. Palliative care teams offer expertise in symptom control and have an increasing role to play in the management of end-stage heart failure.

Further reading

European Society of Cardiology Guidelines for management of acute and chronic heart failure: http://www.escardio.org/knowledge/guidelines/ ACUTE_HEART_FAILURE.htm

http://www.escardio.org/knowledge/guidelines/ Chronic_Heart_Failure.htm

McMurray JJV, Pfeffer MA. Heart failure (Seminar). *Lancet* 2005; 365: 1877–89.

Chapter 10

Valvular heart disease

Function and pathophysiology

In Europe and North America, degenerative valve disease is now more common than valvular heart disease, occurring as a consequence of previous infection (e.g. rheumatic fever, syphilis). In some patients there may be an underlying congenital abnormality of the valve (e.g. bicuspid aortic valve) or an abnormality of connective tissue (e.g. mitral valve prolapse). With the increasing age of the population, 'senile' calcification of a normal valve (e.g. calcific aortic stenosis) presenting in the seventh and eighth decades is a frequent indication for valve replacement. Surgical intervention has modified the 'natural' history of valvular heart disease. Whereas the myocardial component of valvular heart disease has, until recently, been a major cause of mortality, earlier valve repair or replacement at low risk has resulted in the preservation of myocardial function with superior long-term survival.

Rheumatic fever

Incidence

The incidence of rheumatic fever has decreased markedly in Western Europe and North America during the last few decades, due to an improvement in socio-economic conditions, together with the introduction and widespread use of antibiotics.

Nevertheless, worldwide there are 15–20 million new cases of rheumatic fever per year, and in developing countries the condition accounts for 25–50% of all cardiac admissions to hospital. There is recent evidence of an increase in the incidence of rheumatic fever in middle-class populations in both Europe and the USA. Acute rheumatic fever is a disease of childhood, with a peak incidence between the ages of 5 and 15 years; 20% of cases occur in adults.

Pathogenesis

The pathogenesis of rheumatic fever is related to the immunological response to the cell membrane antigens of the Lancefield group A streptococcus. Streptococcal pharyngitis is the only streptococcal infection associated with acute rheumatic fever. A number of factors can influence the susceptibility to cardiac damage including:
- age;
- socio-economic conditions;
- ethnic origin;
- genetic factors;
- climate.

Rheumatic fever involves all layers of the heart (a pancarditis) with a pathognomonic lesion, the Aschoff body, which is a mass of cells, altered collagen and connective tissue components in the subendocardium that heals to form a fibrous scar. Other organs that may be affected by rheumatic fever include the skin, joints, lungs and central nervous system.

Diagnosis

The diagnosis of rheumatic fever may be difficult. The revised Jones criteria (Table 10.1) act as a guide and reduce the chance of overdiagnosis. The presence of two major criteria, or one major and two minor criteria, together with evidence of preceding streptococcal infection is required to make a confident diagnosis of rheumatic fever. However, none of the manifestations specific. As many of the criteria are clinical, the importance of careful and repeated examination of the patient cannot be overemphasized, particularly as some of the signs (e.g. heart murmurs) may be transient.

Treatment

Treatment is aimed at eradicating the streptococcus, controlling pain and reducing the inflammatory process. High dose aspirin (4–8 g/day in adults)

Table 10.1 The revised Jones criteria for the diagnosis of rheumatic fever.

| *Major manifestations* |
| Carditis |
| Polyarthritis |
| Sydenham's chorea |
| Erythema marginatum |
| Subcutaneous nodules |
| *Minor manifestations* |
| Fever |
| Arthralgia |
| Previous rheumatic fever (or rheumatic heart disease) |
| Evidence of preceding streptococcal infection |
| Increased anti-streptolysin O or other streptococcal antibodies |
| Positive throat culture for Group A β-haemolytic streptococci |
| Positive rapid direct Group A streptococcal carbohydrate antigen test |
| Recent scarlet fever |
| Elevated acute-phase reactants (ESR, CRP) |
| Prolonged PR interval |

CRP, C-reactive protein; ESR, erythrocyte sedimentation rate.

is used as the anti-inflammatory agent and is continued until symptoms regress and the acute phase proteins (ESR and CRP) fall. In addition, the patient may require treatment for heart failure and the non-cardiac manifestations of the infection (e.g. chorea) and other complications.

Prevention

There is general agreement that long-term prophylaxis following an attack of acute rheumatic fever reduces both the late mortality and the chance of recurrent infection. In populations where compliance is a problem, IM benzathine penicillin 1.2 MU every 4 weeks is recommended, but the usual regimen is oral penicillin G 0.25 MU twice daily. For patients allergic to penicillin, erythromycin 250 mg twice daily should be given. Antibiotic prophylaxis should be continued for 5 years after the acute attack or until the age of 30 years (whichever is the longer).

Long-term follow-up

With the appropriate treatment, the 10-year mortality has fallen from 25 to 1% compared with the pre-antibiotic era. Furthermore, it can be expected that >90% of the hearts will be normal at 10-year follow-up.

Aortic valve disease

Aortic stenosis

Pathogenesis

The normal aortic valve consists of three semilunar cusps of similar size with a cross-sectional area of 3–4 cm². Obstruction (stenosis) at valve level may be either congenital or acquired. A bicuspid aortic valve is one of the most common congenital abnormalities (0.9–2.5% incidence), with a male preponderance (4:1). The pattern of acquired aortic stenosis in adults is changing because of the decreasing prevalence of rheumatic disease coupled with the increasing age of the population. Aortic stenosis as a consequence of rheumatic fever is uncommon in the UK (2% of cases), and in such cases the mitral valve is frequently involved.

Secondary calcification of a congenitally bicuspid aortic valve (Fig. 10.1) and primary degeneration of a normal valve (Fig. 10.2) account for the majority of cases of adult aortic stenosis. Only 40% of middle-aged patients with aortic stenosis have a bicuspid valve, but this type of aortic stenosis accounts for 70–80% of cases involving elderly patients. Calcification develops first in the free edges of the cusps and progresses towards the base. Approximately 50% of patients with a bicuspid

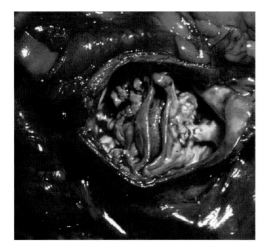

Fig. 10.1 Bicuspid aortic valve.

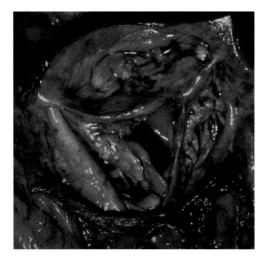

Fig. 10.2 Senile (tricuspid) aortic valve.

aortic valve will develop significant aortic stenosis in later life.

In 'senile' calcification of normal valves, calcium is laid down first in the base of the valve and progresses to involve the free edges. 'Senile' calcification rarely ulcerates or embolizes but may be sufficient to cause an aortic systolic murmur, which reportedly occurs in 65% of normal subjects by the ninth decade.

Aortic stenosis in the adult progresses slowly. The restriction of the orifice produces resistance to left ventricular outflow and a reduction in cusp mobility. As the outflow gradient increases, cardiac output is augmented by compensatory left ventricular hypertrophy. Systolic function is maintained despite the increasing pressure overload, but the ventricle eventually becomes stiff and non-compliant. The resulting impairment of diastolic function increases myocardial oxygen consumption, shortens the period of diastolic coronary artery filling and reduces myocardial perfusion pressure, which leads to subendocardial ischaemia.

Symptoms (see Box 10.1)

Most patients remain asymptomatic until the aortic valve area is reduced to 1.0–1.5 cm^2. Chest pain, syncope and breathlessness are the classic triad of symptoms; once symptoms have developed, the prognosis is poor. The life expectancy for the patient with chest pain or syncope is 3 years, and <2 years in those with breathlessness. Sudden death occurs in all age groups but most frequently in patients who were symptomatic.

Box 10.1 Symptoms in aortic stenosis

- Chest pain
- Exertional syncope
- Breathlessness
- Gastrointestinal bleeding may arise in patients with aortic stenosis in association with angiodysplasia of the colon
- Other complications include infective endocarditis, transient ischaemic attacks (classically amaurosis fugax) and stroke

---

Physical signs (see Box 10.2)

The most important physical sign of aortic stenosis is the character of the pulse, best appreciated by palpating the carotid (or brachial) arteries. The carotid pulse has a small pulse pressure with a slow upstroke caused by prolonged ejection. A palpable (anacrotic) notch in addition to a systolic thrill nearly always indicates severe aortic stenosis.

In the elderly, reduced elasticity of the peripheral arteries may mask pulse abnormalities when the lesion is severe. Calcification and rigidity of the aortic valve reduce the intensity of the aortic second heart sound (A2), and elevation of the left atrial pressure results in an audible fourth heart sound (S4). Because the valve is rigid, the systolic ejection click, so common in children, is rarely heard in the elderly.

The characteristic murmur of aortic stenosis is crescendo–decrescendo ('ejection'), beginning after the first heart sound (S1) and terminating prior to the second heart sound (S2) (Fig. 10.3). Neither the intensity nor the length of the murmur is related to the severity of the valve lesion. Occasionally, patients with critical aortic stenosis have no murmur because of low forward flow, allowing the diagnosis to be easily missed. Many patients with aortic stenosis (of any aetiology) have associated, often mild, aortic regurgitation.

Box 10.2 Signs in aortic stenosis

- Small volume pulse
- Slow upstroke
- Single S2
- Ejection murmur (± EC)

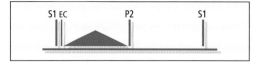

Fig. 10.3 Auscultatory findings in aortic stenosis.

Investigations

Although 70–80% of patients with aortic stenosis have an abnormal electrocardiogram (ECG), a normal ECG does not exclude important aortic stenosis. Left ventricular hypertrophy on voltage criteria may be associated with the so-called 'strain' pattern (Fig. 10.4); T-wave inversion in isolation is an unreliable finding in the elderly.

In uncomplicated aortic stenosis, heart size is normal on chest radiography, but post-stenotic

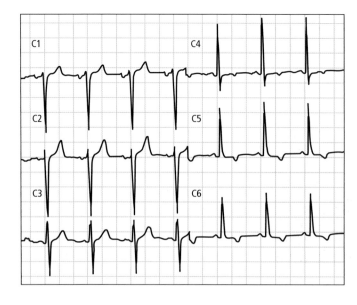

Fig. 10.4 Left ventricular hypertrophy and 'strain' in a patient with aortic stenosis.

dilatation of the ascending aorta is present in 80% of patients (Fig. 10.5). Aortic valve calcification is often visible on the lateral chest radiograph (Fig. 10.6) without a significant gradient; conversely, aortic stenosis without valve calcification is very rare in the elderly.

M-mode and cross-sectional echocardiography are a useful means of assessing the consequences of aortic stenosis, such as left ventricular wall

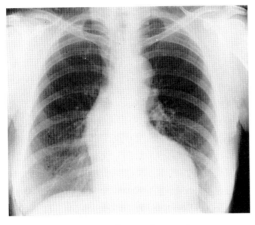

Fig. 10.5 Chest radiograph in aortic stenosis.

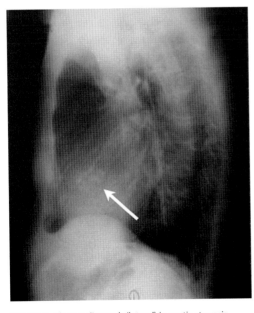

Fig. 10.6 Chest radiograph (lateral) in aortic stenosis.

hypertrophy with a reduced cavity size and impaired diastolic function. Restricted leaflet motion on imaging may indicate aortic stenosis or low forward flow secondary to impaired ventricular function. Multiple echoes may arise from the valve in patients with valve calcification and do not necessarily indicate narrowing of the valve orifice.

Doppler echocardiography has proved invaluable in the assessment of aortic stenosis (see Chapter 3). The maximum systolic pressure difference across the valve (peak instantaneous pressure) can be calculated from the maximum velocity detected by Doppler as gradient $(\text{mmHg}) = 4v^2\,\text{ms}^{-1}$. Estimates are unreliable in patients with a low cardiac output, and in this setting a Doppler gradient of 40–50 mmHg may be significant.

Cardiac catheterization is undertaken predominantly in patients presenting with chest pain to delineate the coronary anatomy.

Differential diagnosis

Other forms of left ventricular outflow obstruction, commonly hypertrophic obstructive cardiomyopathy, may mimic aortic stenosis. Echocardiography and a Doppler examination usually establish the diagnosis, although the presence of an asymmetrical pattern of hypertrophy in some patients with valvular aortic stenosis suggests a degree of overlap.

Management

Medical therapy has little to offer once the patient has become symptomatic. Aortic stenosis is a mechanical problem, and both diuretics and vasodilators may result in a reduction in either preload or afterload, which effectively reduces left ventricular function or increases the gradient.

The asymptomatic patient with aortic stenosis should be followed up at 6- or 12-monthly intervals, using serial electrocardiography and echo-Doppler. When the patient develops symptoms, surgical referral becomes appropriate. A more difficult problem is the management of the patient who remains asymptomatic with a significant aortic gradient. As the aortic gradient is dependent on cardiac output, an absolute valve gradient should not determine the need for surgical intervention; however, a peak instantaneous gradient on Doppler of 70 mmHg or more (equivalent to a peak-to-peak withdrawal gradient of 50 mmHg measured invasively) usually indicates the need for surgery. If the left ventricle is dilated or ventricular function compromised, a lower value may be significant.

Aortic valve replacement

A mechanical prosthesis is appropriate for the majority of patients (Fig. 10.7). A biological valve (porcine xenograft, homograft or pericardial)

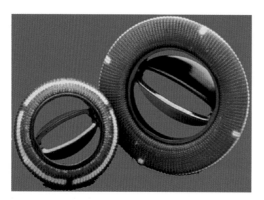

Fig. 10.7 A mechanical valve prosthesis.

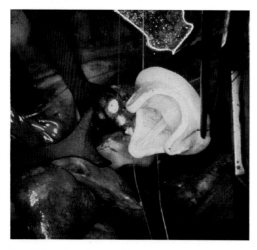

Fig. 10.8 A tissue (xenograft) valve.

(Fig. 10.8) may be implanted in women of child-bearing age or the elderly (>70 years), in whom anticoagulants may be undesirable. Early mortality for aortic valve replacement is now <5%. Incremental risk factors include preoperative functional status and increasing age, although the latter does not appear to be a strong risk factor in experienced centres. Concomitant CABG should not increase the in-hospital mortality and indeed may reduce the early risk. Symptomatic results and late survival rates are excellent and superior to those following mitral valve replacement. Five-year actuarial survival rates of 70–90% with a 10-year survival of 70–75% are typical for reported series.

Balloon aortic valvuloplasty and percutaneous valve replacement

There has been some interest in balloon dilatation of the aortic valve, particularly in the elderly patient with aortic stenosis. Published experience suggests that the procedure is low in risk (~5%), with a worthwhile improvement in symptoms, particularly if the gradient can be reduced by 50% or more. However, in the majority of patients, the procedure is no more than palliative, with recurrent stenosis occurring within 6–18 months after successful balloon dilatation. Furthermore, it appears that the natural history of untreated aortic stenosis is not modified by balloon valvuloplasty. The disappointing results with this technique are not surprising as the cause of flow reduction in the majority of patients is calcification of the valve cusps rather than commissural fusion. There is some early experience with percutaneous aortic valve replacement using stent-mounted valves inserted retrogradely via a femoral artery approach. After an initial learning curve, short-term results appear satisfactory, but more long-term data are required and the criteria for patient selection are as yet uncertain.

Given the low operative risk and excellent functional results of aortic valve replacement, aortic valvuloplasty should be restricted to symptomatic patients with other life-threatening conditions, such as carcinoma.

Aortic regurgitation

Pathogenesis

Several mechanisms may be responsible for the development of aortic regurgitation, depending on whether the disease process affects the valve cusps themselves or the aortic root.

Despite the reduction in the incidence of syphilis, aortic regurgitation as a consequence of an aortopathy appears to be increasing, accounting for one-third of patients coming to surgery.

Acute aortic regurgitation may be due to cusp rupture or perforation secondary to infection, aortic dissection and, rarely, closed chest trauma. Connective tissue diseases (e.g. Marfan syndrome) also occasionally cause acute aortic regurgitation.

Causes of chronic aortic regurgitation are listed in Table 10.2. In diseases of the aortic root, the cusps themselves may appear normal, but an increase in root diameter causes a loss of the usual cusp overlap, leading to the development of a central regurgitant jet.

The severity of the condition depends on the aortic valve area, the heart rate and the diastolic pressure gradient between the left ventricle and the aorta. In early disease, the left ventricle

Table 10.2 Causes of chronic aortic regurgitation.

Cusp abnormality	
Perforation	Infective endocarditis
Reduction in area	Rheumatic disease
	Rheumatoid, ankylosing spondylitis
	Acromegaly
Aortic root disease	
Root distortion	Rheumatoid, ankylosing spondylitis
	Syphilis
	Non-specific urethritis (Reiter syndrome)
	Non-specific aortitis
Root dilatation	Syphilis
	Marfan syndrome
	Ehlers–Danlos syndrome
	Pseudoxanthoma elasticum
	Osteogenesis imperfecta

maintains output by a degree of hypertrophy, but eventually the diastolic overload produces left ventricular dilatation followed by a reduction in forward flow and pulmonary venous hypertension. Changes in heart rate or systemic vascular resistance may alter the regurgitant fraction.

Symptoms (see Box 10.3)

As with mitral regurgitation, aortic regurgitation is well tolerated. The appropriate management is complicated by the late occurrence of symptoms, usually after considerable left ventricular damage has arisen that cannot be reversed by surgical intervention. Restriction of exercise tolerance due to breathlessness and fatigue is followed by orthopnoea and pulmonary oedema as a consequence of pulmonary venous hypertension.

Physical signs (see Box 10.4)

Examination may reveal that the aortic regurgitation is occurring as part of a systemic disorder (e.g. rheumatoid arthritis, ankylosing spondylitis and Marfan syndrome). In acute aortic regurgitation, features of aortic dissection or endocarditis may also be present.

The wide pulse pressure and rapid diastolic run-off give rise to a number of clinical signs, which are reflected in the active, hyperdynamic and often laterally displaced apex beat. Typically, a high-pitched early diastolic murmur commences

---

Box 10.3 Symptoms in aortic regurgitation

- Fatigue
- Breathlessness
- Orthopnoea
- Nocturnal dyspnoea

Box 10.4 Signs in aortic regurgitation

- Wide pulse pressure
- Hyperdynamic apex
- Early diastolic murmur
- ±Mid-diastolic murmur

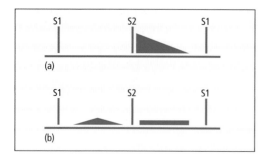

Fig. 10.9 Auscultatory findings in aortic regurgitation. (a) Early diastolic murmur. (b) Systolic flow murmur and mid-diastolic (Austin Flint) murmur.

immediately after A2 and is audible at the left sternal edge and base; the length, rather than the loudness, of the murmur relates to severity. An additional systolic flow murmur is often audible and does not necessarily imply additional aortic stenosis. Similarly, a mid-diastolic flow murmur (Austin Flint murmur) may be present when aortic regurgitation is severe (Fig. 10.9). All these signs may be absent in acute aortic regurgitation because of equalization of the left ventricular end-diastolic and the aortic diastolic pressures. In these circumstances, the patient may appear breathless and unwell, with a sinus tachycardia but otherwise quiet heart.

Investigations

The ECG is rarely normal in chronic aortic regurgitation and often shows marked repolarization changes. In acute aortic regurgitation, the ECG may be normal. Dilatation of the left ventricle leads to progressive cardiac enlargement on the chest radiograph. Although the ascending aorta is often prominent, the aetiology of the valve lesion cannot be determined. On echocardiography, the left ventricular dimensions in early aortic regurgitation are normal, often in association with mild left ventricular hypertrophy. Contractility is well preserved and may be exaggerated. If aortic regurgitation is neglected, left ventricular dilatation ensues with a progressive reduction in systolic function, leading to a left ventricle similar in appearance to that seen in dilated cardiomyopathy. Abnormalities of the aortic root (such as in Marfan syndrome) can also be demonstrated by echocardiography.

Doppler echocardiography, particularly colour-flow mapping, is very sensitive and can detect minor degrees of aortic regurgitation and map the direction of the jet, which may give additional information regarding the severity of the lesion. Most surgeons require the patient to undergo aortography before considering operative intervention. Conventional transthoracic echocardiography (TTE) in adults demonstrates the proximal part of the aortic root on imaging, whereas transoesophageal echocardiography (TOE) visualizes the entire aorta. Similarly, magnetic resonance imaging (MRI) may give the surgeon sufficient information to avoid the need for cardiac catheterization if the coronary anatomy is not required.

Medical management

More than 50% of patients with untreated aortic regurgitation are alive after 10 years; therefore, a conservative policy is usually followed. The asymptomatic patient with mild aortic regurgitation should be followed up at 6- or 12-monthly intervals by serial echo-Doppler. Evidence of left ventricular dilatation with or without a reduction in function suggests surgical intervention is appropriate. Diuretic and vasodilator therapy (e.g. angiotensin-converting enzyme (ACE) inhibitors) may be used as a holding manoeuvre. As these lesions are also prone to infective endocarditis, good dental hygiene is important, and all patients should be given antibiotic cover for dental and other minor operative procedures.

Surgical intervention

The early and late mortality following aortic valve replacement for aortic regurgitation is similar to the results of valve replacement in aortic stenosis (see page 160). In the current era of cardiac surgery, aortic root replacement is no longer a risk factor for early mortality.

Mitral valve disease

Rheumatic mitral valve disease

Pathogenesis

Mitral stenosis is the most common late consequence of rheumatic carditis. A latency period of 20 years between the acute infection and symptomatic valvular dysfunction is not uncommon, with the typical patient presenting in the fourth or fifth decade. In patients from the Far East and South America, severe valvular disease may present in their early twenties.

Pathological abnormalities of the valve include commissural fusion, fibrous scarring and obliteration of the normally layered valvular architecture as a result of healed acute valvulitis and superimposed fibrosis. Progressive fibrous bridging across the valvular commissures may produce a rigid 'fish mouth' deformity resulting in a fixed orifice, which is both stenosed and regurgitant. The valve leaflets become calcified and the chordae tendineae thickened, fused and shortened.

Symptoms (see Box 10.5)

The clinical features of mitral stenosis are determined by the left atrial pressure, cardiac output and pulmonary vascular resistance. As the left atrial pressure increases, pulmonary compliance is reduced, making breathing more laboured. Initially, breathlessness only arises when the heart rate is increased, for example during exercise, stress and fever. As the severity of the lesion increases, the patient becomes orthopnoeic. Prior to the onset of paroxysmal dyspnoea, nocturnal coughing may be the only symptom of an elevated left atrial

pressure. Nowadays, haemoptysis is rarely seen. Palpitation due to atrial fibrillation becomes more common with increasing age; 80% of patients over the age of 50 years have this complication.

Pulmonary arterial pressure rises in parallel with an increase in left atrial pressure, in most patients becoming 10–12 mmHg greater than left atrial pressure. In some patients, particularly those with severe mitral stenosis, pulmonary arterial pressure rises disproportionately, so-called reactive pulmonary hypertension. Right-sided symptoms may predominate in these patients (see also Chapter 16).

Physical signs (see Box 10.6)

The most important and often neglected physical sign in mitral stenosis is accentuation of S1. Sudden tensing of the mitral leaflets by the subvalve apparatus and the halting of the downward movement of the mitral valve causes a high-pitched opening snap in early diastole, 40–120 ms after S2 (Fig. 10.10). If the valve is still mobile, the interval between S2 and the opening snap will vary inversely with the mean left atrial pressure. The classic low-pitched rumbling diastolic murmur is often localized to the apex or axilla; it is short in duration when the valve lesion is mild. The duration, not the loudness of the murmurs relates to lesion severity. Mitral facies are usually indicative of longstanding mitral stenosis associated with pulmonary hypertension. Other physical features include the signs of pulmonary oedema (basal lung crackles),

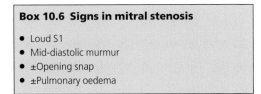

Box 10.6 Signs in mitral stenosis

- Loud S1
- Mid-diastolic murmur
- ±Opening snap
- ±Pulmonary oedema

Box 10.5 Symptoms in mitral stenosis

- Fatigue
- Breathlessness
- Orthopnoea
- Nocturnal dyspnoea
- ±Palpitation (atrial fibrillation)

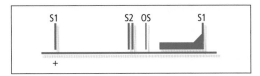

Fig. 10.10 Auscultatory findings in mitral stenosis.

together with fluid retention, hepatic congestion and tricuspid regurgitation.

Investigations

In the majority of patients, mitral valve disease is adequately assessed non-invasively, but occasionally cardiac catheterization and haemodynamic investigation are necessary. The features of mitral stenosis on the ECG are non-specific; if the patient is in sinus rhythm, a broad biphasic P wave is present in 90% of patients with mitral stenosis. P-wave morphology is related to left atrial dilatation rather than hypertrophy.

In pure mitral stenosis, the size of the heart on chest radiography is normal unless long-standing pulmonary hypertension has caused dilatation of the right-sided chambers. The left atrium is selectively enlarged, causing elevation of the left main bronchus, which may be more easily seen on a penetrated film (Fig. 10.11). In the elderly, mitral valve calcification (visible on the lateral view) must be differentiated from mitral annulus calcification. When left atrial pressure rises, there is pulmonary venous distension followed by upper lobe blood diversion and the radiographic signs of interstitial and alveolar oedema. Echocardiography combined with Doppler examination is the single most useful investigation in the patient with mitral valve disease.

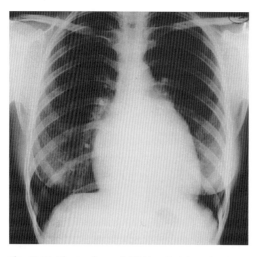

Fig. 10.11 Chest radiograph (PA) in mitral stenosis.

Suitability for a conservative procedure (e.g. valvotomy or valve repair) is best determined by echocardiography. Both M-mode and cross-sectional echocardiography show valve thickening and a reduction in the mid-diastolic closure rate of the anterior leaflet. The posterior leaflet may also be tethered and move anteriorly (instead of posteriorly) during diastole. The left atrial dimension is increased, and occasionally thrombus may be visible in the left atrial appendage. TOE is more reliable in the identification of intracavity thrombus. The pressure drop across the mitral valve using continuous-wave Doppler correlates well with the haemodynamic gradient measured at cardiac catheterization but, as with direct measurement of the gradient, the Doppler gradient is very much dependent on heart rate. The pressure half-time may be a more reliable index of the severity of mitral stenosis (see Chapter 3).

Invasive assessment by cardiac catheterization is limited to certain subgroups of patients, for example to define the coronary anatomy, and is no longer a prerequisite to mitral valve surgery.

Medical management

The objective of drug therapy for mitral stenosis is to control the ventricular rate, reduce left atrial pressure and prevent systemic thromboembolism.

The onset of atrial fibrillation, which usually occurs in the sixth decade, is often associated with rapid symptomatic deterioration. Digoxin is the drug of choice at a dose sufficient to maintain the resting ventricular rate between 60 and 70 bpm, usually 0.125–0.25 mg/day depending on age, body weight and renal function. Although effective at rest, digoxin is often disappointing in controlling the ventricular rate during exertion. Toxicity may occur if the patient is hypokalaemic. Difficulty with rate control may require a small dose of an additional β-blocker (e.g. atenolol 25 mg once daily) or a calcium antagonist (e.g. verapamil 40 mg twice daily). Alternative agents include a β-blocker alone or amiodarone. Electrical or chemical cardioversion rarely restores sinus rhythm long term in the patient with significant mitral stenosis.

Fluid retention responds well to diuretic therapy; however, pulmonary oedema occurs as a consequence of an anatomical obstruction and overvigorous diuretic therapy may result in hypovolaemia, hypokalaemia and pre-renal azotaemia. Large doses of loop diuretics should be avoided in favour of a thiazide or combination diuretic.

In the patient with atrial fibrillation due to rheumatic mitral valve disease, there is a 15- to 20-fold increase in the risk of stroke from systemic thromboembolism, which is highest at the time of onset of atrial fibrillation. Patients with significant mitral stenosis, especially if there is evidence on echocardiography of left atrial enlargement, require anticoagulation with warfarin, aiming to maintain the international normalized ratio (INR) between 2.0 and 2.5.

Mitral valve surgery

If the patient remains significantly limited despite diuretic therapy and control of the ventricular rate, surgical intervention or balloon valvuloplasty should be considered. Occasionally, patients with recurrent thromboembolism, despite adequate anticoagulation, may also require operation. However, it should be borne in mind that the long-term results of mitral valve surgery are less favourable than those of aortic valve replacement, especially as symptomatic deterioration may be very slow in mitral valve disease.

A conservative procedure on the mitral valve is possible in a small minority of patients. Usually they are young, in sinus rhythm and without evidence of involvement of the subvalve apparatus by the rheumatic process on echocardiography. Most of these patients in whom open mitral valvotomy is considered are suitable for balloon mitral valvuloplasty (see below).

Replacement of the mitral valve with a mechanical prosthesis is usually appropriate, as the patient will require anticoagulation in any case for the atrial fibrillation. A tissue valve may be considered for the very elderly or women of childbearing age in whom anticoagulation may be a problem. Early mortality for mitral valve replacement is 6–8%, with a late valve-related mortality of 3–5% per annum, which is not related to valve type. Thromboembolic complications with mechanical valves occur at a rate of 3–5% per patient-year follow-up.

Balloon mitral valvuloplasty

Balloon dilatation of the mitral valve appears to be a suitable alternative to surgery in selected patients. Left atrial thrombus must be excluded by TOE, mitral regurgitation should be minimal and the results are more favourable if the valve is non-calcified without evidence of chordal fusion and shortening. An Inoue balloon is introduced under local anaesthesia from the right femoral vein and via a trans-septal approach from the right to the left atrium; the balloon is dilated sufficiently to cause splitting of the fused commissures (Fig. 10.12). Early mortality is low at <1%, with a morbidity of 2–4%. Early experience suggests that the results match those from mitral valvotomy, even in the elderly.

Degenerative mitral valve disease

Acute mitral regurgitation

Within 14 days of an acute myocardial infarct, 0.4–0.5% of patients die from acute mitral regurgitation secondary to papillary muscle rupture. Sudden, severe mitral regurgitation results in early acute pulmonary oedema and cardiogenic shock; without immediate mitral valve replacement, 75% of patients die within 24 h. Unlike chronic mitral regurgitation, there is insufficient time for compensatory mechanism of left atrial and left ventricular dilatation to adapt to the volume load. Other causes of acute mitral regurgitation include valve destruction (cusp perforation or chordal rupture) by infective endocarditis, partial papillary muscle rupture and spontaneous chordal rupture.

Chronic non-rheumatic mitral regurgitation

Pathogenesis

Myxomatous degeneration of the mitral valve leads to a spectrum of valve abnormalities ranging

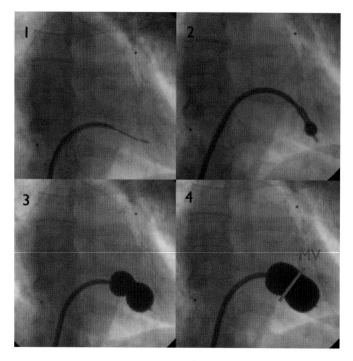

Fig. 10.12 Balloon mitral valvuloplasty.

Box 10.7 Symptoms in mitral regurgitation

- Fatigue
- Breathlessness
- Orthopnoea
- Nocturnal dyspnoea
- Palpitation (atrial fibrillation)

Box 10.8 Signs in mitral regurgitation

- Hyperdynamic apex
- ±Systolic thrill
- Pansystolic murmur
- ±Systolic click(s)

---

from minor degrees of cusp prolapse, present in up to 5% of the population, to a 'floppy valve' due to chordal elongation or rupture causing significant mitral regurgitation.

Symptoms (see Box 10.7)

Many patients remain asymptomatic until the insidious onset of fatigue, breathlessness and palpitation, the latter presenting as a hyperdynamic heartbeat, extrasystoles or atrial fibrillation.

Physical signs (see Box 10.8)

The pulse and venous pressure appear normal in isolated mitral regurgitation, unless there is secondary pulmonary hypertension. Palpation of the precordium is an important means of assessing the severity of mitral regurgitation. If mild, the precordial impulse is quiet but, as the severity increases, the cardiac apex becomes hyperdynamic and displaced laterally, often in association with a systolic thrill.

Mild degrees of mitral regurgitation due to mitral valve prolapse are characterized by a quiet, late systolic murmur, associated with one or more systolic clicks. As the regurgitation becomes more severe, the murmur lengthens, obscuring S2 and the systolic clicks (Fig. 10.13). Murmur location, typically at the apex, may be unreliable because a jet directed anteriorly can be heard at the base and radiates to the neck.

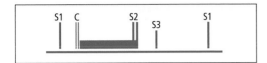

Fig. 10.13 Auscultatory findings in non-rheumatic mitral regurgitation.

Investigations

The ECG may be normal in mild to moderate mitral regurgitation. As the left atrium enlarges, the P waves become biphasic. Later still, when the left ventricle dilates, the anterior voltages become prominent, often in association with T-wave inversion.

In moderate to severe mitral regurgitation, there is evidence of both left atrial and left ventricular dilatation on chest radiography. Left atrial enlargement may reach aneurysmal proportions. Pulmonary venous congestion and interstitial oedema arise late in the course of the disease.

Serial echo-Doppler examinations have largely replaced radiography in the follow-up of the patient with mitral regurgitation. Prolapse of one or both leaflets may be visible, as well as the redundant cusp tissue typical of a 'floppy' valve. Similarly, ruptured chordae can be seen, although there may be difficulty in differentiating between a vegetation and the rolled-up cusp margin seen in partial chordal rupture. In mild disease, the left ventricular and left atrial dimensions are normal but, as the regurgitation increases in severity, left ventricular and septal movement become more vigorous; and eventually the left ventricle dilates with a reduction in systolic function.

Doppler ultrasound is an accurate and sensitive method of detecting mitral regurgitation. Both the direction and the magnitude of the regurgitant jet(s) can be mapped using colour-flow techniques, allowing a semi-quantitative assessment of the severity of the lesion (see Chapter 3).

Haemodynamic assessment is usually only necessary prior to mitral valve surgery, when cardiac catheterization is required to document the coronary anatomy.

Medical management

Patients with mild mitral regurgitation may only require antibiotic prophylaxis (see page 156). As the severity of the disease progresses, a mild diuretic or vasodilators (e.g. an ACE inhibitor) are equally effective. Only if these measures fail to provide symptomatic relief, or if there is echocardiographic evidence of progressive cavity dilatation, should surgical intervention be considered.

Atrial fibrillation should be treated as for mitral stenosis (see page 165). The incidence of systemic thromboembolism is said to be low in isolated mitral regurgitation, but in the patient with atrial fibrillation, treatment with warfarin is recommended.

Surgical intervention

Progressive symptoms of fatigue or breathlessness, or echocardiographic evidence of left ventricular dilatation (even without symptoms), indicate the need for surgical intervention. Reconstruction of the mitral valve has superior long-term results compared with valve replacement, with a similar early mortality of 0–2%. Results are particularly good for repair of posterior leaflet prolapse. Cusp resection is often combined with chordal shortening, reinforced with some type of annuloplasty. Late complications associated with thromboembolism or anticoagulation are avoided with repair. Patients with mitral regurgitation as a consequence of myocardial ischaemia or infarction form a high-risk subgroup, with an early mortality of 10–20% reflecting the associated impairment of ventricular function in these patients. There has been recent interest in the percutaneous approach to mitral valve repair; a variety of techniques are under evaluation, including sutures and clips directly applied to the valve, as well as procedures aimed at reducing mitral annulus dimensions.

Mitral valve prolapse syndrome

Mitral valve prolapse, which is a normal variant occurring in 5–10% of the population at large, may be associated with a more widespread spectrum

of cardiac and extra-cardiac symptoms. These
include:

- chest pain;
- palpitation;
- anxiety;
- fatigue;
- lethargy;
- an inability to concentrate;
- exercise intolerance;
- postural giddiness.

Because of the diverse nature of the symptoms,
there is a tendency for the physician to dismiss the
symptoms as having no organic basis. It is important to take a careful history and to confirm
the diagnosis of mitral valve prolapse on echocardiography. Evidence of pre-excitation or variable
inferior repolarization changes may be present
on the resting ECG, and a 'false-positive'
exercise response is not uncommon. Atrial and
ventricular ectopics may be documented by Holter
monitoring.

The mainstay of treatment is careful explanation
and reassurance. Avoidance of stimulants (e.g. tea
and coffee) may be helpful and, in occasional
patients, a small dose of a β-blocker (e.g. atenolol
25 mg once daily) may be beneficial. Investigations
should usually stop short of invasive testing unless
there is concern that there may be additional coronary artery disease.

Mitral annulus calcification

This is a condition of the elderly in which calcium
is laid down in the mitral annulus and may occasionally spread to involve the conducting tissue,
causing heart block, or the mitral leaflets themselves, causing mitral regurgitation. Females are affected more frequently than males, and there is an
association with hypercalcaemia, diabetes mellitus
and systemic hypertension. Symptoms are unusual, although calcification may act as a source of systemic thromboembolism or be the substrate for
infective endocarditis. The diagnosis can be confirmed by echocardiography or on the lateral chest
radiograph, the calcified annulus appearing as a
curved J- or U-shaped shadow (see Fig. 19.5).

Infective endocarditis

See Chapter 12.

Pulmonary valve disease

See Chapter 18.

Tricuspid valve disease

Pathogenesis and aetiology

The tricuspid valve consists of three leaflets of differing size. The annulus of the valve is a dynamic
structure that changes size during the cardiac
cycle. Most commonly, tricuspid regurgitation
is 'functional', i.e. the valve leaks as a consequence
of right ventricular dilatation secondary to pressure overload, for example from mitral or aortic
valve disease, or cor pulmonale. Other rare
causes of tricuspid regurgitation include right
ventricular infarction, infective endocarditis,
trauma, carcinoid or rheumatic fever. Tricuspid
stenosis is very rare in Europe and North America
and is nearly always associated with mitral valve
disease.

Symptoms

In most patients, the left-side symptoms predominate (breathlessness, orthopnoea, nocturnal dyspnoea). Patients may complain of visible neck
pulsation from the raised venous pressure, fluid
retention (abdominal and lower limb swelling),
right upper quadrant pain (hepatic congestion),
anorexia and weight loss.

Physical signs

A raised venous pressure with a prominent systolic
('v') wave is characteristic, in association with a
pansystolic murmur. The localization of the murmur and the increase in intensity with inspiration
may not be useful in clinical practice. Late in the
disease, hepatic pulsation may be present, reflecting the severity of the regurgitation.

Investigations

Atrial fibrillation on the ECG is the norm, and the chest radiograph nearly always shows cardiac enlargement with additional features of left-sided disease. Echocardiography demonstrates dilatation of the right-sided chambers, often in association with paradoxical septal motion. Organic disease of the valve (e.g. vegetations) may be apparent. Doppler assessment allows a semi-quantitative assessment of the severity of the regurgitation, together with the calculation of right ventricular systolic pressure. Many normal subjects have mild tricuspid regurgitation on colour-flow mapping.

Management

Tricuspid regurgitation is well tolerated. Management of the left-sided problem (e.g. mitral valve replacement) is appropriate, which will usually result in a fall in the right ventricular pressure thereby reducing the severity of the tricuspid regurgitation. An additional tricuspid annuloplasty may be required in severe cases. Tricuspid valve replacement is rarely undertaken today because of problems of valve thrombosis. In patients with infective endocarditis, a conservative approach (e.g. valve debridement and/or annuloplasty) may be required to restore valve competence.

Innocent murmurs

A short innocent or physiological mid-systolic murmur can be heard in ~8% of the normal population. Typically, a well-localized, quiet crescendo–decrescendo ('ejection') murmur is heard at the left sternal edge, and may be augmented by conditions that increase cardiac output (e.g. anaemia, fever, pregnancy). These murmurs are thought to arise from turbulence in the right ventricular outflow tract. The diagnosis is usually clear-cut on clinical examination alone; if necessary, echocardiography and a Doppler examination can confirm the absence of structural heart disease.

Further reading

ACC/AHA 2006 Guidelines for the Management of Patients with Valvular Heart Disease: a report of the American College of Cardiology/ American Heart Association Task Force on Practice Guidelines (Writing Committee to Revise the 1998 Guidelines for the Management of Patients with Valvular Heart Disease). *Journal of the American College of Cardiology* 2006; 48: e1–148.

European Society of Cardiology Guidelines (2007) on Valvular Heart Disease http://www.escardio. org/knowledge/guidelines/Valvular-Heart-Disease.htm?hit=men06

Chapter 11

The endocardium

Function and pathophysiology

The endocardium is a thin layer that invests the entire inner surface of the heart. The structure and thickness of the endocardium vary from one chamber to another and from one region to another within a given chamber. The endocardium is thicker in the atria than the ventricles and thicker in the left-sided chambers compared with the right. The endocardium is well developed in the left ventricular outflow tract, forming five distinct layers: (i) the endothelial layer; (ii) inner connective tissue; (iii) elastic tissue; (iv) smooth muscle; and (v) outer connective tissue layers. The total thickness of the endocardium in the left ventricular outflow tract is 200 μm, but as thin as 50 μm elsewhere in this chamber. The thickest endocardium is found in the left atrium where it may approach 900 μm. With increasing age, the endocardium increases in thickness and becomes more opaque due to a proliferation of elastic tissue and collagen.

The endocardial connective tissue is continuous with that in the myocardial interstitium and valvular leaflets. Integrity of the endocardium is important as a means of reducing platelet deposition and thrombus formation, as well as reducing the likelihood of the deposition and multiplication of the microorganisms that cause infective endocarditis.

Localized thickening of the endocardium may result from haemodynamic derangement of the heart valves; 'jet' lesions may be seen as a result of aortic or mitral regurgitation, and ventricular friction lesions can occur in mitral valve prolapse or in patients with hypertrophic obstructive cardiomyopathy due to systolic anterior movement of the mitral valve.

Carcinoid

Pathology

Carcinoid tumours arise from cells originating in neural crest tissue (Kulchitsky cells). Most commonly, primary tumours arise in the small intestine, especially the terminal ileum and appendix, although carcinoid tumours have been described in the bronchi, pancreatic ducts, ovaries, testicles, rectum and stomach. Carcinoid tumours involving the appendix usually remain localized; the spread of tumour to regional lymph nodes or the liver may result in the carcinoid syndrome.

Carcinoid syndrome

Symptoms of the carcinoid syndrome only occur when a primary tumour has metastasized to the regional lymph nodes or liver. The classic symptom is flushing of the skin that particularly affects the face, head and neck but may progress to involve the whole trunk.

Other features include bronchoconstriction, weight loss, profuse diarrhoea and abdominal pain.

Carcinoid tumours metabolize the amino acid tryptophan, producing the vasoactive amine 5-hydroxytryptamine (5-HT; serotonin) which is thought to be responsible for many of the clinical features of the syndrome. Urinary excretion of 5-hydroxyindole acetic acid (5-HIAA) is a useful marker for the condition, but high levels of this metabolite may occur from the ingestion of foods high in 5-HT (e.g. bananas, pineapples and walnuts). If at all possible, histological confirmation of the diagnosis should be performed with biopsy of either the primary or secondary tumour. Treatment should include the control of diarrhoea (e.g. codeine phosphate, diphenoxylate or with the somatostatin analogue octreotide), together with the administration of 5-HT antagonists (cyproheptadine, methysergide) and β-blockers (e.g. phenoxybenzamine) for symptoms of flushing. The prognosis is variable. Many tumours are slow growing and metastasize late.

Cardiac carcinoid

In carcinoid heart disease there is either focal or diffuse plaque-like thickening of the endocardium, which is nearly always limited to the right heart.

Inactivation of 5-HT by the lungs accounts for the relative sparing of the left-sided valves. Cardiac involvement is seen only in patients with hepatic secondaries or when the venous drainage from the tumour bypasses the liver (e.g. bronchial and ovarian tumours). Deposition of fibrous tissue on the pulmonary valve results in predominant stenosis, although some additional regurgitation may occur. Adherence of the leaflets of the tricuspid valve to the ventricular septum causes tricuspid regurgitation; fibrous deposition of the plaque on the posterior and septal leaflets of the valve can result in tricuspid stenosis. The pathogenesis of the carcinoid plaque is uncertain. Rarely, surgical debridement of the affected valve or valve replacement may be required.

Endomyocardial fibrosis

Endomyocardial fibrosis (EMF) is a condition most frequently seen in the tropics, with sporadic reports from temperate climates. Progressive thickening and fibrosis of the endocardium affecting either the left or, more usually, both ventricles results in haemodynamics indistinguishable from those of a restrictive cardiomyopathy in association with atrioventricular (AV) valve regurgitation.

Apical obliteration of either ventricle by thrombus may result in systemic or pulmonary embolism. A moderate eosinophilia suggests an association with eosinophilic endomyocardial disease (see below) but may merely reflect concomitant parasitic infection found in the tropics. Treatment consists of diuretic therapy, with mitral or tricuspid repair or replacement, together with endocardial resection in selected patients.

Eosinophilic endomyocardial disease

This is a rapidly progressive condition, first described by Loeffler, in which an eosinophilic endomyocarditis is associated with a systemic disorder including anorexia, weight loss, cough and wheezing. Unlike EMF, the condition is seen more frequently in temperate climates.

Three stages of the condition are described: (i) the early necrotic stage; (ii) the thrombotic stage; and (iii) the fibrotic stage. The latter is pathologically indistinguishable from the histology seen in EMF. Endomyocardial biopsy may be diagnostic in the early necrotic stage, showing a combination of myocardial necrosis and an eosinophilic infiltrate. Typically, the peripheral blood eosinophils are degranulated, with the suggestion that the proteins contained within the granules have been released and are cardiotoxic. Early treatment with steroids and immunosuppressive drugs may reduce the level of circulating eosinophils, resulting in resolution of the myocarditis. Occasional patients require AV valve replacement or endocardial resection.

Endocardial fibroelastosis

This is a condition of infancy and childhood of obscure aetiology, characterized by thickening of the endocardium by a white homogeneous glistening material usually involving the left atrium and ventricle.

Haemodynamics are similar to those found in a dilated cardiomyopathy with impaired systolic function, although occasional patients present with a restrictive defect. The differential diagnosis includes storage diseases (e.g. Pompe's), an idiopathic dilated cardiomyopathy, EMF and an anomalous coronary artery. The prognosis is poor.

Infective endocarditis

Clinical presentation

In the past, infective endocarditis was a disease of young adults, but currently the average age is 50–60 years, with males affected more frequently than females (2:1). Factors responsible for the changing pattern of the disease include the widespread and early use of antibiotics, the increasing number of patients undergoing cardiac surgery and the increase in intravenous drug abuse. There is little evidence to suggest that the prognosis is improving, with an overall case fatality rate of approximately 30%. The widespread and indiscriminate use of antibiotics has resulted in an increase in the frequency of culture-negative endocarditis, which is associated with a less favourable prognosis.

Although some forms of endocarditis are more virulent than others, antibiotic therapy has modified the clinical course to such an extent that the terms 'acute' and 'subacute' are no longer applicable. 'Infective' rather than 'bacterial' is the preferred term, as non-bacterial forms (e.g. marantic in advanced malignancy, Libman–Sachs in systemic lupus) may be seen infrequently.

Portal of entry

Microorganisms gain entry to the bloodstream by a variety of routes (Table 11.1), although the mode of access can only be determined in one-third of patients. Less than 15% of patients give a history of prior dental treatment.

Table 11.1 Infective endocarditis: portals of entry.

Portals of entry	%
Dental treatment	<15
Genitourinary tract	4
Gastrointestinal	4
Respiratory	3
Skin	3
Cardiac surgery	3
Vascular surgery	3
Drug abuse	1
Pregnancy	<1
Fractures	<1
Unknown	64

Pathogenesis

Endothelial damage results from turbulence (e.g. bicuspid aortic valve, pulmonary stenosis, mitral valve prolapse) and may also be associated with high-pressure interfaces (e.g. ventricular septal defect (VSD), patent ductus arteriosus (PDA), coarctation of the aorta, hypertrophic cardiomyopathy). Areas of endothelial injury may provide a focus for the formation of a platelet–fibrin aggregate within which a small focus of circulating bacteria becomes entrapped and multiply. A transient bacteraemia complicating, for example, a surgical procedure then leads to tissue destruction, septic emboli and immune complex deposition, the three mechanisms of tissue damage in the patient with infective endocarditis.

Organisms

It is only with knowledge of the organisms responsible for infective endocarditis that the appropriate antibiotic treatment can be started. This is particularly important if therapy needs to be started early because of haemodynamic deterioration, before the organism is isolated. Table 11.2 lists the common organisms causing infective endocarditis. The spectrum of organisms may be different in some subgroups of patients. In recent years, the HACEK (*Haemophilus*, *Actinobacillus*, *Cardiobacterium*, *Eikenella*, *Kingella* spp.) group of organisms has become an increasingly recognized cause of infection. Intravenous drug abusers are infected with

Table 11.2 Common organisms causing infective endocarditis.

Organisms	%
Staphylococcus aureus	32
Streptococcus viridans	18
Enterococci	11
Staphylococcus spp. (coagulase negative)	11
Culture negative	8
Streptococcus bovis	7
Streptococcus spp. (others)	5
Non-HACEK Gram-negative spp.	2
Fungi	2
HACEK	2
Polymicrobial	1
Others	3

HACEK, *Haemophilus, Actinobacillus, Cardiobacterium, Eikenella, Kingella* spp.

Box 11.1 Symptoms in infective endocarditis

- Malaise
- Anorexia
- Weight loss
- Sweats
- Rigors

Box 11.2 Signs in infective endocarditis

- Fever
- Anaemia
- Clubbing (late)
- Heart murmur
- Splenomegaly
- Immune complex deposition
- Thromboembolism

---

staphylococcal spp. in 50% of cases, *Pseudomonas* spp. in 15% and fungi (frequently *Candida* spp.) in 5%. In patients with early prosthetic heart valves, infection with *Staphylococcus* spp. accounts for the majority of cases.

Culture-negative endocarditis occurs most frequently (>60% of cases) as a result of prior antibiotic treatment. Other causes include anaerobic (e.g. *Bacteroides* spp.) or other fastidious organisms (e.g. *Brucella* spp.), non-bacterial endocarditis (e.g. *Coxiella burnetii* or 'Q' fever), fungal infection (e.g. *Candida, Aspergillus* spp.) or non-infective (thrombotic) endocarditis. Endocarditis in HIV-seropositive patients usually relates to intravenous drug abuse or infection of indwelling venous catheters and, therefore, is caused by staphylococcal spp. in the majority of patients.

Symptoms (see Box 11.1)

Infective endocarditis is a diagnosis that is frequently missed due to the insidious nature of the disease. General malaise, anorexia, weight loss, headache, sweats and rigors for a period of 4–8 weeks have often been attributed to a protracted 'viral illness'. Other symptoms relate to systemic thromboembolism affecting any major vessel or immune complex deposition causing vascular injury in the skin, joints, kidney and the central nervous system (CNS).

Destruction of valve tissue can cause symptoms due to a raised pulmonary venous pressure including breathlessness, orthopnoea or nocturnal dyspnoea. Symptomatic deterioration may be particularly rapid when the aortic valve is infected.

Physical signs (see Box 11.2)

General physical signs include asthenia, fever and anaemia. Many of the peripheral manifestations of the condition result from immune complex deposition in the skin (e.g. petechiae, subungal 'splinter' haemorrhages (Fig. 11.1), Osler's nodes, Roth spots and Janeway lesions). Other classic features include finger clubbing (Fig. 11.2), splenic enlargement and haematuria.

Many of these clinical features may be absent, hence the late appreciation of the diagnosis in many patients. The clinical course in elderly patients may be very atypical, and the patient may remain afebrile throughout the illness.

The cardiac manifestations include a tachycardia related to fever and anaemia, together with new or changing murmurs. Involvement of the mitral

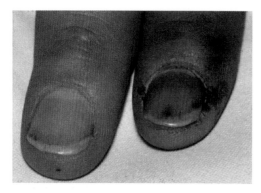

Fig. 11.1 Splinter haemorrhages.

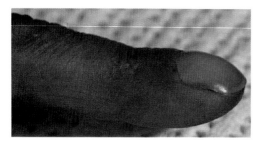

Fig. 11.2 Finger clubbing.

valve occurs in 30–45% of patients and the aortic valve in 15–25%. The characteristic signs of mitral and aortic regurgitation may not be obvious due to the rapid onset of tissue destruction. Occasionally, patients present with severe valve regurgitation with no detectable murmur. Other murmurs relate to the underlying heart lesion (e.g. PDA, VSD).

In 10–15% of patients with infective endocarditis the presenting symptom is neurological, and CNS complications occur in 15–30% of patients during the course of their illness. Mortality in this subgroup is double that of those without neurological complication. CNS complications of infective endocarditis include cerebral abscess, mycotic aneurysm, meningitis, cerebritis and subarachnoid haemorrhage.

Investigations

A high erythrocyte sedimentation rate (ESR) (50–100 mm/h) and C-reactive protein (CRP) are typical, in association with a mild leucocytosis and a normochromic normocytic anaemia. Rarely, a haemolytic anaemia or thrombocytopaenia may be seen.

Bacteraemia in infective endocarditis is continuous, therefore blood cultures timed to coincide with peaks of fever are unnecessary. Furthermore, there is no advantage in taking arterial blood, central venous blood or bone marrow for culture. Six sets of blood cultures taken over a 60-min period will suffice. Aerobic and anaerobic cultures are set up, and additional cultures containing penicillinase if penicillin has been administered within the previous 48 h.

Close co-operation between the clinician and the hospital microbiology department is important for the optimum management of the patient with endocarditis. The microbiologist can offer advice regarding cultures, choice of antibiotic, monitoring antibiotic levels and the response of the organism *in vitro*. In a regional centre, the microbiologist will also liaise with the referring hospital and arrange for transfer of the organism if necessary.

In cases of culture-positive endocarditis, the organism will be isolated from the first blood culture in 60–90% of cases within 48 h.

Circulating immune complexes are present in 80–95% of patients, and levels of haemolytic complement (C_3, C_4, CH_{50}) are reduced in 30% of patients. Urine microscopy reveals microscopic haematuria (red cell casts) and proteinuria in at least 50% of patients.

Echocardiography is the mainstay of investigation, in the diagnosis of infective endocarditis, in the monitoring of treatment and in the timing of surgery. Echocardiography allows delineation of the anatomy including the presence of valvular regurgitation, chordal rupture and cusp perforation, vegetations, abscess formation, abnormal connections (shunts) and the overall haemodynamic effects on ventricular function. Transthoracic echocardiography should be supplemented by transoesophageal studies, which increase both sensitivity and anatomic detail (see Chapter 4). The yield for visualization of vegetations increases from approximately 65 to 95% using the transoesophageal approach.

Antibiotic treatment

Antibiotic therapy should be tailored to the culprit organism (if known) (Tables 11.3 and 11.4). In general, combination intravenous antibiotics are used for a period of 4 weeks, with the monitoring of the antibiotic level against the organism *in vitro* in the laboratory. For sensitive organisms including *Streptococcus* spp., penicillin G 12–18 million U/24h in divided doses is combined with gentamicin 1 mg/kg every 8h, to maintain a trough concentration <1 µg/mL. The aminoglycoside can be discontinued after 2 weeks. Vancomycin 30 mg/kg per 24h in two equally divided doses is recommended for patients allergic to β-lactam antibiotics. For *Entero-* *cocci* spp., ampicillin 12 g/24 h in divided doses is combined with gentamicin (dosing as above). *Staphylococcus* spp. should be treated with a combination of flucloxacillin 2 g every 4 h combined with gentamicin (dosing as above). Methicillin-resistant *Staphylococci* spp. should be treated with vancomycin (dosing as above). In the presence of prosthetic material (e.g. a heart valve), a combination of gentamicin, vancomycin and rifampicin 300 mg orally every 8 h is recommended. HACEK organisms are best treated with a combination of cefotaxime 2 g IV once daily, together with ampicillin 12 g/24 h in divided doses and gentamicin (dosing as above). Culture-negative endocarditis should be treated with a combination of

Table 11.3 Current recommendations for antibiotic treatment of infective endocarditis.

Organism	Antibiotic regimen

Viridans streptococci
Streptococcus oralis, mitis,
    sanguis, mutans, salivarius
	Fully sensitive to penicillin (MIC <0.1 mg/L)
	Benzylpenicillin 7.2 g daily IV in six divided doses for 2/52, **plus**
	    gentamicin 80 mg IV in two doses (NB: monitor blood levels)
	Reduced sensitivity to penicillin (MIC >0.1 mg/L)
	Benzylpenicillin 7.2 g daily IV in six divided doses for 4/52 **plus**
	    gentamicin 80 mg IV in two doses for 4/52 (NB: monitor blood levels)

Streptococcus bovis
Enterococci
Enterococcus faecalis,
    faecium
	As above
	Gentamicin-sensitive or low-level resistant (MIC >0.1 mg/L)
	Ampicillin or amoxycillin 12 g daily IV in six divided doses for 4/52, **plus**
	    gentamicin 80 mg IV in two doses for 4/52 (NB: monitor blood levels)
	Gentamicin highly resistant (MIC >16 mg/L)
	Ampicillin or amoxycillin 12 g daily IV in six divided doses for 6/52, **plus**
	    vancomycin initially 1 g IV over 100 min twice daily for 4/52 (NB: monitor
	    blood levels to achieve a 1 h post-infusion peak level of 30 mg/L and a trough
	    level of 5–10 mg/L)

Staphylococci
Staphylococcus aureus,
    lagdunensis
	Penicillin-sensitive
	Benzylpenicillin 7.2 g daily IV in six divided doses for 4/52, **plus**
	    gentamicin 80–120 mg IV in three doses for 1/52 (NB: monitor blood levels)
	Penicillin-resistant, methicillin-sensitive
	Flucloxacillin 12 g IV in six divided doses for 4/52, **plus**
	    gentamicin 80–120 mg IV in three doses for 1/52 (NB: monitor blood levels)
	Penicillin- and methicillin-resistant
	Vancomycin initially 1 g IV over 100 min twice daily for 4/52 (NB: monitor
	    blood levels to achieve a 1 h post-infusion peak level of 30 mg/L and a
	    trough level of 5–10 mg/L), **plus**
	    gentamicin 80–120 mg IV in three doses for 1/52 (NB: monitor blood levels)

MIC, minimum inhibitory concentration.
Adapted from the Guidelines for the antibiotic treatment of endocarditis in adults: report of the Working Party of the British Society of Antimicrobial Chemotherapy. *Journal of Antimicrobial Chemotherapy* 2004; 54: 971–81.

Table 11.4 Treatment regimens for adults allergic to penicillin.

Organism	Antibiotic regimen
Viridans streptococci	Vancomycin initially 1 g IV over 100 min twice daily for 4/52 (NB: monitor blood
Streptococcus oralis, mitis,	levels to achieve a 1 h post-infusion peak level of 30 mg/L and a trough level
sanguis, mutans, salivarius	of 5–10 mg/L), **or**
Streptococcus bovis	Teicoplanin 400 mg IV 12 hourly for three doses and then a maintenance dose of
	400 mg daily, **plus**
	gentamicin 80 mg IV in two doses for 2/52 (NB: monitor blood levels)
Enterococci	Vancomycin initially 1 g IV over 100 min twice daily for 4/52(NB: monitor blood
Enterococcus faecalis,	levels to achieve a 1 h post-infusion peak level of 30 mg/L and a trough level
faecium	of 5–10 mg/L), **plus**
	gentamicin 80 mg IV in 2 doses for 4/52 (NB: monitor blood levels)
Staphylococci	Vancomycin initially 1 g IV over 100 min twice daily for 4/52 (NB: monitor blood
Staphylococcus aureus,	levels to achieve a 1 h post-infusion peak level of 30 mg/L and a trough level
	of 5–10 mg/L), **plus**
Lagdunensis	gentamicin 80–120 mg IV in three doses for 1/52 (NB: monitor blood levels)

Adapted from the Guidelines for the antibiotic treatment of endocarditis in adults: report of the Working Party of the British Society of Antimicrobial Chemotherapy. *Journal of Antimicrobial Chemotherapy* 2004; 54: 971–981.

ampicillin, flucloxacillin and gentamicin (dosing as above). Antibiotic doses assume normal hepatic and renal function. Doses may be reduced in the elderly and according to lean body mass.

Surgical intervention

Surgical intervention should be considered in high-risk groups of patients. High risks include:
- infection on prosthetic heart valves;
- haemodynamically significant aortic or mitral regurgitation;
- infection with *Staphylococcus* spp.;
- fungal endocarditis;
- shunts;
- abscess formation;
- atrioventricular block;
- large (>10 mm diameter) vegetations.

The timing of surgery is crucial and depends on clinical judgement, which should include the assessment of the whole patient. In general, surgical intervention should be undertaken early, before the advent of renal impairment, antibiotic resistance/toxicity and intracardiac extension of infection. Aortic regurgitation, in particular, should be treated with valve replacement prior to haemodynamic deterioration. In the setting of infective endocarditis, aortic valve replacement is associated with a perioperative mortality of 4–8%, mitral valve replacement with a mortality of 5–10%, and a re-operation rate of 5–10%. There is some evidence that valve replacement using tissue valves is superior to prosthetic valves in the setting of active infection. Patients operated on early after a cerebral complication (abscess, thromboembolic stroke, cerebritis) do particularly poorly.

Prognosis

In the majority of patients, fever and constitutional upset resolves within 1 week of the commencement of antibiotics. Fevers persisting more than 2 weeks may indicate resistant organisms, an inappropriate antibiotic regimen, ongoing immune complex deposition or focal sepsis. Persistent fever is associated with a poor prognosis and may be an indication for surgical intervention. A fever that settles and then recurs after 2–3 weeks usually indicates a reaction to an antibiotic; the fever may be associated with a second elevation in ESR or CRP. Both the temperature and the abnormal inflammatory markers normalize promptly once the antibiotic has been discontinued.

There is little evidence that the prognosis in infective endocarditis has improved over the last 25 years, with an overall mortality of 15–30% in reported series. An adverse prognosis is associated with *Staphylococcus* spp., *Enterococcus* spp. and culture-negative endocarditis. Other significant factors include increasing age, renal impairment, involvement of the aortic valve and cerebral complications.

Table 11.5 Indications for antibiotic prophylaxis.

Dental treatment
Extractions, scaling or periodontal disease (dental treatment likely to breach the gum margin)
Surgery or instrumentation of the upper respiratory tract
Tonsillectomy, adenoidectomy, nasal packing, tongue piercing, laryngoscopy
Genitourinary surgery or instrumentation
Cystoscopy, prostatectomy, urethral dilatation, trans-rectal prostatic biopsy
Obstetric and gynaecological procedures
Caesarean section, vaginal hysterectomy (NB: not vaginal delivery)
Gastrointestinal procedures
Treatment of oesophageal varices (sclerotherapy), oesophageal stricture (dilatation), oesophageal laser therapy, endoscopic retrograde cholangio-pancreatography, hepatic/biliary surgery, gallstone lithotripsy, surgery involving the intestinal mucosa, colonoscopy

Adapted from the Guidelines for the prevention of endocarditis: report of the Working Party of the British Society of Antimicrobial Chemotherapy. *Journal of Antimicrobial Chemotherapy* 2006; 57: 1035–42.

Table 11.6 Current recommendations for antibiotic prophylaxis against infective endocarditis*.

Treatment	Antibiotic regimen
Dental treatment Upper respiratory tract procedures	Amoxycillin 3 g single oral dose 1 h before treatment

Dental treatment (allergic to penicillin)
Upper respiratory tract procedures (allergic to penicillin)
	Erythromycin stearate 1.5 g orally 1–2 h before treatment, **plus**
	  erythromycin stearate 0.5 g orally 6 h later, **or**
	  clindamycin 600 mg single oral dose 1 h before treatment
	Amoxycillin 1 g IM just before induction, **plus**
	  gentamicin 120 mg IM just before induction, **then**

Special risk patients: 1. Patients with prosthetic valves who are to have a general anaesthetic 2. Patients who are to have a general anaesthetic and who are allergic to penicillin or who have had penicillin in the previous month 3. Patients who have had a previous attack of infective endocarditis 4. Patients undergoing genitourinary procedures 5. Patients undergoing obstetric and gynaecological procedures 6. Patients undergoing gastrointestinal procedures	Amoxycillin 0.5 g orally 6 h later
Special risk patients (as above) (allergic to penicillin)	Vancomycin 1 g by slow IV infusion over 1 h, **plus** gentamicin 120 mg IM just before induction

*NB: reduce doses proportionately for children.
Adapted from the Guidelines for the prevention of endocarditis: report of the Working Party of the British Society of Antimicrobial Chemotherapy. *Journal of Antimicrobial Chemotherapy* 2006; 57:1035–42.

Antibiotic prophylaxis

The British Society of Antimicrobial Chemotherapy has produced a set of guidelines relating to the appropriate use of antibiotic prophylaxis for patients at risk from infective endocarditis. Table 11.5 lists the indications for endocarditis prophylaxis and Table 11.6 lists the current drug regimen.

Further reading

Baddour LM, Wilson WR, Bayer AS, Fowler VG Jr, Bolger AF, Levison ME, Ferrieri P, Gerber MA, Tani LY, Gewitz MH, Tong DC, Steckelberg JM, Baltimore RS, Shulman ST, Burns JC, Falace DA, Newburger JW, Pallasch TJ, Takahashi M, Taubert KA. Infective endocarditis: diagnosis, antimicrobial therapy, and management of complications: a statement for healthcare professionals from the Committee on Rheumatic Fever, Endocarditis, and Kawasaki Disease, Council on Cardiovascular Disease in the Young, and the Councils on Clinical Cardiology, Stroke, and Cardiovascular Surgery and Anesthesia, American Heart Association: endorsed by the Infectious Diseases Society of America. *Circulation* 2005; 111: e394–434. http://circ.ahajournals.org/cgi/content/full/111/23/e394

Elliott TS, Foweraker J, Gould FK, Perry JD, Sandoe JA; Working Party of the British Society for Antimicrobial Chemotherapy. Guidelines for the antibiotic treatment of endocarditis in adults: report of the Working Party of the British Society for Antimicrobial Chemotherapy. *Journal of Antimicrobial Chemotherapy* 2004; 54: 971–81. http://jac.oxfordjournals.org/cgi/content/full/54/6/971

Gould FK, Elliott TSJ, Foweraker J, Fulford M, Perry JD, Roberts GJ, Sandoe JAT, Watkin RW. Guidelines for the prevention of endocarditis: report of the Working Party of the British Society for Antimicrobial Chemotherapy. *Journal of Antimicrobial Chemotherapy* 2006; 57: 1035–42. http://jac.oxfordjournals.org/cgi/content/full/57/6/1035

Horstkotte D, Follath F, Gutschik E, Lengyel M, Oto A, Pavie A, Soler-Soler J, Thiene G, von Graevenitz A, Priori SG, Garcia MA, Blanc JJ, Budaj A, Cowie M, Dean V, Deckers J, Fernandez Burgos E, Lekakis J, Lindahl B, Mazzotta G, Morais J, Oto A, Smiseth OA, Lekakis J, Vahanian A, Delahaye F, Parkhomenko A, Filipatos G, Aldershvile J, Vardas P. Task Force Members on Infective Endocarditis of the European Society of Cardiology; ESC Committee for Practice Guidelines (CPG). Guidelines on prevention, diagnosis and treatment of infective endocarditis executive summary; the task force on infective endocarditis of the European Society of Cardiology. *European Heart Journal* 2004; 25: 267–76. http://eurheartj.oxfordjournals.org/cgi/content/full/25/3/267

Ramsdale DR, Turner-Stokes L. Prophylaxis and treatment of infective endocarditis in adults: a concise guide. Advisory Group of the British Cardiac Society Clinical Practice Committee; RCP Clinical Effectiveness and Evaluation Unit. *Clinical Medicine* 2004; 4: 545–50.

Chapter 12

The pericardium

Anatomy and function

The pericardial sac surrounds the heart in the mediastinum. It encloses:
- the aortic root;
- the main pulmonary artery;
- the origin of the pulmonary veins and the venae cavae.

These vessels' adventitia is anchored by the pericardium and its ligamentous extensions into the sternum, vertebral column and diaphragm, also anchoring the heart during changes in body position. The pericardium has visceral and parietal aspects. The visceral pericardium is a serous membrane, applied to the surface of the heart and composed of a single layer of mesothelial cells. It reflects on itself so lining the inner surface of the parietal pericardium, which is fibrous tissue made up of collagen and elastin fibres. A thin film of fluid is secreted into the space between the two pericardial layers, lubricating the epicardial surface of the heart, facilitating motion within the pericardial sac and reducing friction with the surrounding organs. Absence of pericardium (congenital or after surgical removal) does not significantly impair cardiac function.

Acute pericarditis

Aetiology

- Idiopathic.
- Viral infection (especially Coxsackie) — usually rapid onset.
- Bacterial infection (especially tuberculosis) — usually insidious onset.
- Myocardial infarction.
- Autoimmune disease (systemic lupus erythematosus (SLE), rheumatoid, systemic sclerosis).
- Uraemia.
- Neoplasia.
- Trauma.

An autoimmune process can be triggered by exposure of cardiac antigens to the immune system, as may occur after cardiac surgery (postcardiotomy syndrome) or myocardial infarction (Dressler syndrome).

Clinical features

Symptoms

1 Left precordial pain:
- persistent;
- usually positional (relieved by sitting forward and exacerbated by lying supine); and
- usually sharp and radiating to the neck or shoulders.

2 Dyspnoea (often the consequence of shallow breathing or may indicate the development of a pericardial effusion).

3 Systemic features of inflammation (such as fever, malaise and arthralgia).

Physical signs

- May be none.
- Auscultation of a 'pericardial rub' (high-pitched, scratching sound) with audible

components throughout the cardiac cycle, intensity varying with position, and often evanescent.

Clinical features of cardiac tamponade may appear if a pericardial effusion significantly elevates the intrapericardial pressure.

Investigations

The electrocardiogram (ECG) may show the characteristic change of convex upward elevation of the ST segment in all leads (Fig. 12.1). In the absence of a significant pericardial effusion, the chest radiograph and echocardiogram are unhelpful. Virology or autoimmune screening may demonstrate an underlying cause. Antistreptolysin-O (ASO) titres are elevated in rheumatic fever and cold agglutinins in mycoplasma infection. Thyroid function tests should be performed to exclude hypothyroidism, and an estimation made of renal function (uraemic pericarditis). If there has been recent cardiac surgery or myocardial infarction, cardiac-specific antibodies may be detected. Elevation of

cardiac enzymes is common and reflects a degree of underlying subepicardial myocarditis. Aspiration of pericardial fluid, when present in sufficient amount, may sometimes be undertaken in order to diagnose a bacterial or fungal aetiology.

Management

Treatment is directed to the underlying condition and for control of symptoms. Response to non-steroidal anti-inflammatory drugs or culchicine is usually dramatic. The illness usually subsides over the course of 7–14 days, although in a small minority chronic or relapsing pericarditis may follow. If pain is not rapidly controlled, steroid therapy should be considered. Steroid treatment should be avoided unless directed at an underlying connective tissue disease.

Complications

Haemorrhage into the pericardial sac may occur, particularly in patients on anticoagulants. An acute

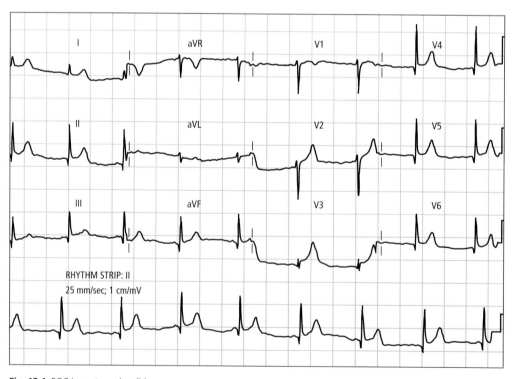

Fig. 12.1 ECG in acute pericarditis.

haemorrhagic episode may progress to pericardial tamponade, constrictive pericarditis or chronic (relapsing) pericarditis. The latter may recur over months and years, and may require long-term steroid or immunosuppressive therapy.

Constrictive pericarditis

Pathophysiology

Constrictive pericarditis is often of unknown aetiology, although in many cases it begins with an episode of acute pericarditis. Fibrotic thickening of the pericardial sac impairs filling of the cardiac chambers during diastole. Calcification or fibrosis of the pericardium may limit diastolic filling which abruptly terminates during early diastole at the volume set by non-compliant pericardium. Progressive restriction results in most ventricular filling occurring at the beginning of diastole with abrupt cessation. There are high, usually equal, diastolic pressures in all four cardiac chambers.

Aetiology

- Idiopathic (probably following an episode of unrecognized acute pericarditis).
- Tuberculosis (silent acute pericarditis with silent progression to constriction).
- Autoimmune causes of acute pericarditis and systemic sclerosis.
- Malignant disease (malignant infiltrations or radiotherapy).
- Post-cardiac surgery.

Clinical features (Box 12.1)

1 Those of the underlying condition.
2 Those related to elevation of right and left atrial filling that produce symptoms of:
- abdominal discomfort (with hepatic and gut engorgement);
- head muzziness;
- dyspnoea; and
- reduced exercise tolerance.

The venous pressure may be elevated well above the jaw and, unless the patient is examined sitting up, this clinical sign may be missed. There is a rapid early phase of diastolic filling followed by its sudden cessation due to the inability of the cardiac chambers to dilate further, producing a rapid 'x' and 'y' descent and positive Kussmaul's sign when examining the jugular venous pressure. A diastolic pericardial knock (filling sound), occurring earlier than the third heart sound (S3), may be heard.

> **Box 12.1 Clinical findings in constrictive pericarditis**
>
> - Rapid 'x' and 'y' descent in venous pressure
> - Positive Kussmaul's sign
> - Pericardial knock

Investigations

The **chest radiograph** may be normal, but pericardial calcification (best seen on lateral films) or an increased heart size may be apparent. ECG changes are non-specific and include atrial fibrillation, low-voltage complexes and ST/T wave abnormalities. **Echocardiography** may show abnormal diastolic function. Visualization of thickened pericardium is unreliable. Computed tomographic (**CT**) scanning is usually the best means of imaging the pericardium, but magnetic resonance imaging (**MRI**) is a good alternative and may better demonstrate cardiac function.

On **cardiac catheterization** simultaneous intracavitary pressure recordings during diastole show equilibrium of pressure in all four cardiac chambers. There is a **rapid 'x' and 'y' descent** of the right atrial waveform, and ventricular diastolic filling may show the 'square root' sign. There may be modest elevation of pulmonary artery pressure and pulmonary venous (pulmonary capillary wedge) pressures. Infusion of intravenous saline may be necessary to demonstrate these haemodynamic features.

Management

Most symptomatic patients become progressively more disabled without surgical resection of the parietal pericardium. This is a major and often difficult surgical procedure. The alternative of palliation with diuretic therapy is short lived.

Pericardial effusion and cardiac tamponade

Aetiology

Pericardial effusion may develop in response to any parietal pericardial inflammation. When pericardial fluid accumulates under pressure (due to large volume or indistensible pericardium, or both), the right atrial and right ventricular diastolic pressures may be exceeded by the intrapericardial sac pressure. The transmural pressure gradient declines to zero and tamponade occurs, causing:

- a fall in diastolic filling;
- a fall in stroke volume;
- a fall in cardiac output;
- impairment of venous return.

In contrast to pericardial constriction, ventricular filling is impaired throughout diastole.

Often a pericardial effusion is not clinically apparent but, as it enlarges, cardiac tamponade ensues. Symptoms occur if the volume of the effusion is large or if a more moderate volume accumulates sufficiently rapidly, without there being time for distension of the pericardial sac, or if the pericardium is abnormal and indistensible. The normal pericardial sac contains 15–30 mL of fluid. Up to 2 L of effusion may be present without haemodynamic features of tamponade if the effusion accumulates gradually, but as little as 250 mL of rapidly accumulated fluid may have haemodynamic consequence. After cardiac surgery there may be blood and clot in the pericardial space. The osmotic effects of clotted blood may cause rapid filling of the pericardial sac.

Clinical features (Box. 12.2)

Moderate effusions, especially when chronic, may produce no signs but, as the volume accumulates, the patient will become breathless, have a reduced exercise tolerance and may notice venous neck engorgement. Systemic arterial pressure falls, the venous pressure is elevated, **the 'y' descent is**

> **Box 12.2 Clinical findings in cardiac tamponade**
>
> - No 'y' descent and exaggerated 'x' descent in venous pressure
> - Quiet heart sounds
> - Pulsus paradoxus

---

abolished and the 'x' descent exaggerated. The heart sounds are quiet, the respiratory rate and pulse rate are increased and pulsus paradoxus may be present (arterial pressure drop >10 mmHg during breathing).

Investigations

- The chest radiograph may show an increased heart size if >250 mL of pericardial fluid is present, often giving a rather globular appearance to the heart.
- The ECG may have features of pericarditis or, when the effusion is large, electrical alternans of the QRS may occur (due to beat-to-beat alteration of the right and left ventricular filling) and the voltages may be small.
- Echocardiography shows diastolic collapse of the right ventricle and right atrium early in tamponade. The absence of an effusion excludes the diagnosis, but a loculated posterior pericardial effusion may be difficult to image on transthoracic echocardiography, particularly in the postoperative patient.
- Cardiac catheterization has little role, although it can quantify haemodynamic impairment. If the diagnosis of effusion is made on echocardiographic findings and clinical features of tamponade are present, then pericardiocentesis is required.

Management

Pericardiocentesis (tapping of pericardial fluid) relieves the haemodynamic embarrassment. This is usually performed as a percutaneous technique, a needle passing into the pericardial space under fluoroscopic or ultrasound control, and the Seldinger technique, adapted for passage of a drainage catheter into the pericardial space over a guide wire using either a subxiphoid or transthoracic approach. Recurrent effusions, as occur with malignant tumour involvement of the pericardium, may require a window to be created between the pericardial and pleural or abdominal space, using a formal surgical approach with a mini-thoracotomy. Alternatives to formal surgery, using specialized equipment to facilitate pericardial drainage, may occasionally be required in individuals where respiratory disease precludes surgery. Injection of sclerosing agents into the pericardial space after drainage is of limited value in preventing reaccumulation.

Further reading

Baue AE, ed. *Glenn's Thoracic and Cardiovascular Surgery*. Tsamford, CT: Appleton and Lange, 1996.

Grossman W, Baim DS, eds. *Cardiac Catheterization, Angiography, and Intervention*. London: Lea & Febiger, 1991.

Spodick DH. *The Pericardium: A Comprehensive Textbook*. New York: Marcel Dekker, 1997.

Chapter 13

Electrophysiology

Introduction

Cardiac myocyte contraction generates the mechanical force of atrial and ventricular systole.

• Individual myocyte contraction is the end result of a complex of ionic fluxes that cause cell membrane depolarization and repolarization.

• The transmembrane voltage changes (the consequence of ionic flux across the cell membrane) which occur during this process can be recorded using specialized techniques and are depicted as the action potential (Fig. 13.1).

Cell membrane depolarization and repolarization trigger activation and subsequent relaxation of the actin–myosin complex. Co-ordination of myocyte mechanical activity through the heart is achieved by the cardiac conduction system, itself a complex arrangement of cells that depolarize and repolarize. Potential gradients, created by myocardial depolarization, can be detected by body surface electrodes. These may be translated into an electronic or pen and ink inscription showing potential gradient variation with time in any given recording electrode. Recording electrodes may be bipolar or unipolar, and potential differences recorded in a standardized way, in either frontal or coronal planes. Thus, summation of the electrical activity of the heart is used to generate the surface electrocardiogram (ECG; see Chapter 3).

Arrhythmia

Abnormalities of cardiac rhythm

• **Bradycardia**: abnormally slow rate (defined as <60 cardiac bpm).

• **Tachycardia**: abnormally fast rate (defined as >100 bpm).

• **Irregularity of rhythm**.

Symptoms

• **Palpitation**: awareness of the heart beating, often due to an abnormality of rhythm, but sometimes an exaggerated awareness of sinus rhythm, or an increase in stroke volume (e.g. aortic or mitral regurgitation) or a sinus tachycardia (e.g. anxiety, fever, hyperthyroidism). Not all patients associate tachycardia with palpitation and may use the term to describe the irregularity of heart beat which comes, for example, with ventricular ectopic activity.

• **Dizziness, presyncope or syncope** can occur with systemic arterial hypotension causing hypoperfusion of the brain. Although an assessment of these symptoms requires exclusion of non-cardiac causes, systemic arterial hypotension may be the consequence of tachycardia, bradycardia, intravascular volume depletion, arterial vasodilatation or low cardiac output.

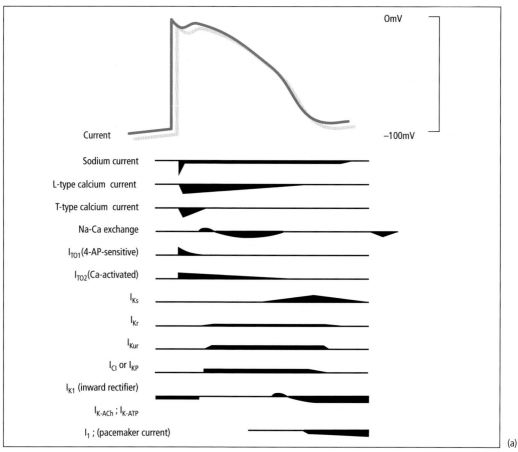

Current

Sodium current

L-type calcium current

T-type calcium current

Na-Ca exchange

I_{TO1} (4-AP-sensitive)

I_{TO2} (Ca-activated)

I_{Ks}

I_{Kr}

I_{Kur}

I_{Cl} or I_{KP}

I_{K1} (inward rectifier)

I_{K-ACh} ; I_{K-ATP}

I_1 ; (pacemaker current)

(a)

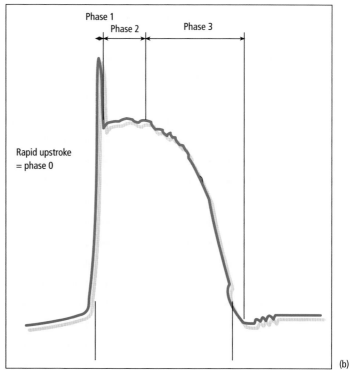

Phase 1

Phase 2

Phase 3

Rapid upstroke = phase 0

(b)

Fig. 13.1 (a) The relationship between transmembrane voltage gradient and time inscribes the action potential, the component currents of which are shown. Outward currents are grey, inward currents, black. (b) A schematic of the phases of the action potential.

Box 13.1 Electrophysiological investigations

- ECG
- Signal-averaged ECG
- 24-hour tape and patient-activated recorders
- Implantable loop recorder
- Tilt table test
- Carotid sinus massage
- EP study

- **Non-specific symptoms** such as malaise, poor exercise tolerance and dyspnoea may occur with persistent bradycardia. Dyspnoea and chest pain, often anginal in character, may occur in tachycardia.

Electrophysiological investigations

(Box 13.1)

Surface ECG

See Chapter 3.

Signal-averaged ECG

This employs computer analysis of ECG recordings to identify late potentials in electrical activity related to myocardial depolarization in regions of myocardial abnormality, which may be the substrate for re-entry ventricular arrhythmia.

Ambulatory ECG monitoring

These devices (Holter monitors) are mini-ECG recorders, about the size of a small personal stereo. They continuously record two ECG leads via electrodes attached to the anterior chest wall over a 24-hour period, during which time the patient continues with their usual activities. They keep a diary of any symptoms which can be correlated with the ECG.

Patient-activated recorders

Patient-activated devices will record a single ECG lead which can be analysed later or transmitted by telephone to a central recording station. Their particular value is in the assessment of patients whose symptoms are infrequent, but the ECG recordings are often of poor quality.

Implantable recording devices

Small subcutaneous recording devices can be implanted as a minor procedure. ECG is stored in the device prior to patient activation so that events which give rise to immediate loss of consciousness can be recorded after the event. This feature and long device life facilitate capture of infrequent events.

Tilt table testing and carotid sinus massage

Patients lie on a couch which can be tilted (head up) to 60°. Continuous monitoring of blood pressure, heart rate and ECG is performed. Tilting usually continues for 45 min but is stopped if bradycardia (cardioinhibition) or hypotension (vasodepression) occurs. In some centres there may be additional use of sublingual nitrates or intravenous isoprenaline to stress vagotonic reflexes. Patients with carotid sinus hypersensitivity syndrome may also have vagal cardioinhibition on inadvertent stimulation of the carotid sinus. Carotid sinus massage under controlled conditions and after assessment of carotid artery disease may unmask this.

Exercise stress testing

Exercise stress testing will demonstrate inability of the sinus node (SN) to mount a tachycardia in response to physiological demand (chronotropic incompetence).

Electrophysiology study

Catheters mounted with recording electrodes are introduced through the femoral or subclavian veins using a standard Seldinger technique under local anaesthetic. These are passed to the heart using standard cardiac catheterization techniques and positioned in the atria, at the atrioventricular node (AVN) and in the RV. Electrical activity from the endomyocardium apposed to the electrodes is filtered, amplified and recorded in unipolar or bipolar configurations as electrograms. The timing of electrical activity recorded from the endocardial surface (electrograms) at these sites and the response of electrical activity to cardiac pacing and extrastimulation (addition of premature paced beats during steady rate pacing) allow assessment of sinus and AV nodal activity and the integrity of the conduction system. Extrastimulation techniques are also used to assess inducibility and mechanism of tachycardias.

Bradycardia

Bradycardia may be arbitrarily defined as a heart rate below 60 bpm but in many individuals, particularly those who are fit, this may be entirely normal. Electrocardiograms showing examples of various bradycardias can be found in Chapter 3.

Bradycardia may be secondary to a number of non-cardiac disorders such as hypothyroidism, raised intracranial pressure or severe jaundice, but is most commonly due to some form of intrinsic heart disease.

Causes of bradycardia

Sinus node disease
(see Fig. 3.8, Chapter 3)

This may be due to degenerative disease of the SN, which is more common with increasing age, ischaemic heart disease, viral infection or autoimmune disease such as lupus. The SN may depolarize slowly or there may be a delay in electrical activity leaving the SN ('exit block').

Atrioventricular node disease and conduction disease

AVN disease causes heart block. This may be caused by or follow:
- ischaemic heart disease;
- autoimmune disease (e.g. lupus);

- aortopathy in Reiter's or ankylosing spondylitis sarcoidosis;
- destruction by infection (aortic root abscess);
- prosthetic aortic or mitral valve replacement.

Interruption of AVN conduction may be incomplete and produce various degrees of block.

First degree heart block
(see Fig. 3.10b, Chapter 3)

Prolongation of the PR interval >0.2 s on the surface ECG. It is indicative of AVN disease. In isolation it requires no treatment, but it may be the only manifestation of conduction disease in a patient with higher degrees (second or third) of heart block.

Second degree heart block
(see Fig. 3.10c and d, Chapter 3)

- Type 1: there is prolongation of successive PR intervals with failure of conduction of the ultimate P wave of a series (P wave not succeeded by a QRS complex). Again, as an isolated finding it requires no treatment, but may be the only manifestation of conduction disease in patients with symptomatic intermittent higher degree heart block.
- Type 2: there is intermittent but regular failure of P waves to conduct through the AVN with consequent bradycardia, the ventricular rate being 1/2, 1/3 or 1/4, etc. of the atrial rate. Prophylactic pacemaker implantation is indicated regardless of symptomatic status, as progression to complete heart block with the risk of a slow ventricular escape rhythm, or even asystole, is common.

Complete heart block (third degree heart block) (see Fig. 3.10e, Chapter 3)

There is failure of atrioventricular nodal conduction so that there is complete AV dissociation. The ventricular rate is always slower than the atrial rate (note that AV dissociation is not complete heart block when the atrial rate is slower than the ventricular rate). If the atrial rate is very slow, as can occur with increased vagal tone, the automaticity of the ventricles results in a ventricular escape rhythm which is faster than the slow atrial rate and dissociated from it.

Bundle branch block (see Chapter 3)

Conduction disease distal to the AVN may give rise to either impairment of AV conduction or an altered pattern of ventricular depolarization with altered left or right bundle branch conduction. Right bundle branch block may occur in the normal heart. Left bundle branch block is regarded as usually indicating underlying cardiac disease, although it may be difficult to determine the cause. Isolated bundle branch block has no effect on cardiac rate and requires no treatment as a lone finding. Disease of the right bundle and left anterior fascicle with first degree heart block (so-called 'trifascicular block') carries a high risk of development of complete heart block and is usually considered an indication for prophylactic ventricular pacemaker implantation.

Vasovagal syndrome

A complex inter-relationship between cardiac rate and vasomotor tone normally exists to maintain systemic arterial pressure. When there is an imbalance in either or both of these, patients may experience syncope or presyncope. A sudden increase in vagal tone can cause a precipitous fall in arterial pressure whether as a result of bradycardia (due to cardioinhibition) or of vasodilation (due to depression of vasomotor tone) or a combination of both. In susceptible individuals, increased vagal tone may follow external stimuli such as exposure to needles or the sight of blood, or it can occur spontaneously, when it is termed vasovagal syndrome. **Carotid sinus syndrome** is a similar entity. Sensitivity of the carotid sinus to mechanical pressure causes a surge in vagal tone, in turn causing cardioinhibition and vasodepression, and profound systemic arterial hypotension.

Investigations for bradycardia

Ambulatory (Holter) monitoring or patient-activated recorders (See page 186)

Holter monitors provide limited information in individuals who have symptoms infrequently. In these situations, a patient-activated recorder allows the symptoms to be recorded when they occur. Typically a patient may keep one of these with them for 2–4 weeks at a time.

Implantable recorder (See page 186)

Activation of the device using a hand-held, patient-activated control unit allows the storage of the ECG data related to the patient-identified episodes, up to a total of 42 min recording.

Electrophysiology study

Invasive electrophysiology study can assess the performance of the SN, AVN and conduction systems. It is unusual to need to do this solely for bradycardias as most relevant information can be obtained through ambulatory monitoring.

Treatment

Drug therapy

Treatment with anticholinergics (atropine) or sympathomimetics (isoprenaline) is often useful acutely in the management of a bradycardia but is inappropriate for longer-term treatment of symptomatic SN or conduction disease because of a combination of side-effects (anticholinergic — dry eyes, mouth, urinary retention, constipation), impracticability (isoprenaline is given intravenously) and limited efficacy. Pacemaker implantation is usually the treatment of choice. Although somewhat counterintuitive because of their rate-slowing effect (negative chronotropism), β-blockers may nevertheless help partially alleviate vasovagal syndrome.

Cardiac pacemakers (Fig. 13.2)

Permanent pacemaker implantation was first performed in a human in 1958. Since then it has become the principal treatment for bradycardia, with >25 000 devices implanted annually in the UK. Pacemakers may be implanted to correct symptomatic bradycardia or to act as prophylaxis against asystolic sudden death (AV block without a ventricular escape rhythm). Pacemakers are classified according to their mode of operation (see Table 13.1), with four letters relating to options in each of the four columns.

Depolarization of ventricular myocardium is achieved by delivery of electrical charge via unipo-

lar or bipolar pacing electrodes. A potential difference as small as 0.1 mV is often sufficient to achieve a propagating activation wavefront.

Single chamber pacemakers

These sense and pace a single cardiac chamber (either RA or RV). It is unusual to pace just the atrium unless the only condition the patient has is related to the SN, and AVN/His bundle conduction can be shown to be normal.

Dual chamber pacemakers

These pacemakers maintain AV synchrony. Thus, both atrium and ventricle can be either sensed, paced, or both, depending on pacemaker programming and spontaneous cardiac activity. The interval between atrial and ventricular pacing (AV delay) can be set to optimize cardiac function as there is evidence that the duration of the AV delay can influence the dynamics of ventricular filling and may favourably affect ventricular function.

Additional features

The choice of pacemaker is tailored to the individual patient according to the particular features offered by the specific pacemaker:
• Rate responsive — these increase their pacing rate in response to physical activity. This is achieved either by use of a device that generates current in response to vibration (e.g. piezoelectric crystal) or by the action of an accelerometer which increases pacing rate in response to a sensed

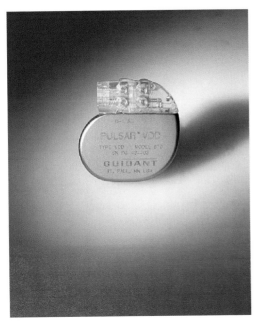

Fig. 13.2 Cardiac implantable pacemaker.

Table 13.1 Classification of pacemakers.*

Paced chamber	Sensed chamber	Effect of sensing	Programming/rate responsiveness
0 = none	0 = none	0 = none	0 = none
A = atrium	A = atrium	T = triggered	P = simple
V = ventricle	V = ventricle	I = inhibited	M = multiprogrammable
D = dual (A+V)	D = dual (A+V)	D = dual (T+I)	C = communicating
			R = rate responsive

* For example a DDDR device will both pace and sense electrical activity in both chambers, with the response being to trigger or inhibit depending on what is sensed. It also has the ability to increase the heart rate depending on the patient's activity level ('rate responsive').

physiological event, such as a shortening of the QT interval which occurs with increased sympathetic tone or changes in respiratory rate. Programmability of the relationship between an increase in heart rate and the 'sensed' physiological parameter activity allows the pacing rate to be adjusted to suit the physiological demands of the individual.

• Mode-switching—if an atrial arrhythmia is detected, such as atrial fibrillation, the pacemaker will switch from a dual to a single chamber (ventricle) mode.

• Atrial arrhythmia prevention—various algorithms exist to prevent episodes of AF. Some of these attempt to reduce pauses that may be the precursor for AF.

Temporary pacemakers

Complete heart block (CHB) complicating myocardial infarction may be temporary, with return of AV conduction up to 1 week later. If a patient is in heart block and haemodynamically compromised, temporary cardiac pacing of the RV (and RA) can be performed via temporary pacing lead(s) to the right heart, connected to an external pacing generator which the patient carries until permanent pacemaker implantation or AV conduction recovery. Surgeons will often leave pacing wires attached to the epicardium at the end of cardiac operations if heart block is anticipated, allowing temporary pacing by external, rather than endocardial, stimulation. CHB is more common following an inferior myocardial infarction as the right coronary artery usually supplies the AV node. It is usually transient and often there is no need for a temporary pacemaker. CHB following an anterior myocardial infarction implies a large myocardial infarction and usually requires temporary pacing.

Pacing for vasovagal syndrome

When bradycardia is a major component of vasovagal syndrome, implantation of a pacemaker may cure or ameliorate symptoms. Similarly, increased vagal tone may follow stimulation of a hypersensitive carotid sinus. This phenomenon is common in elderly patients, and carotid sinus massage is an important investigation in elderly syncopal or presyncopal patients or patients with a history of unexplained falls.

Cardiac resynchronization therapy (CRT)

Biventricular cardiac pacing, with appropriate modulation of timing of chamber contraction by pacing settings, can offset some of the adverse haemodynamic consequences of ventricular dysfunction. Left ventricular pacing is achieved by access of the coronary venous system via the coronary sinus. Transvenous epicardial pacing is then used to stimulate the LV. CRT is appropriate for some patients with heart failure who have:

• severely impaired LV function (EF <35%);
• NYHA II–IV;
• LBBB.

In patients who have an indication for CRT, many will also benefit from implantable cardiac defibrillator therapy (ICD) to reduce the risk of sudden cardiac death. Hence ICD function is frequently incorporated into biventricular (resynchronization) pacing devices (CRT-D).

Choice of pacing electrode

Pacemaker leads and pacemaker programming output may be either bipolar or unipolar.

Unipolar leads have a terminal electrode and use the pacemaker generator box as the other pole of the circuit. Bipolar leads have two electrodes close to their tip, which helps to minimize the inappropriate detection of far-field signals.

Pacemaker implantation

Under local anaesthetic, and fluoroscopic X-ray control, electrodes are inserted transvenously (usually via cephalic or subclavian vein) into the right ventricle and/or right atrium. Single chamber pacemakers require only a single pacing wire; most dual chamber pacemakers require two. The leads are attached proximally to a pacemaker generator box, weighing about 20 g, which itself is implanted subcutaneously below either the left or right clavicle

Box 13.2 Parameters tested at pacemaker implantation

- Sensed R or P wave amplitude
- Pacing threshold (in mV or mA at 0.05 ms pulse width)
- Pacing lead impedance
- Pacing lead stability on deep inspiration/ coughing
- Muscle stimulation/diaphragm stimulation at maximum device output

on the anterior chest wall. Testing of pacemaker electrodes is performed at the time of implantation (Box 13.2).

Pacing wire and electrode construction

Wires are fixed into the RV trabeculations or RA appendage, either by the 'passive' anchoring action of tines (terminal plastic flanges) or by extendable 'active fixation' screw mechanisms at the tip of the electrode. Most electrodes are constructed of titanium with an outer surface of polyurethane. The tip electrode is metal but may have steroid-eluting tip properties to help reduce the endocardial inflammatory response to wire implantation, which can otherwise interfere with pacing characteristics.

Pacemaker complications

Although uncommon, the following may occur associated with pacemaker implantation:
- Haematoma.
- Pneumothorax.
- Infection.
- Pacemaker lead displacement.
- Subclavian vein thrombosis.
- Pericardial effusion.
- Pacemaker syndrome — symptoms occurring with single chamber pacing when the atria dysnchronously contract against a closed tricuspid valve. This is corrected by upgrading to a dual chamber pacemaker.
- 'Twiddlers' syndrome — patient manipulation, often inadvertent, of the pacemaker generator leading to retraction of the leads out of the heart.

Pacemaker follow-up

Pacemaker longevity varies between types of pacemakers and how much the device is used. Generator battery life may be up to 10 years. After implant, it is customary practice to check pacemaker function at 1 month and thereafter annually. The interval is determined both by the battery capacity and by the electrical properties of the pacemaker. Deterioration may also occur in the pacing leads, due either to a gradual degradation of the lead structure or to alteration of the lead–endocardial interface so that lead electrical properties or pacing thresholds may change and become unacceptable. Infrequently, lead breaks may occur due to fracture of the pacing wire, usually at points of frequent stress such as under the clavicle or across the tricuspid valve.

Driving after pacemaker implantation

The Driver and Vehicle Licensing Agency (DVLA) is responsible for regulation of driving licence holders in the UK. At present, pacemaker patients are not allowed to drive for a period of 1 week from device implant.

Tachycardia

Sinus tachycardia

This may be a physiological response to exercise or stress, but abnormal automaticity, either of the SN or an ectopic focus in either atrium or ventricle, or a re-entry excitation mechanism may cause non-physiological tachycardia.

Automatic tachycardias are due to abnormal pacemaker properties in either diseased specialized pacemaker tissue or ordinary cardiac tissue which develops pacemaker properties as a consequence of disease. Examples are ectopic atrial tachycardias occurring in children with congenital heart disease or VT complicating acute myocardial ischaemia.

A re-entry circuit is illustrated in Fig. 13.3. For re-entry to occur, a circuit must have an anatomical barrier to electrical conduction and a zone of

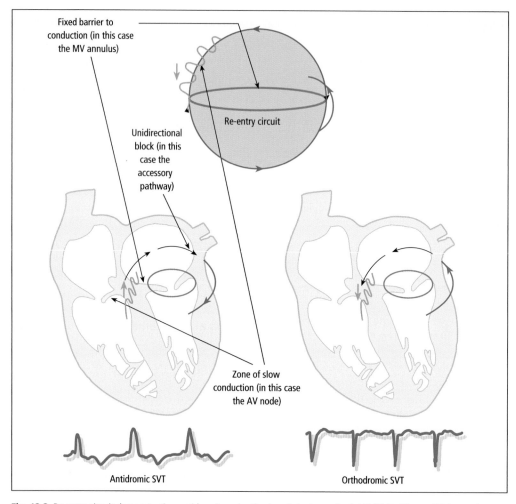

Fixed barrier to conduction (in this case the MV annulus)

Re-entry circuit

Unidirectional block (in this case the accessory pathway)

Zone of slow conduction (in this case the AV node)

Antidromic SVT

Orthodromic SVT

Fig. 13.3 Re-entry circuit demonstrating antidromic and orthodromic tachycardias in Wolff–Parkinson–White syndrome.

slowed conduction, so that the refractory period (time to recovery of excitability after depolarization) is shorter than the total conduction time around the re-entry circuit. In this way, myocardium is again available for depolarization by the time the circular excitation wave front completes the circuit. Re-entry circuits may be the tachycardia mechanism for either supraventricular (SVT) or ventricular tachycardias (VT).

Tachycardias may be classified as SVT or VT (Box 13.3).

- SVT either originate or require participation in the re-entry circuit of cardiac tissue above the AV rings.

Box 13.3 Classification of tachycardias

Supraventricular
- Triggered: ectopic atrial tachycardia/focal AF
- Re-entry: AF/macro re-entrant atrial tachycardia
- A-V re-entrant tachycardia
- A-V nodal re-entrant tachycardia

Ventricular
- Triggered: idiopathic left VT/right ventricular outflow tachycardia/ventricular ectopic activity/torsades de pointes
- Micro re-entrant: fascicular tachycardia
- Macro re-entrant: VT (monomorphic or polymorphic)/ventricular fibrillation

• Ventricular arrhythmias originate in ventricular myocardium, and maintenance of the tachycardia does not require the involvement of conducting tissue in the AV rings.

Treatments for tachycardia

Treatments include anti-arrhythmic drug therapy, device therapy (antitachycardia pacemaker, implantable defibrillator) and curative ablative therapy (either surgical or using catheter ablation techniques).

Anti-arrhythmic drug therapy

The use of anti-arrhythmic drugs is discussed in relation to each type of tachycardia in subsequent sections. A classification of anti-arrhythmic drugs by Vaughan-Williams (Table 13.2) has been the cornerstone of the clinical approach to anti-arrhythmic drug choice. In many conditions, anti-arrhythmic drug therapy is secondary or adjunctive to ablative or device therapy.

Catheter ablation techniques

Following accidental induction of complete heart block during a cardiac catheterization procedure, the therapeutic possibilities of minimally destructive ablative procedures were appreciated. **Ablation** procedures damage a small area of myocardium, critical to an arrhythmia mechanism using an endocardial percutaneous catheter approach and radiofrequency energy. Radiofrequency energy requires low-voltage, high-frequency current to ablate myocardium via a steerable catheter with a tip-mounted electrode. The target tissue

Table 13.2 The Vaughan-Williams anti-arrhythmic drug classification.

Class	Action	Prototype agent
I	Local anaesthetic action reducing Na current	Quinidine
II	β-blockade	Propanolol
III	Action potential prolongation	Amiodarone
IV	Calcium channel blockade	Verapamil

is either critical to an arrhythmia substrate or part of the conduction system.

Damage to AV node and specialized conduction system tissue reduces the ventricular response rate to atrial activity or, in the case of AVN ablation, creates iatrogenic complete heart block. An implanted pacemaker is required to maintain an adequate ventricular rate, because an escape ventricular rhythm is usually slow or may be absent.

Device implantation for tachycardia

Anti-tachycardia pacemakers are able to pace-terminate certain types of SVT and VT. Ablation procedures have superseded the use of anti-tachycardia pacemakers in the treatment of SVT and anti-tachycardia pacing, of VT carries the risk of tachycardia acceleration, or even the induction of ventricular fibrillation. Thus, anti-tachycardia pacing devices for pace-termination of VT are usually combined with the ability to deliver defibrillation shocks — the automatic implantable cardiac defibrillator (ICD) (see page 202).

Supraventricular tachycardias

Sinus node re-entry, intra-atrial re-entry and ectopic atrial tachycardias

With the exception of 'common' atrial flutter, these are all rare tachycardias. Intra-atrial re-entrant circuits can be located anywhere in the atrium. Generally circuits can be divided into those which generate an atrial depolarization pattern which is very close, and sometimes identical, to that generated by the SN (SN re-entry) and those which do not (intra-atrial re-entry).

SN re-entry usually generates a tachycardia of around 130 bpm and has the following diagnostic features:
• initiated by atrial or ventricular pacing, and by atrial or ventricular premature extrastimuli; or electrophysiology study
• the same atrial activation pattern as sinus rhythm;
• unaffected by AV nodal blocking manoeuvres but slows in response to vagal tone.

Intra-atrial re-entry tachycardia involves atrial myocardium distant from the SN. It is:
- rarely induced by ventricular extrastimulation;
- associated with intra-atrial conduction delay (unlike SN re-entry), necessary for the induction of intra-atrial re-entry;
- different in atrial activation pattern from that in sinus rhythm;
- usually faster than SN re-entry (around 140–240 bpm);
- less responsive to vagal manoeuvres than SN re-entry.

Ectopic atrial tachycardia is:
- usually associated with organic heart disease or metabolic derangement;
- more common in children;
- not reliably initiated by pacing techniques;
- different in atrial activation patterns from sinus rhythm;
- not responsive to vagal manoeuvres;
- sometimes suppressed by overdrive pacing.

All of the above rarely respond to antiarrhythmic medication. Catheter ablation can successfully treat these arrhythmias.

Atrial fibrillation

AF may be the consequence of primary electrical disease of the atrium (in particular, 'focal' AF is thought to be the consequence of abnormal 'triggering' ectopic foci), secondary to structural heart disease causing atriopathy, or complicating systemic conditions such as hyperthyroidism.

AF is classified as:
- paroxysmal (spontaneous return to sinus rhythm);
- persistent (sinus rhythm achievable with intervention);
- permanent (sinus rhythm not achieveable even with intervention).

In general, paroxysms of AF become more frequent, and ultimately established, as atrial disease progresses. Atrial hypertrophy and dilatation secondary to structural heart disease is often the substrate for AF, but it may occur in structurally normal hearts. Micro re-entry circuits or focal triggering sites in the atria cause repetitive excitation of atrial myocardium. The atria cease to contract in a co-ordinated fashion. Frequent and irregular atrial activation result in bombardment of the AVN by depolarization wavelets. Due to its specialized conduction, the AVN cannot depolarize in response to each wave of excitation, and so the ventricular response rate to AF is determined by its conduction properties.

The causes of AF include:
- triggering foci (idiopathic);
- atrial myopathy;
- atrial pressure or volume overload due to structural heart disease.

Anti-arrhythmic drug therapy may be directed to control of the ventricular response rate to AF by impairing the conduction properties of the AVN (digoxin, verapamil, β-blockers), or to stabilization of the atrium to prevent AF occurring — amongst other properties, sotalol and amiodarone all prolong the action potential and thus increase refractoriness in the atrial myocardium, making atrial re-entry circuits less sustainable. Class 1 drugs slow intra-atrial conduction and by this mechanism may also help maintain sinus rhythm. If the ventricular response rate to AF cannot be controlled by AVN-blocking agents, drug side-effects are unacceptable or the subjective sensation of AF is unacceptable to the patient, then AVN conduction can be permanently interrupted by ablation. Permanent pacing is then required to maintain an adequate ventricular rate, and there is a long-term risk of morbidity or death associated with the procedure. AVN 'modification' may reduce ventricular response rate to AF without complete interruption of AV conduction, and so avoid the need for permanent pacing, but may still leave the patient with the sensation of palpitation due to the persistence of an irregular ventricular beat.

Anticoagulation and antiplatelet drugs

AF renders the atria and particularly the left atrial appendage susceptible to intra-atrial thrombus formation. This can give rise to embolism, the most dangerous consequence of which is a cerebrovascular accident (stroke). The risk is greatest in patients with:

- accompanying mitral valve disease;
- enlargement of the LA or other structural heart disease;
- a history of previous systemic embolism, diabetes mellitus or hypertension, and in those over 65 years old.

In these high-risk groups, anticoagulation with warfarin (INR 2–3) reduces stroke risk 5-fold. In other low-risk patient groups (paroxysmal AF in the structurally normal heart), treatment with aspirin alone may be sufficient. Transoesophageal echocardiography may have a role in identifying patients with intra-atrial thrombus, although its value in guiding management of patients in whom atrial thrombus is not seen, is undecided.

There are alternative anticoagulants to warfarin under development. However, unexpected and unacceptable side-effects have been seen, and for the moment there is no suitable alternative to warfarin.

Cardioversion

External DC countershock is used to convert persistent AF to sinus rhythm when it is felt likely that the patient will remain in sinus rhythm for the long term, with or without additional drugs to stabilize the atrium and reduce the likelihood of reversion to AF. This is performed under general anaesthesia and shocks of between 50 and 360 J are delivered. High energy levels (>300 J) are often required to terminate AF. Biphasic shocks have been shown to have increased defibrillation efficacy at lower energy levels, and most commercially available external defibrillators deliver this type of waveform.

The use of digoxin is not a contraindication to cardioversion, although in the presence of digoxin toxicity, DC shock is said to increase the risk of VF. Because of the risk of embolization, patients are anticoagulated for 6 weeks prior to attempted cardioversion. Even if cardioversion successfully restores sinus rhythm, anticoagulation should be continued for a further 2 weeks as atrial 'stunning' leaves even patients in sinus rhythm susceptible to further intra-atrial thrombus formation during this time.

Atrial fibrillation ablation

Uptake of AF ablation by percutaneous ablation techniques is rapidly increasing. Surgical creation of linear scars within the atrial myocardium to prevent sustenance of re-entry circuits by atrial compartmentalization can abolish AF, and it is a well established but little used therapy because of concomitant patient morbidity. There has been interest in minimally invasive surgical approaches. However, the procedures for catheter ablation of triggering foci for AF or to create long linear lesions to emulate surgical compartmentalization are now widely used. It has become clear that many patients with AF in the context of structurally normal hearts develop the arrhythmia because of triggered (ectopic) activity emanating from the pulmonary veins. Myocardial sheaths invaginating the pulmonary veins are the source of this activity. A range of technologies and techniques have been developed to abolish this activity, which results in cure of AF in the majority of patients who present with 'lone' AF; however, up to 30–40% may require multiple procedures to achieve 'pulmonary vein isolation'. Extension of the approach with creation of extensive endocardial 'linear lesions' may abolish AF even in the presence of structural heart disease, but the evidence base for long-term success is less compelling. Novel catheter guidance systems are in development to better facilitate endocardial lesion creation for the purpose of AF ablation in the broad population of atrial fibrillation sufferers.

Atrial flutter

Atrial flutter needs classification as there is a series of macro re-entrant circuits that can give rise to this arrhythmia (Box 13.4). Typically the atrial flutter rate is 300 bpm; 2:1 conduction through the AVN will give a ventricular response rate of 150 bpm. Anti-arrhythmic drug therapy may modify either the ventricular response or the atrial flutter rate. Counterclockwise macro re-entrant atrial tachycardia (CCMAT) or **'common flutter'** constitutes about 90% of atrial flutter cases, the typical 'saw-tooth' atrial flutter pattern being apparent in the inferiorly oriented standard and augmented leads (II, III and AVF) on the ECG (Fig. 13.4a). The re-entry circuit involves an isthmus of tissue in low-RA between the ostium of the coronary sinus and septal leaflet of the tricuspid valve. Otherwise atrial flutter (10% cases) is termed 'uncommon', and differently oriented circuits are used which do not give the typical saw-tooth ECG appearance.

'Incisional tachycardia' is a macro re-entry atrial circuit that revolves around scar tissue created by surgical entry to the atrium, and may be amenable to ablation treatment. It most commonly manifests as a type of atrial flutter in patients with congenital heart disease after palliative surgery.

Atrial flutter is usually paroxysmal but may become 'incessant'. When this occurs, reduction of the ventricular response rate by AVN-blocking drugs is often ineffective because even reduction to 3:1 block may give a tachycardia of 100 bpm. Patients usually undergo DC cardioversion, and atrial stabilizing drugs (sotalol and amiodarone) may prevent or reduce the frequency of recurrence. For incessant or frequent paroxysmal CCMAT, when drug therapy is unsatisfactory, ablation of the re-entry circuit is the treatment of choice by creation of a linear lesion at a critical location in the atrial flutter circuit, usually at the tricuspid valve–inferior vena cava isthmus.

Atrioventricular re-entry tachycardia

Accessory AV connections are muscle bundles connecting atrial and ventricular myocardium across the AV ring. Though they develop during embryogenesis and are present from birth, paroxysms of tachycardia may not occur until late childhood, teenage years or even adulthood. Although present in as many as 1 in 3000 individuals,

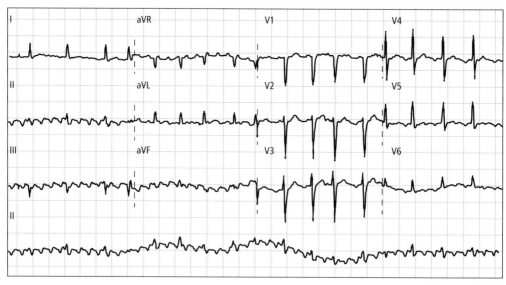

Speed: 25mm/sec Limb:10mm/mV Chest:10 mm/mV

Fig. 13.4 (a) Atrial flutter ECG. Note the characteristic 'saw-tooth' pattern in inferior leads.

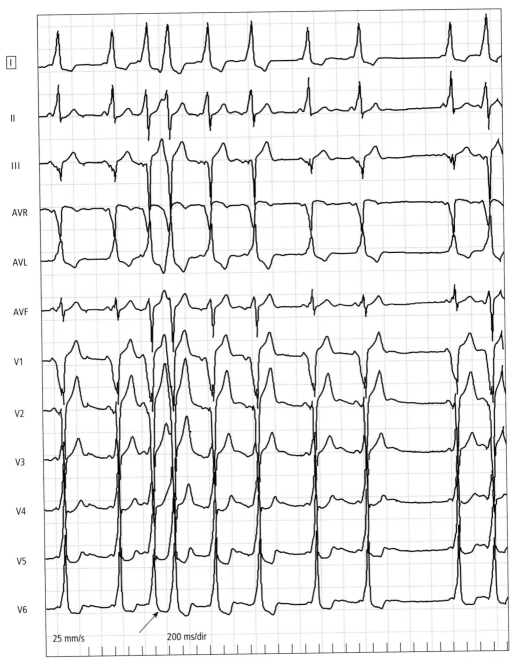

Fig. 13.4 (b) Pre-excitation on surface ECG of patient with Wolff–Parkinson–White syndrome. The pathway is located on the right free wall. Note the slurred upstroke of the QRS (so-called delta wave of pre-excitation) which is exaggerated after the atrial premature beat indicated by the arrow due to the greater proportion of the ventricular mass activated via the connection (slowed AV node/His–Purkinje conduction after premature extrastimulation).

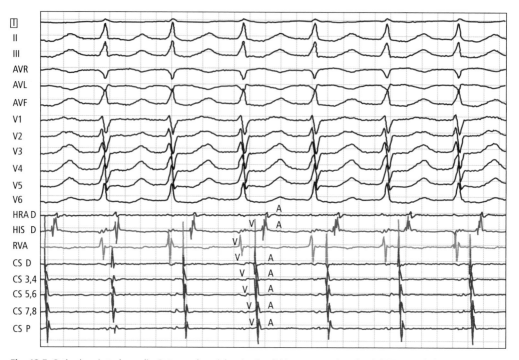

Fig. 13.5 Orthodromic tachycardia. Retrograde atrial activation (A) in coronary sinus leads (ESP→CSD) shows atrial activation occurs earliest in left atrium in SVT (compare to A in high right atrium HRAD) and area of the His bundle (HISD). This confirms a left-sided accessory pathway.

estimates vary widely as to the proportion (10–95%) of such individuals who will experience symptomatic AVRT. Pathways that are able to conduct anterogradely (atrium to ventricle) are usually evident on the resting surface ECG (pre-excitation) (Fig. 13.4b). A portion of the ventricular mass is excited by the excitation front traversing the accessory pathway. This portion of the ventricular mass depolarizes early relative to the remaining ventricular mass, which is depolarized via the normal conduction system, because unlike the AVN there has been no delayed conduction in the accessory pathway. Thus, in sinus rhythm, the PR interval is short. However, this pre-excited portion of the ventricle spreads the excitation wavefront via slowly conducting myocardium, giving rise to a slurred deflection at the beginning of the QRS complex (the delta wave). Pathway conduction during tachycardia may be from atrium to ventricle (antidromic AVRT) with retrograde conduction through the AVN. This is uncommon

and produces a broad complex tachycardia. More usually, conduction is retrograde in the accessory pathway and anterograde through the AVN, resulting in a narrow complex tachycardia (Fig. 13.5).

Some patients can display both types of AVRT, and approximately 10% of patients with AVRT have multiple pathways with complex mechanisms of tachycardia. In addition to re-entry tachycardia, the presence of an accessory pathway predisposes to AF. AF can be life-threatening in some patients with pre-excitation if the accessory pathway has rapid anterograde conduction characteristics which allow very rapid ventricular response rates to AF (the ventricle losing its usual protection from the slow conduction properties of the AVN) and ventricular fibrillation can ensue. Although uncommon, this is the mechanism where sudden death occurs in patients with accessory pathways. Mahaim pathways are uncommon connections between AV nodal tissue and RV. Tachycardia mechanisms are similar. Accessory pathways are common in Ebstein's anomaly.

Treatment

Anti-arrhythmic drugs can be used to modify the conduction properties of the AVN or accessory pathway so as to render the re-entry circuit unsustainable. Thus, drugs which slow AV nodal or accessory connection conduction (β-blockers, calcium anatagonists, class 1 drugs or amiodarone), may reduce the ventricular rate when paroxysms of tachycardia occur, or the frequency of attacks. Complete freedom from paroxysms of tachycardia is difficult to achieve using drug therapy. Catheter ablation of accessory pathways is now the treatment of choice in symptomatic patients and has a high primary success rate (about 95%) and a low associated morbidity.

Atrioventricular nodal re-entry tachycardia

The substrate for this re-entry tachycardia is again present from birth, but may not cause symptomatic tachycardia until adult life. It is more common in young females and is a more common tachycardia than AVRT. The re-entry circuit exists within, or is intimately related to, the AVN and its associated tissues but is independent of the ventricle. AV conduction during normal rhythm occurs through two 'pathways' which have differing conduction characteristics:

- one pathway has a slow conduction velocity but short refractory period;
- the other pathway has a faster conduction velocity but longer refractory period.

The re-entry circuit uses these fast and slow conduction limbs (Fig. 13.6).

Treatment

Drugs which influence AV nodal conduction may modify the properties of the re-entry circuit (principally calcium antagonists, β-blockers and class 1 drugs), but complete freedom from tachycardia is difficult to achieve. Ablation procedures are now

the treatment of choice. Catheter ablation of either the slow or fast pathway (both termed AV nodal 'modification') can be achieved by selective destruction of a portion of the AVN or tissues adjacent to it. Complete heart block occurs in up to 1% of cases and requires permanent pacing.

Sudden cardiac death

Sudden cardiac death is defined as death from a cardiac cause within 1 h of the onset of symptoms. It is a major cause of mortality in the Western world, being responsible for up 60 000 deaths per annum in the UK. Although a proportion of such deaths follow acute myocardial infarction, some deaths are due to a primary arrhythmia unrelated to infarction. As many as two-thirds of sudden cardiac deaths may be due to ventricular arrhythmia, the substrate being a scarred myocardium which generates VT, which may then degenerate to ventricular fibrillation. Risk stratification for those considered susceptible to ventricular arrhythmias involves Holter monitoring, a signal-averaged ECG, electrophysiological study and assessments of ventricular function. The signal-averaged ECG is a technique involving computer analysis of surface ECG lead recordings to identify depolarization in the later portion of the QRS (late potentials), thought to be indicative of slowed myocardial conduction and the presence of an arrhythmia substrate. All the above investigations have relatively low sensitivity and specificity. Patients rescued from sudden cardiac death have a poor prognosis, with a 30% 2-year mortality. They should be investigated for possible underlying coronary artery disease and considered for treatment with an ICD.

Ventricular ectopics

Although a common and largely benign phenomenon, frequent ventricular ectopic activity may indicate underlying structural heart disease. There is no evidence that suppression of ventricular ectopic activity by anti-arrhythmic drug treatment improves the prognosis of the underlying disease or reduces the risk of sudden death. Indeed, drug

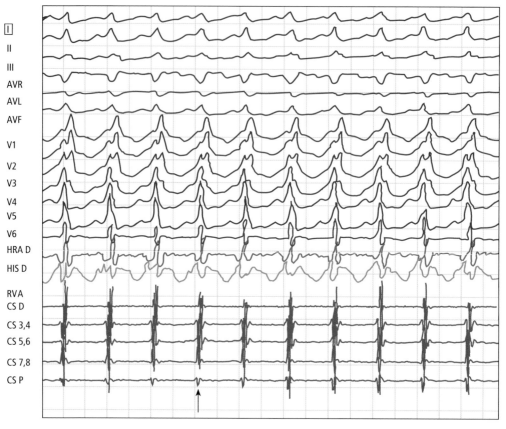

Fig. 13.6 Re-entry circuit in AV nodal re-entry tachycardia. Arrow indicates simultaneous nature of atrial activation (from atrial electrogram pattern) in both right and left atria due to spread of activation from the AVRNT re-entry circuit in the AV node/triangle of Koch. Note also rate related right bundle branch aberrancy in the surface ECG in this patient.

trials to assess the impact of ectopic activity suppression by Class Ic drugs after myocardial infarction have shown an increased sudden death rate in 'successfully' treated groups. This may reflect the pro-arrhythmic potential of some anti-arrhythmic drugs.

Ventricular tachycardia

Monomorphic VT has a constant QRS morphology (Fig. 13.7) but polymorphic VT has continuous variation in the QRS morphology. Sustained tachycardia continues for a minimum of 30 s, and non-sustained tachycardia self-terminates within 30 s. ECG differentiation from other broad complex tachycardias is illustrated in Fig. 13.8.

Mechanisms

Re-entry (see Fig. 13.3) in and around scarred myocardium is the most common mechanism of recurrent monomorphic sustained VT. However, acute severe metabolic changes in myocardium, including those caused by acute ischaemia, can cause spontaneous cell membrane depolarization. Thus, 'early after-depolarizations' are caused by abnormality of ionic flux during the repolarization phase which may then generate polymorphic VT.

Electrophysiology study of VT

Standard electrophysiological 'induction protocols' have been shown reliably to initiate VT in patients

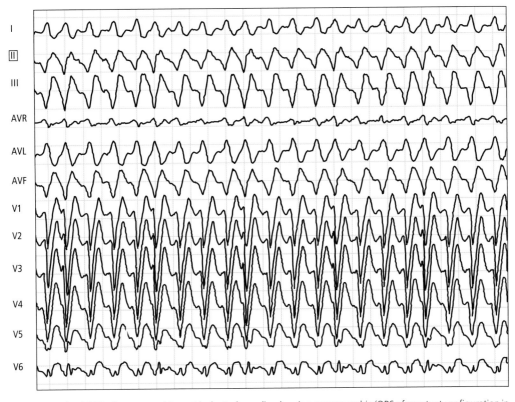

Fig. 13.7 12 lead ECG of monomorphic ventricular tachycardia, showing monomorphic (QRS of constant configuration in a given ECG lead other than for occasional complexes when there is fusion with activation via the His Purkinje system) sustained (lasting longer than 30 s) VT at 25 mm/s paper speed. Tachycardia rate is 190 bpm.

who have the necessary arrhythmia substrate. However, the reproducibility, sensitivity and specificity of ventricular extrastimulation studies have been best characterized in patients with ventricular arrhythmias complicating healed myocardial infarction. Their value in assessing prognosis or symptomatic efficacy of drug or other therapies in dilated, arrhythmogenic or hypertrophic cardiomyopathies is uncertain. A typical induction protocol uses constant ventricular pacing at the right ventricular apex at a drive rate of 100 bpm for seven beats (drive train), with delivery of a single premature extrastimulus following each drive train. The intervals between the last beat of the drive train and the premature extrastimulus is decrementally decreased in small steps (usually 10 ms) until the extrastimulus fails to generate a QRS complex, indicating failure to capture local ventricular myocardium. A

second, and subsequently a third, extrastimulus is introduced and then the process is repeated at a faster drive rate (usually 150 bpm). This scheme is used at both right ventricular apical and right outflow tract pacing sites. Some protocols also involve the use of isoprenaline or other pro-arrhythmic drugs. Study end-points are the induction of ventricular arrhythmia or completion of the study protocol without arrhythmia induction.

However, induction of polymorphic VT or ventricular fibrillation may be non-specific and not reproducible. Thus the relevance of these types of arrhythmia to a given clinical scenario is difficult to determine. Induction of monomorphic VT confirms the presence of a substrate for VT, whether or not the induced VT has the same QRS morphology as the clinically documented tachycardia. Inducibility can then be used as a guide to arrhythmia

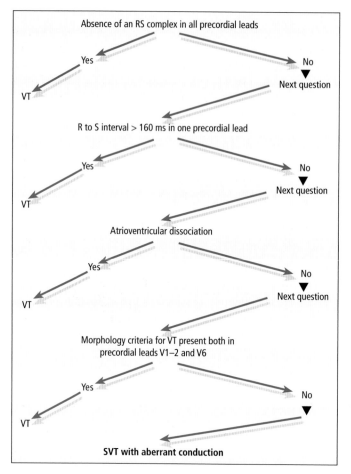

Absence of an RS complex in all precordial leads

Yes → No → Next question

VT

R to S interval > 160 ms in one precordial lead

Yes → No → Next question

VT

Atrioventricular dissociation

Yes → No → Next question

VT

Morphology criteria for VT present both in precordial leads V1–2 and V6

Yes → No

VT

SVT with aberrant conduction

Fig. 13.8 ECG diagnosis of VT.

suppression by the drug(s), or the induced tachycardia can be 'mapped' to identify the re-entry circuit location with a view to either catheter ablation or surgical resection. The choice of therapy will in part be determined by the underlying disease. Most ventricular arrhythmias are the consequence of myocardial scarring complicating coronary artery disease and myocardial infarction. Anti-arrhythmic drugs and device therapy may be used whatever the aetiology of the arrhythmia substrate, while surgical and ablation treatments are limited in their application.

Drug treatment

With current ICD indications, there is no role for serial electrophysiological studies to assess antiar-rhythmic drug efficacy, as such an approach has been shown not to enhance patient survival. Holter monitoring in highly selected patients may be as accurate as electrophysiology study in predicting anti-arrhythmic drug efficacy. Amiodarone may improve prognosis in some particular patient groups (e.g. hypertrophic cardiomyopathy) but, for most patients with ventricular arrhythmias, it confers no prognostic benefit although it is commonly prescribed empirically in UK practice. The data with respect to prognostic benefit conferred by amiodarone therapy for all disease substrates giving rise to ventricular arrhythmia are complex and unclear. However, drug manufacturers of anti-arrhythmic drugs in general and amiodarone in particular are unable to claim prognostic benefit as a drug therapy indication. Class I, II and III drugs (see Table 13.2) may all be used to reduce frequency of symptomatic palpitation.

The failure of drug therapy to improve prognosis in carefully designed drug trials has stimulated the search for other treatments. These now include catheter ablation techniques, surgical resection of the arrhythmia substrate and ICD implantation. Anti-arrhythmic drug therapy still has an important role as an adjunct to these interventional therapies.

ICD treatment

The ICD was conceived by Dr M. Mirowski in the USA, with the first implant performed in a human in 1982. These are sophisticated devices which are able to sense and terminate VT or fibrillation. The devices are able to pace-terminate VT (Fig. 13.9), cardiovert VT or defibrillate from ventricular fibrillation. They offer tiered therapy and programmable, sophisticated arrhythmia sensing.

First-generation devices required the placement of epicardial defibrillation patch electrodes at formal thoracotomy, but recent innovations now allow endocardial placement of shock electrodes in a manner analogous to the implantation of a pacemaker device. Also, the devices were originally implanted in abdominal pouches with electrodes tunnelled subcutaneously from the portal of venous entry (usually subclavian), whereas devices are now sufficiently small to allow routine prepectoral subcutaneous implantation. Innovations include the combination of a full range of pacemaker functions for bradycardia within AICD units and increased capability for telemetry.

Indications for ICD implantation have greatly increased in recent years and are summarized in Table 13.3. In particular there is increased use of ICDs for 'primary prophylaxis' of sudden cardiac death in patients considered to be at high risk based on risk stratification assessments, including a left ventricular ejection fraction <30%.

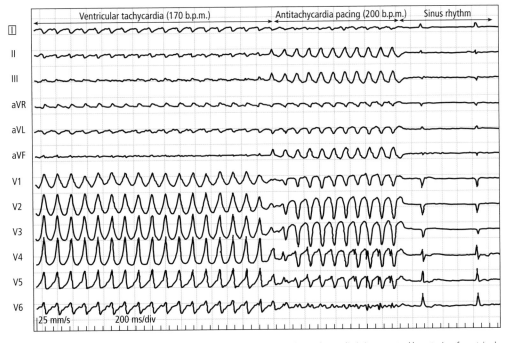

Fig. 13.9 Termination of ventricular tachycardia by overdrive pacing. The tachycardia is interrupted by a train of ventricular pacing at a rate faster than the spontaneous ventricular tachycardia. Note the pacing spikes and changed QRS morphology during ventricular pacing.

Table 13.3 Summary of currently agreed indications for ICD implantation in patients with either coronary artery disease or idiopathic dilated cardiomyopathy

Survivor of SCD	Presentation with haemodynamically unstable VT	Prior MI	Revascularization indicated	LVEF	Underlying disease	VT induced at EPS	NYHA class
√		√	No	√	CAD		
	√	√	No		CAD		
√	√			√	IDC		
√	√			≤40%	Heart failure		
		>40 days	No	≤30–40%	CAD		II or III
				≤30–35%	IDC		II or III
	√	> 3 months		<35%	CAD	√	

Most patients requiring ICDs do so on the background of these conditions, but there are other indications (see hypertophic cardiomyopathy and 'channelopathies').

CAD, coronary artery disease; EPS, electrophysiology study; IDC, idiopathic dilated cardiomyopathy; LVEF, left ventricular ejection fraction; MI, myocardial infarction; SCD, sudden cardiac death; VT, ventricular tachycardia

Arrhythmia surgery

Surgical removal of scar tissue together with deeper endomyocardial incisions or application of cryoprobes to interrupt re-entry circuits can result in cure of VT complicating healed myocardial infarction. This approach requires open heart surgery and is associated with significant morbidity and mortality, and risks causing further impairment of ventricular function. Thus, to be a candidate for this therapy, patients must have well-preserved ventricular function and the VT must be amenable to mapping techniques to allow the electrophysiologist to guide the surgical approach. Patients with multiple VT circuits, which are poorly tolerated haemodynamically, and with severe impairment of ventricular function will not be suitable for surgical therapy. Only a minority of patients with VT will be suitable for surgical intervention, and most will have coronary artery disease.

Catheter ablation of VT

Current technology offers only limited curative success for ablation of the arrhythmia substrate of ventricular arrhythmias in the context of coronary artery disease. Although ablation techniques are increasingly employed with success rates enhanced by technological advancement in mapping and lesion creation techniques, evolution of the arrhythmia substrate leaves individuals at ongoing risk of sudden cardiac death. Therefore, ablation is most often performed as an adjunct to ICD therapy to reduce the burden of ICD therapy experienced by a patient. Specific ventricular tachycardias may be amenable to curative ablation (see below).

Other ventricular arrhythmias

Ventricular fibrillation

VF commonly complicates acute myocardial ischaemia or infarction (reflecting electrical instability caused by biochemical derangement in the myocardium). Monomorphic and polymorphic VT can degenerate into VF, leading to death. However, outside the context of acute myocardial ischaemia, VF is less common than VT as a primary event. VF is likely to be the underlying arrhythmia in the majority of patients with sudden cardiac death.

Right ventricular outflow tract tachycardia

The arrhythmia substrate is located in the right ventricular outflow tract and probably is a localized re-entry circuit. There is usually no obvious

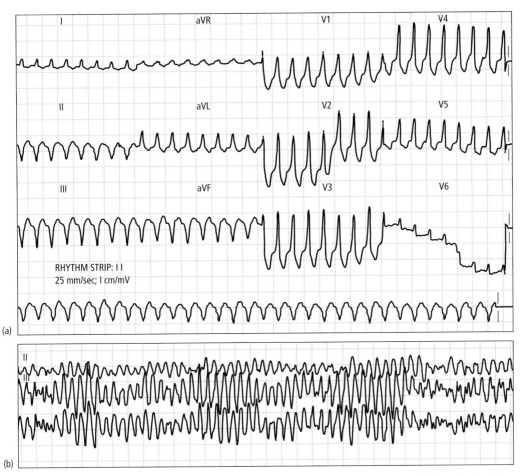

(a)

(b)

Fig.13.10 (a) Fascicular tachycardia. Note left axis deviation and right bundle branch block pattern. (b) Torsades de pointes tachycardia. Note characteristic 'complementary' and continuing axis change.

underlying structural heart disease on investigation. It is a benign arrhythmia and amenable to catheter ablation.

Fascicular tachycardia

This condition complicates some types of congenital heart disease and coronary artery disease. It is a relatively benign type of VT and is amenable to catheter ablation. The substrate is probably a micro re-entry circuit involving the left posterior hemifascicle, producing a characteristic surface ECG configuration during the tachycardia of right bundle branch morphology and superior axis (Fig. 13.10a).

Bundle branch re-entry tachycardia

This tachycardia is caused by a re-entry circuit involving conduction bundle tissue as part of the re-entry circuit. Catheter ablation of the bundle branch limb of the circuit can abolish the arrhythmia.

'Channelopathies' and idiopathic polymorphic ventricular tachycardia

Long QT syndrome

Sympathetic drive and variation in cardiac rhythm are known precipitants of torsades de pointes tachycardia in patients with the cell membrane ionic transport abnormalities that are thought to underlie long QT syndrome. The characteristic ECG features of this type of polymorphic VT (Fig. 13.11b) are associated with prolongation of the QT interval in sinus rhythm and are linked to abnormal repolarization mechanisms. It can be a component of a hereditary syndrome associated with deafness (Romano–Ward) but can complicate the use of anti-arrhythmic drugs which prolong myocardial repolarization (class III action). A genetically determined abnormality of sodium and postassium cell membrane ion pump chanels ('channelopathy') creates an electrophysiological milieu that facilitates ventricular arrhythmogenesis.

Brugada syndrome

This is another similar 'channelopathy' specifically linked to the SC5NA gene which codes for features of sodium ion pumps in cardiac cell membranes. It commonly results in a characteristic right bundle branch pattern with coved ST segment elevation in the anterior chest leads of the resting surface ECG, despite structural normality of the heart. Individuals may be at high risk of polymorphic ventricular tachycardia and sudden death.

Further reading

Benditt DG, Benson DW, eds. *Cardiac Pre-excitation Syndromes: Origins, Evaluation and Treatment*. Dordrecht: Kluwer Academic Publishers, 1986.

Ellenbogen KA, Kay GN, Wilkoff BL, eds. *Clinical Cardiac Pacing and Defibrillation*. London: WB Saunders Co., 2000.

Huang S, Wood MA. *Catheter Ablation of Cardiac Arrhythmias*. Philadelphia, PA: Saunders Elsevier, 2006.

Josephson ME. *Clinical Cardiac Electrophysiology: Techniques and Interpretation*, 2nd edn. London: Lea & Febiger, 1993.

Zipes DP, Jalife J, eds. *Cardiac Electrophysiology: From Cell to Bedside*, 3rd edn. London: WB Saunders Co., 2000.

Chapter 14

Cardiopulmonary resuscitation

Introduction

Cardiopulmonary resuscitation (CPR) aims to restore adequate oxygen delivery to vital organs following cessation of spontaneous cardiac output. It describes a continuum of care, beginning with basic life support, progressing to defibrillation and advanced life support, and includes post-resuscitation care.

Cardiac arrest is the only medical condition that affects everyone. Its aetiology changes with age; cardiac arrest in children is usually due to hypoxia, in young adults due to trauma and in older adults due to cardiac ischaemia (Box 14.1). CPR is usually required because of a sudden cessation of adequate blood flow to vital organs. In ischaemic heart disease, this is usually due to acute myocardial ischaemia, as occurs with an acute coronary syndrome. It may also result from major obstruction to blood flow through the central circulation (e.g. acute massive pulmonary embolus) or in the context of more chronic obstruction (e.g. valvular stenosis). Respiratory pathology can also cause cardiac ischaemia, which if severe may progress to cardiac arrest.

Cardiac arrest may occur out of hospital or in hospital. The incidence of out-of-hospital cardiac arrest is approximately 50 per 100 000 population, whereas in hospital it is approximately 2–3 per 1000 admissions (excluding arrest in the Emergency Department and patients where resuscitation is inappropriate). Irrespective of the aetiology or location of the cardiac arrest, the principles and practice of cardiopulmonary resuscitation generally remain the same.

The sequence of actions in cardiopulmonary resuscitation has been described as the Chain of Survival (Fig. 14.1). The four links are early recognition of the emergency and activation of the emergency services, early CPR, early defibrillation and post-resuscitation care. All must be performed promptly and effectively if CPR is to be translated into patient survival.

The outcome from cardiac arrest is generally poor, with survival to discharge from out-of-hospital cardiac arrest averaging no more than 5%. However, most patients who suffer a cardiac arrest undergo a period of deterioration prior to collapse. Out-of-hospital, ambulance paramedic training emphasizes the need to recognize this deterioration, and in hospital, activation of medical emergency teams to critically ill patients reduces the incidence of patients progressing to cardiac arrest.

External chest compression and early defibrillation are the only two interventions that have been proven to improve survival after a cardiac arrest. All other interventions are based on conclusions drawn from basic physiological principles and limited research studies in animals and humans. When a cardiac arrest does occur, survival is associated with the following:

Box 14.1 Review of possible causes

Possible cause of arrest	Action
Acute myocardial infarct	? Thrombolysis
Severe valvular disease	? Urgent surgery
Aortic dissection	? Refer to cardiothoracic unit
Tamponade	Pericardiocentesis
Acute massive pulmonary embolus	? Thrombolysis or embolectomy
Pneumothorax	Chest drain
Airway obstruction	? Bronchodilators/bronchoscopy
Haemorrhage	Blood transfusion, consider source of bleeding
Cerebrovascular event	? Refer to neurosurgical unit
Septic shock	? Vasoconstrictors/antibiotics
Anaphylactic shock	Adrenaline/steroids
Addisonian crisis	Corticosteroids
Drug toxicity (e.g. β-blockers)	? Antidotes/increase excretion (aminophylline or glucagon raise cAMP)
Electrolyte/glucose disorder	Correct as appropriate

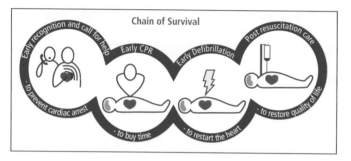

Fig. 14.1 Chain of Survival. Courtesy of the European Resuscitation Council.

- witnessed collapse;
- bystander CPR;
- arrhythmia associated with electrical activity (e.g. ventricular fibrillation as opposed to asystole);
- early defibrillation.

The resuscitation guidelines outlined in this chapter were published in November 2005 following an evidence-based review of all resuscitation science by the International Liaison Committee on Resuscitation, of which the European Resuscitation Council and Resuscitation Council (UK) are represented. They supersede the 2000 guidelines and are scheduled for a further revision in 2010.

Basic life support

Basic life support (BLS) refers to the maintenance of an airway, and support of breathing and circula-tion without equipment (other than a simple airway or protective airway barrier device). The BLS algorithm is shown in Fig. 14.2. Although the actions follow the well-known ABC sequence, it is important to note that for adult cardiac arrest, chest compressions are now recommended before any rescue breaths.

Airway

- Open the airway by tilting the head backwards and lifting the chin.
- **Look** for chest movement, **listen**, and **feel** for exhaled air with your cheek.

Breathing

- Observe for no more than 10s before deciding breathing is absent.

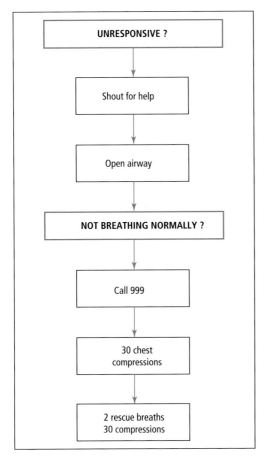

UNRESPONSIVE ?

↓

Shout for help

↓

Open airway

↓

NOT BREATHING NORMALLY ?

↓

Call 999

↓

30 chest
compressions

↓

2 rescue breaths
30 compressions

Fig. 14.2 Algorithm for basic life support. Courtesy of the Resuscitation Council (UK).

- If present, turn the patient on their side in the recovery position.
- If absent, progress to external chest compression.

Circulation

- If possible, move the patient onto a firm surface.
- Commence external chest compression (cardiac massage) by placing the heel of one hand in the centre of the patient's chest and the other hand on top. Give **30 chest compressions at a rate of 100 per min**, depressing the sternum 4–5 cm, ensuring that it recoils fully between compres-

sions. The compression and relaxation phases should be of equal duration.

- When 30 chest compressions have been completed, give two rescue breaths (mouth-to-mouth): open the airway again as described. Pinch the soft part of the victim's nose and seal your lips around the patient's open mouth. Blow steadily into the patient's mouth and watch for the chest to rise. This usually requires a tidal volume of around 400–600 mL in an adult. Take about 1 s to make the chest rise. Repeat once more.
- Once two rescue breaths have been completed, immediately recommence 30 chest compressions. Continue the 30:2 cycle until the patient starts breathing.

Precordial thump

The electrical threshold for defibrillation rises rapidly during cardiac arrest. However, the mechanical energy of a thump may generate sufficient current to cardiovert ventricular fibrillation (VF)/ventricular tachycardia (VT) to sinus rhythm if performed immediately. It is delivered by giving a sudden firm blow to the front of the victim's chest using a clenched fist. A precordial thump may cause pulsatile VT to convert to pulseless VT or VF, or convert VF to asystole. It is therefore only recommended for a witnessed, monitored arrest.

Physiology of blood flow during external chest compression

Two theories have been proposed to explain blood flow generated by external chest compression.

- The **cardiac pump** theory proposes that sternal compression results in ventricular compression and ejection of blood into the pulmonary artery and aorta. Echocardiography has shown that the cardiac valves may remain open in the early stages of cardiac arrest, lending support to this theory.
- The **thoracic pump** theory proposes that chest compression increases intrathoracic pressure, causing collapse of the thin-walled veins with blood being ejected through the stronger-walled arteries that remain open. This is the mechanism

by which coughing alone is thought to be able to generate life-sustaining circulation during early cardiac arrest or profound bradycardia.

Even when performed optimally, chest compressions do not achieve more than 30% of normal cardiac output. Mechanical devices that perform external chest compression may be more effective than manual compression, but further studies on long-term survival are awaited.

Choking

Foreign-body airway obstruction is an uncommon but potentially treatable cause of accidental death, causing approximately 150 deaths per annum in the UK. Because eating is usually witnessed, most cases are potentially treatable while the victim is still responsive.
• Coughing is the most effective method of removing the foreign body; encourage the victim to do so if they are able.
• If the victim shows signs of severe airway obstruction and is conscious, give five back blows, alternating with five abdominal thrusts. In children <1 year of age, chest thrusts should replace abdominal thrusts because of the risk of traumatizing abdominal viscera.
• If the patient has suffered a cardiac arrest, use the standard BLS and advanced life support (ALS) algorithms.
• A cricothyroidotomy to bypass the obstruction may be necessary if the patient cannot be intubated and ventilated by the usual methods.

Defibrillation

Defibrillation is the passage of an electrical current of sufficient magnitude to depolarize a critical mass of myocardium and enable restoration of co-ordinated electrical activity. The probability of successful defibrillation and subsequent survival to hospital discharge declines rapidly with time, and the ability to deliver early defibrillation is one of the most important factors in determining success. For every minute that passes following collapse, mortality increases 7–10% in the absence of bystander CPR.

External defibrillator technology has progressed considerably over recent years. The older monophasic waveform has now been superseded by a biphasic waveform which is more effective at cardioversion of both atrial and ventricular arrhythmias at lower energy levels. Both waveforms, however, remain in use while new technology replaces old.

Single shock strategy

The practice of giving three successive shocks has now been replaced by a single shock strategy. This is because if a biphasic shock has been unsuccessful, further shocks are unlikely to succeed without a period of CPR.

Treat VF/pulseless VT with a **single** shock, followed by immediate resumption of CPR (30 compressions to two ventilations) because, even if a perfusing rhythm is achieved, myocardial contractility will initially be inadequate to generate adequate blood pressure. CPR should only be interrupted to check the rhythm and give another shock (if indicated) after 2 min.

Energy levels

Monophasic defibrillators
First shock: 360 J (increased from previously recommended 200 J which had a poor first shock efficacy for termination of VF).
Second and subsequent shocks: 360 J.

Biphasic defibrillators
• First shock: 150–200 J.
• Second and subsequent shocks: 150–360 J.

CPR before defibrillation

In the seconds and minutes following cardiac arrest, the metabolic state of myocardial cells deteriorates rapidly. A brief period of chest compression will deliver oxygen and energy substrates and increase the probability of restoring a perfusing rhythm after shock delivery if the patient has been collapsed more than 4–5 min. Therefore, the following is recommended:

- In an unwitnessed out-of-hospital cardiac arrest (i.e. collapse likely to be >4–5 min), give CPR for 2 min before attempting defibrillation.
- Do not delay defibrillation if an out-of-hospital arrest is witnessed (i.e. has occurred within 4–5 min of defibrillation being available).
- Do not delay defibrillation for in-hospital cardiac arrest (where it is also assumed that collapse has occurred within 4–5 min of defibrillation being available).

Defibrillation technique

Self-adhesive pads vs. manual paddles. Self-adhesive defibrillation pads are safe and effective and are an acceptable alternative to standard defibrillation paddles. They enable the operator to defibrillate from a safe distance, rather than leaning over the patient as occurs with paddles.

Paddle position. The right (sternal) electrode is placed to the right of the sternum, below the clavicle. The apical paddle is placed in the midaxillary line, approximately level with the position of a V_6 ECG electrode. This anterolateral position should be clear of any breast tissue. Other acceptable pad positions which may be used if the anterolateral placement fails include:

- standard apical position and the other on the right or left upper back;
- one anteriorly over the left precordium, and the other posteriorly just below the left scapula.

Implantable medical devices (e.g. permanent pacemaker, implantable cardioverter defibrillator (ICD)) may be damaged during defibrillation unless the defibrillation electrodes are placed away from these devices.

Transdermal drug patches may cause arcing and burns if the defibrillator pad/paddle is placed directly over the patch during defibrillation. Remove and wipe the area before applying the pads/paddles.

Oxygen is usually in use during defibrillation and, in an oxygen-enriched atmosphere, sparks from a poorly applied defibrillator electrode may cause a fire. The following precautions will minimize this risk:

- Remove any oxygen mask or nasal cannulae and place at least 1 m away from the patient.
- A ventilation bag connected to the tracheal tube may be left. Alternatively, disconnect the ventilation bag from the tracheal tube and move it at least 1 m from the patient's chest.
- Self-adhesive defibrillation pads, rather than manual paddles, may minimize the risk of sparks.

Defibrillation safety

Paddles charged to 360 J deliver approximately 3000 V. Charged paddles should never be removed from a patient's chest. Discharge the paddles first if defibrillation is not indicated. When defibrillating, make sure all those attending keep clear and have no contact with the patient, bed or connected equipment.

Advanced life support

The resuscitation process is a continuum; the division between BLS and ALS is arbitrary and the two overlap. The algorithm for ALS is shown in Fig. 14.3.

The priority at any stage of CPR is to ensure chest compressions are given with minimal interruption. Feel for a carotid pulse and look for signs of life for no more than 10 s. If signs of an adequate circulation are absent, continue 30 chest compressions followed by two ventilations.

- Maintain the airway and ventilate the lungs with the most appropriate equipment available and use high-flow oxygen. A self-inflating bag and mask or equivalent should be used while a laryngeal mask airway (LMA) or endotracheal tube is prepared. Tracheal intubation should be attempted only by those who are competent. Confirm correct placement using a stethoscope.
- Once intubated, ventilate the lungs at a rate of 10/min. It is important not to hyperinflate the patient as this increases intrathoracic pressure, reduces venous return and decreases cardiac output. Oxygenation is the primary objective, and 100% inspired oxygen should be given. Adequate minute

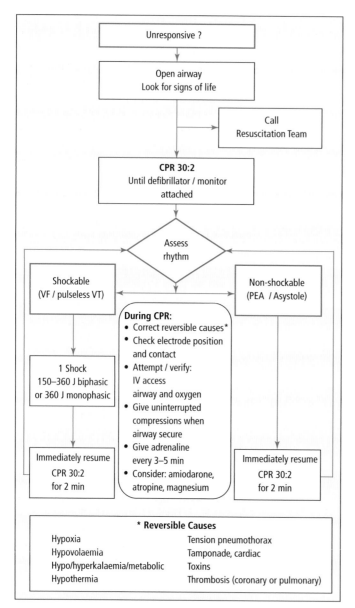

```
                    ┌─────────────────────────┐
                    │      Unresponsive ?      │
                    └─────────────────────────┘
                                │
                    ┌─────────────────────────┐
                    │       Open airway        │
                    │   Look for signs of life │
                    └─────────────────────────┘
                                │
                                │        ┌─────────────────────────┐
                                ├───────▶│          Call           │
                                │        │   Resuscitation Team     │
                                │        └─────────────────────────┘
                    ┌─────────────────────────┐
                    │        CPR 30:2          │
                    │ Until defibrillator/monitor │
                    │        attached          │
                    └─────────────────────────┘
                                │
                            ◇ Assess ◇
                            ◇ rhythm ◇
```

Shockable (VF / pulseless VT) ⟷ **Non-shockable** (PEA / Asystole)

1 Shock 150–360 J biphasic or 360 J monophasic

During CPR:
- Correct reversible causes*
- Check electrode position and contact
- Attempt / verify: IV access airway and oxygen
- Give uninterrupted compressions when airway secure
- Give adrenaline every 3–5 min
- Consider: amiodarone, atropine, magnesium

Immediately resume CPR 30:2 for 2 min

Immediately resume CPR 30:2 for 2 min

* Reversible Causes	
Hypoxia	Tension pneumothorax
Hypovolaemia	Tamponade, cardiac
Hypo/hyperkalaemia/metabolic	Toxins
Hypothermia	Thrombosis (coronary or pulmonary)

Fig. 14.3 Algorithm for advanced life support. Courtesy of the Resuscitation Council (UK).

volume is also important to clear CO_2 and prevent respiratory acidosis, especially after the administration of CO_2-producing buffers such as sodium bicarbonate. Gas exchange across the lungs is suboptimal because of an increase in dead space, reduced pulmonary blood flow, pulmonary oedema and, in some patients, pulmonary aspiration.

- Chest compression should continue without interruption (except for defibrillation or pulse checks when indicated), at a rate of 100/min.

- Apply the self-adhesive pads or defibrillator paddles to the patient and pause briefly to analyse the rhythm. If indicated, attempt external defibrillation. After the defibrillation attempt, do not pause to analyse the rhythm or feel for a pulse, but recommence chest compressions immediately, pausing to analyse the rhythm only after a further

2 min of CPR. The person providing chest compressions should be changed every 2 min to avoid fatigue.
- Once external chest compression, ventilation and defibrillation have commenced as appropriate, consider intravenous cannulation (see later).
- Arterial blood gases (radial or femoral) should be taken for estimation of blood gases, pH, electrolytes and glucose every 10–15 min.
- The best signs of restoration of oxygenated blood flow to the tissues are spontaneous movement by the patient, respiratory effort and small pupil size (NB: atropine and catecholamines cause pupillary dilation and may be given during the arrest, so dilation does not always signify brain death).

Shockable rhythms (ventricular fibrillation/pulseless ventricular tachycardia)

- Patients with shockable rhythms are treated with a 2 min cycle of CPR (as above) followed by a short pause to check the ECG and pulse, and perform defibrillation if indicated. If VF/VT persists after the first two shocks, give adrenaline 1 mg IV followed immediately by a third shock (150–360 J biphasic or 360 J monophasic) and resume CPR (drug–shock–CPR–rhythm check sequence). Adrenaline that is given immediately before the shock will be circulated by the CPR that follows the shock. Regardless of the arrest rhythm, give adrenaline 1 mg IV every 3–5 min until return of spontaneous circulation (ROSC) is achieved; this will be once every two loops of the algorithm.
- After drug delivery and 2 min of CPR, analyse the rhythm and deliver another shock immediately if indicated. If VF/VT persists after the third shock, give amiodarone 300 mg IV. Inject the amiodarone during the brief rhythm analysis before delivery of the fourth shock.

Non-shockable rhythms (asystole/ pulseless electrical activity)

Pulseless electrical activity (PEA) is defined as cardiac electrical activity in the absence of any palpable pulse. These patients often have myocardial contractions that are too weak to produce a detectable pulse or blood pressure. Asystole and PEA have a much poorer prognosis than VF/VT, with survival rates of <5%. Survival following cardiac arrest with asystole or PEA is unlikely unless a reversible cause can be found and treated effectively, though survival is better in the context of cardiac arrest due to drowning, hypothermia or drug overdose.
- A straight line on the monitor may indicate faulty equipment or connections, rather than asystole. Check, without stopping CPR, that the leads are attached correctly. If there is doubt as to whether the ECG shows asystole or fine VF, treat as a non-shockable rhythm. A period of CPR may coarsen the VF and improve the chance of successful defibrillation.
- Use the same 2 min cycle of CPR (as above) followed by a short pause to check the ECG and pulse. If the initial monitored rhythm is PEA or asystole, start CPR 30:2 and give adrenaline 1 mg IV, and repeat every 3–5 min until ROSC is achieved; this will be once every two loops of the algorithm.
- Give atropine 3 mg IV to block vagal tone if there is asystole or the rhythm is slow (rate <60/min). 'P' wave asystole may respond to cardiac pacing, although there is no benefit from attempting to pace true ventricular asystole.
- In atropine-resistant bradycardia, consider sympathomimetics (adrenaline, dopamine, isoprenaline) or temporary pacing. Pacing can be achieved by transvenous insertion of an intracardiac pacing wire (usually under X-ray screening), or be performed using an external pacing system, an option which is available on some defibrillators.
- If the rhythm changes to a shockable rhythm, change the algorithm pathway to follow that for shockable rhythms. If a pulse becomes palpable, continue post-resuscitation care and/or treatment of peri-arrest arrhythmias.

Causes of pulseless electrical activity

The potentially reversible causes of PEA (four Hs, four Ts) are listed in Box 14.2.

Intravenous access and drugs

(see Table 14.1)

Drug delivery

Intravenous (IV) drug administration is the route of choice. Peripheral access is usually the quickest, but central venous access is the optimal route. Flush all intravenous drugs with 20 mL of 0.9% saline IV. Insertion must not interrupt chest compression or delay defibrillation more than briefly.

Box 14.2 Causes of pulseless electrical activity

- Hypothermia
- Hypoxia
- Hypovolaemia
- Hyperkalaemia, hypokalaemia, hypocalcaemia
- Tension pneumothorax
- Tamponade (cardiac)
- Toxins
- Thromboembolism

Intraosseous (IO) drug administration can be used and achieves plasma levels of drugs comparable with the IV route. Marrow aspirate can be used for venous blood gas analysis and measurement of electrolytes and haemoglobin.

Endotracheal drug delivery should be regarded as a last resort because of unpredictable and poor drug absorption. Agents that can be given by this route include adrenaline, lidocaine (lignocaine) and atropine. Doses used should be three times the standard venous doses, and agents should be diluted up to a volume of at least 10 mL with saline. After administering a drug into the trachea, give five ventilations to increase dispersion into the bronchial tree, which will assist absorption.

Vasopressors

Although not of proven benefit, vasopressors continue to be recommended with the aim of increasing cerebral and coronary perfusion.

Table 14.1 Cardiovascular drugs.

Drug	Intravenous dose	Infusion dose*
Adrenaline (epinephrine)	1 mg	1–20 mcg/min
Aminophylline		500 mcg/kg/h
Amiodarone	300 mg	900 mg/24 h
Atropine	3.0 mg maximum	
Calcium chloride (10%)	10 mL	
Digoxin	0.5 mg	0.5–1.0 mg/day
Dobutamine		2.5–10.0 mcg/kg/min
Dopamine		1–20 mcg/kg/min
Flecainide	100–150 mg	100–250 mcg/kg/h
Glucagon	2–10 mg	
Glyceryl trinitrate (GTN)		10–200 mcg/min
Labetalol	50–200 mg	0–2 mg/min
Lidocaine (lignocaine)	100 mg	1–4 mg/min
Noradrenaline (norepinephrine)	100–200 mcg	1–20 mcg/min
Phenylephrine	50–100 mcg	1–20 mcg/min
Propranolol	1–10 mg	
Salbutamol	250 mg	3–20 mg/min
Sodium bicarbonate (8.4%)	50 mL repeated as necessary	
Verapamil	5–15 mg	

*Infusion doses only apply to the first few hours and should be reviewed thereafter.

Adrenaline

The α-adrenergic effects of **adrenaline** cause systemic peripheral vasoconstriction, and its β-adrenergic actions increase heart rate and contractility, both of which may improve cerebral and coronary perfusion.

Indications
- First drug used in cardiac arrest of any aetiology, being given every 3–5 min of CPR.
- Treatment of anaphylaxis.
- Cardiogenic shock.

Dose
- During cardiac arrest give adrenaline 1 mg IV or IO. Give 3 mg if administered via the endotracheal route.
- During severe anaphylaxis, give adrenaline 1 mg IM.

Use
Adrenaline is available in two dilutions. Great care must be taken to give the correct dose.
- 1 in 10000 (10 mL of this solution contains 1 mg of adrenaline)
- 1 in 1000 (1 mL of this solution contains 1 mg of adrenaline).

Side-effects
- Adrenaline increases myocardial oxygen consumption which may worsen myocardial ischaemia. Following return of spontaneous circulation, even small doses (0.5 mg) of adrenaline may induce tachycardia, VT or VF. Intravenous doses of 50–100 μ IV are usually sufficient to maintain adequate blood pressure in the post-resuscitation phase. An infusion provides more stable haemodynamic effects.
- Pupillary dilation (also caused by atropine or cerebral hypoxia).
- Sympathomimetic agents should be used with caution where cardiac arrest is the result of solvent abuse, cocaine or other sympathomimetic drugs, all of which cause vasoconstriction.

Vasopressin

Vasopressin is a naturally occurring antidiuretic hormone. In very high doses it is a powerful vasoconstrictor which acts by stimulation of smooth muscle V_1 receptors. The benefits of vasopressin found in small clinical trials have not been repeated in a large CPR trial. Its routine use is therefore not recommended.

Antiarrhythmics

Amiodarone

Amiodarone is a class III antiarrhythmic drug which achieves membrane stabilization by prolonging the plateau phase of the action potential, thus lengthening the refractory period. In shock-refractory VF, amiodarone improves survival to hospital discharge compared with placebo or lidocaine.

Indications
- Shock-refractory VF/VT.
- Frequent multifocal premature ventricular beats compromising blood pressure.
- Haemodynamically stable VT and other resistant tachyarrhythmias, polymorphic VT and wide-complex tachycardia of uncertain origin.
- Paroxysmal supraventricular tachycardia (SVT) uncontrolled by adenosine, vagal manoeuvres or atrioventricular (AV) nodal blockade.

Dose
- During cardiac arrest, give amiodarone 300 mg IV as a single bolus. A further dose of 150 mg IV may be given for recurrent or refractory VF/VT, followed by an infusion of 900 mg IV over 24 h.

Side-effects
- Amiodarone can cause hypotension and bradycardia, which can be prevented by slowing the rate of drug infusion, or can be treated with fluids and/or inotropic drugs. The side-effects associated with prolonged oral use (abnormalities of thyroid function, corneal microdeposits, peripheral neuropathy and pulmonary/hepatic infiltrates) are not relevant in the acute setting.

215

Lidocaine (lignocaine)

Lidocaine is a class I antiarrhythmic drug which acts by increasing the myocyte refractory period. It decreases ventricular automaticity, and its local anaesthetic action suppresses ventricular ectopic activity. Lidocaine suppresses activity of depolarized, arrhythmogenic tissues while interfering minimally with the electrical activity of normal tissues. Lidocaine raises the threshold for ventricular fibrillation. Its use has been superseded by amiodarone but is still indicated if amiodarone is unavailable.

Dose

Give 100 mg IV if the patient remains in VF/VT following three shocks. Excessive lidocaine causes paraesthesia, hypotension, convulsions and coma. The maximum safe dose is 3 mg/kg over the first hour.

Magnesium

Magnesium is an important constituent of enzyme systems involved with ATP generation. It improves myocardial contractility and limits infarct size by an unknown mechanism. The normal plasma range of magnesium is 0.8–1.0 mmol/L. Hypomagnesaemia may contribute to arrhythmias or cardiac arrest either directly or by accelerating digoxin uptake to cardiotoxic levels. Hypomagnesaemia may occur in chronically ill patients and is associated with hypokalaemia, hypophosphataemia, hyponatraemia and hypocalcaemia.

Indications

- Shock-refractory VF in the presence of possible hypomagnesaemia.
- Ventricular tachyarrhythmias in the presence of possible hypomagnesaemia.
- Torsades de pointes.
- Digoxin toxicity.

Dose

In shock-refractory VF, give an initial dose of 2 g IV (4 ml (8 mmol)) of 50% magnesium sulphate)

peripherally over 1–2 min; it may be repeated after 10 – 15 min.

Side-effects

Side-effects associated with hypermagnesaemia are rare. Magnesium inhibits smooth muscle contraction, causing vasodilatation and a transient dose-dependent hypotension, which usually responds to intravenous fluids and vasopressors.

The antiarrhythmic drugs listed are the first-line drugs during cardiac arrest. **Flecainide**, **β-blockers** and **calcium channel blockers** may all have a role to play in the management of peri-arrest arrhythmias, but it is beyond the scope of this chapter to discuss these drugs in detail (see http://www.resus.org.uk).

Other drugs

Atropine

Cardiac arrest is associated with increased vagal tone, which may cause bradycardia or asystole. Atropine antagonizes the action of the parasympathetic neurotransmitter acetylcholine at muscarinic receptors. It therefore blocks the effect of the vagus nerve on both the sinoatrial node and the AV node, increasing sinus automaticity and facilitating AV node conduction. The benefit of atropine in cardiac arrest is not proven.

Indications

- Asystole.
- PEA with a rate <60/min.
- Sinus, atrial or nodal bradycardia causing haemodynamic instability.

Dose

For asystole, give 3 mg IV as a single bolus. Smaller doses (0.6–1.8 mg) may be adequate to treat bradycardia.

Side-effects

Pupillary dilation (also caused by sympathomimetics or cerebral hypoxia). Blurred vision, dry mouth, urinary retention and acute confusional states are not an issue in the acute setting of a cardiac arrest.

Calcium

Many intracellular mechanisms, particularly those involving myocardial contraction, are regulated by calcium. The benefit of calcium in cardiac arrest is not proven.

Indications
- Hyperkalaemia.
- Hypocalcaemia.
- Overdose of calcium channel-blocking drugs.

Dose
A 10 mL dose of 10% calcium chloride can be given, and repeated if necessary. Do not give calcium solutions and sodium bicarbonate simultaneously by the same route (precipitates as calcium carbonate). Calcium chloride is preferable to calcium gluconate because blood levels of ionized calcium are more predictable.

Buffers

The cessation of pulmonary gas exchange and increased anaerobic cellular metabolism during cardiac arrest leads to a progressive respiratory and metabolic acidosis, respectively. Artificial ventilation and effective cardiac massage may limit the degree of acidosis. Cellular homeostasis is disrupted by relatively small changes in acid–base balance, and acidosis may reduce tissue oxygen delivery and cause impaired myocardial contractility. Measurement of arterial blood gases gives a limited indication of tissue acid–base balance because stagnant arterial blood may have undergone little gas exchange compared with stagnant capillary blood which will undergo rapid oxygen depletion and acidosis. Analysis of central venous blood may provide a better estimation of tissue pH. The most commonly used buffer for correction of acid–base imbalance is sodium bicarbonate. Studies examining the benefits of buffers in cardiac arrest remain inconclusive.

Indications
Arterial blood pH <7.1, or base excess more negative than –10 mmol/L during or following resuscitation from cardiac arrest.

Dose
- Titrate 50 mL boluses of 8.4% sodium bicarbonate IV, according to acid–base measurements.
- Consider for life-threatening hyperkalaemia, severe metabolic acidosis or tricyclic overdose.
- Routine use during cardiac arrest is not recommended.

Side-effects
- Sodium ions are osmotically active and may exacerbate fluid overload in a struggling circulation. Carbon dioxide generated from bicarbonate diffuses rapidly into cells, which may exacerbate intracellular acidosis.
- As the bicarbonate ion is excreted as carbon dioxide via the lungs, ventilation needs to be increased.
- Severe tissue damage may be caused by subcutaneous extravasation of sodium bicarbonate.

Other
Acidosis causes hyperkalaemia. If severe (K^+ >6.0 mmol/L), give insulin (10 IU, IV) and glucose (10 g IV), and repeat as necessary, according to regular measurement of plasma pH, potassium and glucose.

Thrombolytics

Commonly, adult cardiac arrest results from myocardial ischaemia following coronary artery thrombotic occlusion. More rarely, cardiac arrest may result from pulmonary embolus. Several small studies have shown promising results of thrombolytics when arrest occurs in these settings.

Indications
- Consider when cardiac arrest is thought to be due to acute pulmonary embolus.
- Consider in adult cardiac arrest on a case-by-case basis following initial failure of standard

resuscitation in patients in whom an acute thrombotic aetiology for the arrest is suspected.

Side-effects
• Ongoing CPR is not a contraindication to
thrombolysis.
• Risk of haemorrhagic stroke should be considered, but is small compared with the risks of
cerebral ischaemia from cardiac arrest.

Practical considerations
• Following thrombolysis during CPR for
acute pulmonary embolism, survival and good
neurological outcome have been reported in cases
requiring in excess of 60 min of CPR. If a thrombolytic drug is given in these circumstances, consider
performing CPR for at least 60–90 min before termination of resuscitation attempts.
• The optimal choice or dose of thrombolytic
agent is unknown.

Intravenous fluids

Intravenous fluids are not generally indicated in
cardiac arrest secondary to myocardial ischaemia.
Excessive intravenous fluids may precipitate pulmonary oedema and heart failure once spontaneous circulation is established. If hypovolaemia is
thought to be a contributing factor to the cardiac
arrest, establish good intravenous access early and
infuse IV fluids rapidly. In the initial stages of resuscitation, use 0.9% saline or Hartmann's solution. Avoid dextrose, which is rapidly redistributed
from the intravascular space and causes hyperglycaemia, which may worsen neurological outcome
after cardiac arrest.

Post-resuscitation care

The final link in the Chain of Survival is post-resuscitation care. In patients in whom the above procedures generate a return of spontaneous circulation,
optimization of haemodynamic, respiratory and
metabolic parameters is vital in order to achieve
discharge home of a neurologically intact patient.
In patients with more than the briefest of cardiac
arrest who can usually be managed on a Coronary

> **Box 14.3 Post-resuscitation investigations**
>
> • **Chest radiograph**: consider pneumothorax, aspira-
> tion, pericardial effusion, position of endotracheal and
> nasogastric tubes, central venous line and pacing wire
> • **ECG**: consider myocardial infarction, pulmonary em-
> bolism, rhythm disturbance, conduction disease
> • **Echocardiogram**: consider tamponade, left ventricu-
> lar dysfunction, valve disease
> • **Arterial pH and gases**: confirm adequate gas ex-
> change and acid–base status
> • **Electrolytes**: consider hyperkalaemia, hypokalaemia,
> hypomagnesaemia
> • **Glucose**: consider hypoglycaemia, hyperglycaemia
> • **Full blood count**: consider haemorrhage

Care Unit, many patients will require admission to
an Intensive Care Unit for specialist care (see Box
14.3). In addition to the general principles of intensive care management, several specific therapeutic interventions have been demonstrated to
have a significant effect on outcome.

Temperature control

Hyperpyrexia

A period of hyperthermia is common following
cardiac arrest and, if uncontrolled, risks a poor neurological outcome. Any pyrexia occurring in the
immediate 72 h post-arrest must be treated aggressively with anti-pyretics (e.g. paracetamol) and active cooling.

Therapeutic hypothermia

Reperfusion of tissue following cardiac arrest results in inflammatory reactions that produce cyto-
toxic molecules such as free radicals and excitatory
amino acids. A period of mild therapeutic hypothermia suppresses this inflammatory cascade and
has been shown to limit cerebral and myocardial
damage, both experimentally and clinically in
some situations. External and/or internal cooling
techniques can be used to initiate cooling. An
infusion of 30 mg/kg of 4 °C saline decreases core
temperature by 1.5 °C. Intravascular cooling en-

ables more precise control of core temperature than external methods, but it is unknown whether this improves outcome. Unconscious adult patients with spontaneous circulation after out-of-hospital VF cardiac arrest should be cooled to 32–34 °C. Cooling should be started as soon as possible and continued for at least 12–24 h. Induced hypothermia might also benefit unconscious adult patients with spontaneous circulation after out-of-hospital cardiac arrest from a non-shockable rhythm, or cardiac arrest in hospital. This degree of hypothermia requires the patient to be sedated and ventilated in an intensive care setting. At the end of this period, rewarm the patient slowly (0.25–0.5 °C/h) and avoid hyperthermia. Complications of mild therapeutic hypothermia include increased infection, hyperglycaemia and coagulopathy, but benefits of this treatment outweigh these side-effects.

Blood glucose control

There is a strong association between hyperglycaemia and poor outcome after cardiac arrest. Studies of stroke patients show that tight glucose control improves neurological recovery, and animal studies following cardiac arrest demonstrate the same. The optimal level for blood glucose control has not been determined, but maintaining blood glucose from 4.4 to 6.1 mmol/L using insulin reduces hospital mortality in critically ill adults, and a similar range has been recommended for adults in the immediate post-arrest period. Unrecognized hypoglycaemia is also harmful, and careful glucose control in comatose patients is essential for optimal neurological recovery.

Prognostic indicators of survival

Neurological assessment after a successful resuscitation can be difficult. At 72 h post-arrest, the absence of pupillary light reflexes or an absent motor response to pain is predictive of a poor outcome (death or vegetative state) with very high specificity. Grossly abnormal EEG and median nerve somatosensory evoked potentials (SSEPs) are also of use in predicting poor outcome.

Stopping or with holding resuscitation

Stopping resuscitation

Before stopping attempts at resuscitation, the person leading the management of the arrest should be satisfied, as far as possible, that the likely cause of the arrest is known, has been reversed if possible and that no further specific treatment is indicated. Successful resuscitation in these circumstances is unlikely after 20 min of asystole. Exceptions to this are arrests associated with drowning, hypothermia and certain drug overdoses, when survival may occur after even longer resuscitation periods.

Withholding resuscitation

'Do not attempt resuscitation' (DNAR) orders are becoming increasingly common when a patient does not wish to have CPR, or will not survive even if CPR is attempted. If there is any doubt as to the DNAR status, commence resuscitation, but attempt to establish the status as soon as possible. Futile resuscitation attempts are of no benefit to the patient, relatives or staff.

Further reading

Handley AJ, Koster R, Monsieurs K, Perkins GD, Davies ES, Bossaert L. European Resuscitation Council Guidelines for Resuscitation 2005. Section 2. Adult basic life support and use of automated external defibrillators. *Resuscitation* 2005; 67: Suppl 1: S7–23.

Deakin CD, Nolan JP. European Resuscitation Council Guidelines for Resuscitation 2005. Section 3. Electrical therapies: automated external defibrillators, defibrillation, cardioversion and pacing. *Resuscitation* 2005; 67: Suppl 1: S25–37.

Nolan JP, Deakin CD, Soar J, Bottiger B, Smith G. European Resuscitation Council Guidelines for Resuscitation 2005. Section 4. Advanced life support. *Resuscitation* 2005; 67: Suppl 1: S39–86.

Soar J, Deakin CD, Nolan JP, Abbas G, Alfonso A, Handley AJ, Lockey D, Perkins GD, Thies K. European Resuscitation Council Guidelines for Resuscitation 2005. Section 7. Cardiac arrest in special circumstances. *Resuscitation* 2005; 67: Suppl 1: S135–70.

Detailed resuscitation guidelines are available at the Resuscitation Council (UK) website (www.resus.org.uk)

Chapter 15

Diseases of the aorta

Introduction

The aorta is the principal artery connecting the heart to the systemic arterial system. Its wall has three layers:

1 tunica intima (thin layer of endothelial cells);
2 tunica media (spirally arranged laminated elastic tissue); and
3 tunica adventitia (principally collagen but also containing adventitial vessels and lymphatics).

In the media, spirally aligned elastic tissue predominates, giving the aorta a high tensile strength and elasticity, allowing it to expand during systole (storing kinetic energy) and recoil during diastole (releasing energy), which in turn results in forward aortic flow during diastole.

Aortic blood pressure (BP) during systole is determined by the amount of blood ejected during cardiac systole, the compliance of the aorta itself and resistance of the smaller peripheral arterial system (systemic vascular resistance; SVR). SVR and heart rate are indirectly influenced by specialized sensory cells in the ascending aorta and the aortic arch, afferent signals being sent to the central vasomotor centre in the brainstem via the vagus nerve. A rise in BP tends to cause a reflex bradycardia and fall in SVR; a fall causes tachycardia and vasoconstriction.

The aorta has thoracic and abdominal components, with the thoracic portion being divided into ascending, arch and descending components.

• The root of the **ascending aorta** is normally 3–3.5 cm in diameter and comprises the supporting tissue for the aortic valve, the three sinuses of Valsalva which allow space for systolic excursion of the valve cusps (the right and left coronary arteries arise from two of these sinuses), and above these the sinotubular junction, which is a circular ridge between the root and the rest of the ascending aorta. The proximal part of the ascending aorta lies within the pericardium, which is why cardiac tamponade may occur if the aortic wall is breached (e.g. aortic dissection).

• The **aortic arch** gives off the brachiocephalic vessels (innominate, left carotid and left subclavian arteries) and over its course in the superior mediastinum gradually turns from a cranial to caudal direction, in an anteroposterior and slightly leftwards direction.

• The **descending thoracic aorta** runs caudally in the posterior mediastinum from the aortic arch, giving off intercostal and spinal arteries, becoming the abdominal aorta at the diaphragm.

Acute aortic dissection

This is a catastrophic disorder often leading to sudden death. A tear in the aortic intima allows it to be dissected or stripped of its subintimal layers, destroying the media. The process may be initiated by spontaneous haemorrhage within a diseased area of aortic wall with subsequent intimal tearing, or the tear may be caused by shear forces from within the aortic lumen.

Aetiology

There is weakness of the aortic media with breakdown of elastic and collagen tissues (cystic degeneration). Age-related degeneration, often accelerated by hypertension, is the most common process but Marfan, Ehlers–Danlos and Noonan syndromes may be complicated by aortic dissection because of their involvement of connective tissue. Occasionally, dissection follows disruption of atheromatous plaque, aortic arteritis, or occurs in pregnancy.

Clinical features

Patients are most commonly (66%) male, in the sixth or seventh decades. Symptoms are:
- sudden, severe pain (tearing in character, interscapular or anterior chest);
- nausea;
- vomiting;
- sweating;
- syncope.

Dissection involving a coronary artery may cause myocardial ischaemia, and rupture into the pericardium causes acute tamponade. These are the two most common causes of death.

Physical findings

- Hypertension is common, due to pain and frequently a past history of high blood pressure.
- Hypotension suggests tamponade.
- Absence or diminution of pulses is common (mainly in head, neck and arm vessels).
- Aortic regurgitation (AR) may occur, either acutely due to disruption of the aortic ring by dissection of the ascending aorta, or chronically due to root dilatation.
- Pleural effusion may indicate rupture into a pleural space.

Occasionally, an acute aortic dissection may go unrecognized and, if the patient survives, the diagnosis may be made some years later because of increasing AR or an incidental observation on a chest X-ray or other investigation.

Investigations

- Routine laboratory investigations are often unhelpful. An elevated creatinine may be due to pre-existing renal disease, often due to chronic hypertension, but may also occur acutely due to abdominal extension of the dissection involving the renal arteries.
- A chest X-ray will often show a widened mediastinum, although an anteroposterior portable film will tend to exaggerate its dimension.
- Transthoracic or transoesophageal echocardiography may show an abnormal aortic root or the presence of an intimal flap, but these are poor techniques for imaging the arch or descending aorta.
- Magnetic resonance (MRI) or computed tomographic (CT) imaging (Fig. 15.1) provide excellent images of the whole aorta, and are particularly useful if surgery is considered. Patient co-operation and haemodynamic stability are required; not always achievable if the patient is distressed or hypotensive.

Contrast aortography, previously the gold standard investigation, has been superseded by the use of echo, MRI and CT, and is now rarely used.

Classification

Prognosis and management of aortic dissection are related to whether the ascending aorta is involved, because of its association with death due to coronary involvement and/or tamponade. The Stanford classification (Fig. 15.2) simply divides dissections into:
- **Type A**—proximal to the left subclavian artery, involves ascending aorta.
- **Type B**—distal to the left subclavian artery, ascending aorta is spared.

Management

The patient should be given adequate analgesia. Hypertension is rigorously controlled using combinations of intravenous and oral medication:

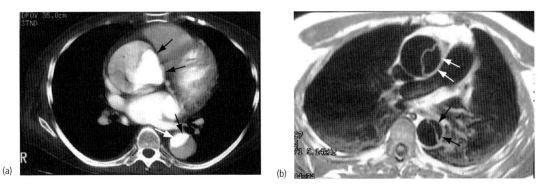

Fig. 15.1 Type A aortic dissection: (a) CT scan; (b) MRI scan. Arrows indicate 'false' lumen in ascending and descending thoracic aorta.

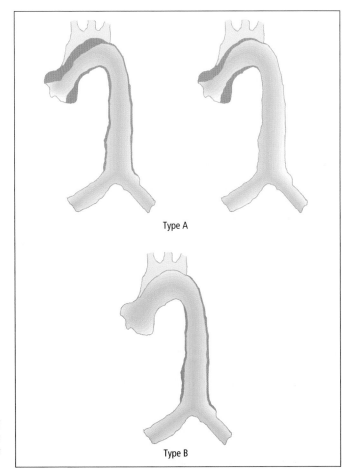

Type A

Type B

Fig. 15.2 Stanford classification of aortic dissection. Type A involves ascending aorta, type B involves only descending aorta.

- β-blockers to lower blood pressure and reduce the rate of rise of aortic blood flow
velocity — dV/dT);
- vasodilators such as hydralazine, nitrates
and some of the calcium antagonists (nifedipine,
amlodipine), and the α-blocker prazosin;
- labetalol, a combined α- and β-blocker;
- intravenous sodium nitroprusside, which is
frequently used as a short-term measure;
- centrally acting agents, such as methyldopa,
which are used occasionally.

Angiotensin-converting enzyme (ACE) inhibitors are best avoided until involvement of the
renal arteries has been excluded. Long-term
antihypertensive therapy is indicated for all
patients.

Surgery

In type A dissection, surgery improves survival and
should be performed urgently as early mortality
is high. Aortic valve replacement, aortic root
replacement with coronary re-implantation and
various forms of aortic reconstruction may be required. Medical therapy is preferred for type B dissections since routine surgery does not improve
overall survival. However, some type B patients
may require surgery for vital organ compromise
(e.g. kidneys, intestines), haemorrhage or evidence
of further dissection. When surgery involves the
descending thoracic aorta, spinal cord ischaemia
and paraplegia may occur due to involvement of
the spinal arteries. Surgery involving the aortic
arch obviously risks ischaemia to the head and
neck circulation.

Aneurysms of the aorta

A 'true' aneurysm is a localized dilatation of the
aorta where the walls of the aneurysm have all the
normal layers of the aortic wall. Atherosclerotic
aortic degeneration, often associated with chronic
hypertension, is the most common cause of thoracic aortic aneurysms, but localized aortic root
dilatation is also common. Although often idiopathic, it is assumed to be due to an abnormality of
medial connective tissue, and is often seen as part
of connective tissue syndromes such as Marfan
syndrome.

Aortic aneurysms gradually enlarge, although
their rate of dilatation varies considerably. The
larger the aneurysm, the greater the risk of rupture.
The most common locations for aneurysms are
ascending aorta (45%), descending thoracic
aorta (35%), arch (10%) and thoracoabdominal
(10%).

Aortitis is now an uncommon cause of aneurysm formation in developed countries due to the
fall in the prevalence of syphilis, but may be associated with rheumatoid disease, Reiter syndrome
and giant cell arteritis.

A **'false' aneurysm** is really a contained rupture,
with the wall of the aneurysm being made up of
adventitia and peri-aortic fibrous tissue. This may
result from previous trauma (aortic transection) or
chronic dissection.

Clinical features

Patients with true aneurysms are often asymptomatic. When symptoms do occur, pain is the most
common manifestation and may be acute or
chronic. Its position depends on the location of
the aneurysm but is frequently precordial and may
radiate to the neck and jaw when the thoracic aorta
is involved, or interscapular if the aneurysm is
in the descending aorta. Symptoms may follow
compression of adjacent structures, and stretching
of the recurrent laryngeal nerve in aneurysms
of the arch may cause hoarseness. Frequently,
there are no physical signs but co-existing hypertension is common. When the ascending aorta is
involved, aortic root dilatation may result in aortic
regurgitation.

Imaging techniques

A plain chest X-ray may suggest the diagnosis, but
more detailed assessment of the aneurysm's location, size and the involvement of major vessel
branches are all critical to the management of these
conditions. The investigations of choice are MRI
and CT scanning, which are also used for follow-up
after surgical intervention.

Management

Patients with asymptomatic dilatation of the aortic root >5 cm, or thoracic aorta elsewhere of >6 cm, should be considered for surgery because rupture may occur. Surgical techniques vary but include replacement of the affected segment of the aorta by synthetic graft. Surgical mortality varies from 5 to 50%, with the greatest risk being for aneurysms of the aortic arch. The most common causes of morbidity are neurological sequelae, particularly paraplegia and paraparesis when aneurysms involve the descending thoracic aorta, cerebral damage with aneurysms of the aortic arch, and renal failure after repair of descending thoracic or thoracoabdominal aorta. Re-operation during follow-up may be required, due to aneurysmal dilatation at the site of anastomosis between synthetic graft and native aorta. Recent advances offer the possibility of new surgical and interventional approaches using endovascular grafts which can be deployed percuataneously.

Marfan syndrome

This is a genetic disorder of connective tissue caused by mutations in the gene that encodes fibrillin-1. It is autosomal dominant but can occur as a spontaneous mutation. The nature of the connective tissue abnormality varies as >100 distinct mutations have been characterized so far. The range of clinical features include:
- skeletal abnormalities;
- arachnodactyly;
- lens subluxation;
- aortic and mitral valvular regurgitation.

Susceptibility to aneurysmal dilatation of the aorta, particularly of the aortic root, and aortic dissection are the principal features of aortic disease. Aortic root dilatation needs to be carefully monitored and aortic root replacement undertaken when dilatation progresses. Absolute aortic root dimensions may not be a particularly accurate guide to risk of aortic rupture, but wall tension is proportional to vessel diameter (Laplace's Law), and most clinicians would recommend surgery if the aortic root diameter exceeds 5 cm.

Takayasu's aortitis

This disease, although rare, occurs worldwide but has a predominance in young oriental females (M : F ratio 1 : 9). The aetiology is unknown but has been related to connective tissue disease and autoimmune disorders. Aortic histological features include marked intimal proliferation and fibrosis, medial elastic fibre degeneration, round cell infiltration, thickened adventitia and destruction of the vasa vasora.

Aneurysm formation, arterial stenoses, poststenotic dilatations and obliterative changes in the aorta and its branches occur. Presentation is often in the teenage years, with a malaise, fever, arthralgia, night sweats and pleuritic chest pain. The complications of the condition relate to the consequences of impaired arterial blood supply to vital organs, which may be accompanied by systemic hypertension. Treatment is directed towards suppression of its presumed immune aetiology with steroids or immunosuppressants, and management of the arterial complications as they arise.

Giant cell arteritis

This predominantly occurs in the sixth decade onwards. Its aetiology is unknown, but the disease mainly involves medium-sized arteries. The aorta and its main branches can be involved in a minority of cases. Characteristically, there is granulomatous infiltration of the arterial media, often with inflammatory eosinophilic cell infiltrate. Fever, malaise and headaches may occur. Weakening of the aortic wall can occasionally lead to aneurysm formation.

Syphilitic aortitis

Syphilis is now a rare cause of aortitis. Spirochaetal infection of the aortic media, usually during the secondary phase of syphilitic infection, sets up a chronic inflammation which results in weakening and destruction of the muscular and elastic components of the aortic wall, and aneurysmal dilatation most commonly of the ascending aorta.

Characteristically, the overlying intima becomes thickened and has a ridged appearance of 'tree bark'. The symptoms and signs are those of any aortic aneurysm and the underlying condition. Tests for syphilitic serology should routinely be performed in patients with ascending aortic dilatation and, if positive, antibiotics (usually benzyl penicillin) are indicated, though there is no evidence that this reverses or halts progression of the aortic disease. Surgery may be required for expanding aneurysms or for aortic regurgitation.

Traumatic injury of the aorta

Aortic rupture (transection) is seen with deceleration injuries, usually due to chest trauma. The diagnosis is usually suspected as a result of investigations undertaken for the patient's injuries. Mediastinal widening and distortion of the aorta may be apparent on the chest radiograph. Thoracic aortography is the investigation of choice. The most common site for aortic transection is at its point of attachment to the ligamentum arteriosum, the remnant of the ductus arteriosus, and is usually just distal to the origin of the left subclavian. Immediate death is the most common outcome of this injury, as a result of massive haemorrhage, but some survive due to containment of the rupture by the aortic adventitia. Undiagnosed, this may lead to chronic false aneurysm formation.

When diagnosed, immediate surgical repair is essential unless contraindicated due to the extent of the patient's other injuries, particularly neurological.

Aortic embolism

Most aortic emboli (90%) originate from the left heart, precipitating conditions being recent myocardial infarction with mural thrombus, left ventricular dilatation or aneurysm, atrial fibrillation with structural cardiac disease, or prosthetic cardiac valves. The remaining 10% come from unknown sources, at least some of which are probably from atheromatous disease of the aortic wall. Although these emboli originating in the aorta are usually small, they may cause stroke, especially if the aorta has been cross-clamped during surgery.

When large emboli lodge in the aorta or its major branches, clinical features are those of sudden ischaemia affecting tissues distal to the obstruction (pain, pallor, paraesthesia, pulselessness, paralysis or cerebrovascular). In about 25% of cases, the embolism lodges at the aortic bifurcation (saddle embolism).

Depending on the site and size of the thrombus, embolectomy may be undertaken with a Fogarty balloon catheter or under direct vision by surgical dissection (operative mortality 15–20%). Due to the risk of recurrent embolism, patients should receive long-term oral anticoagulants.

Chapter 16

Pulmonary hypertension and pulmonary thromboembolism

Pulmonary hypertension

Introduction

The pulmonary circulation is a low pressure system, with mean pulmonary artery pressure (PAP) at rest being <20 mmHg and, whereas systemic arterioles respond to hypoxia by vasodilatation, pulmonary vessels vasoconstrict. Pressures will be temporarily increased on exercise or at altitude, but when mean PAP is consistently >25 mmHg at rest, pulmonary hypertension (PHT) exists. PHT may occur in the absence of any definable cause or may be associated with, or secondary to, other conditions (see Box 16.1).

The first half of this chapter is concerned mainly with idiopathic (previously called 'primary') PHT, although an understanding of underlying principles is helpful in the management of patients with PHT of whatever aetiology. Further information on cardiological conditions causing secondary PHT can be found in other chapters.

The second part covers pulmonary embolism and the PHT that can be associated with this condition.

Epidemiology

Idiopathic PHT (IPHT) is a rare condition, affecting women at least twice as often as men and usually presenting in the second or third decades. Its incidence is unknown because it is usually not considered separately from other, more common causes of PHT (annual death rates due to all-cause PHT are around 50 per million). Its rarity, and lack of a single specific diagnostic test, also means that clinical trials usually involve a relatively small number of patients, and may include heterogeneous patient groups, making interpretation of the findings more difficult.

Pathophysiology

The normal pulmonary circulation reacts to the increased blood flow associated with exercise by vasodilatation and recruitment of vessels which are not perfused at rest. This reduction in pulmonary vascular resistance (PVR) allows the normal right ventricle to accommodate large changes in venous return without increasing its pressure. A rise in PVR stimulates the development of right ventricular (RV) hypertrophy and, for some time, normal pulmonary blood flow can be maintained at the expense of PHT. The increasingly hypertrophied RV demands higher myocardial blood flow, and develops increased wall stress, both of which may precipitate myocardial ischaemia and anginal chest pain. As the PHT worsens so the RV dilates and fails to maintain normal pulmonary flow. Cardiac output falls and exercise tolerance deteriorates progressively until symptoms are present at rest. Advanced PHT may cause atrial (atrial fibrillation) and ventricular (ventricular tachycardia,

Box 16.1 Clinical classification of pulmonary hypertension

Pulmonary arterial hypertension (PHT)

a Idiopathic (IPHT) (including familial)
b Associated with other conditions:
   i Collagen vascular disease
   ii Congenital systemic-to-pulmonary shunts
   iii Portal hypertension
   iv HIV infection
   v Drugs and toxins
      Amphetamines (e.g. appetite suppressant fenfluramine)
      Cocaine
      Some chemotherapeutic agents
      L-tryptophan
      Toxic oil syndrome
c Associated with pulmonary venous or capillary involvement
   i Pulmonary veno-occlusive disease
   ii Pulmonary capillary hemangiomatosis
d Persistent PHT of the newborn

PHT with left heart disease

a Left-sided atrial or ventricular heart disease
b Left-sided valvular heart disease

PHT associated with lung diseases and/or hypoxaemia

a Chronic obstructive pulmonary disease
b Interstitial lung disease
c Sleep-disordered breathing
d Alveolar hypoventilation disorders
e Chronic exposure to high altitude

PHT due to chronic thrombotic and/or embolic disease

a Thromboembolic obstruction of pulmonary arteries
b Non-thrombotic pulmonary embolism (tumour, parasites, foreign material)

Modified from: Clinical classification of pulmonary hypertension. *Journal of the American College of Cardiology* 2004; 43: 10S.

ventricular fibrillation) arrhythmias, and patients are at risk of sudden death. Slow pulmonary blood flow and polycythaemia secondary to hypoxaemia increase the risk of pulmonary thrombosis *in situ*.

Most cases of IPHT are sporadic, but a **familial predisposition** has been observed (5–10% of cases), probably transmitted as an autosomal dominant inheritance with incomplete penetrance. In-terestingly, similar genetic defects are seen in 25% of sporadic cases of PHT, suggesting there may be an underlying unifying mechanism by which idiopathic PHT is generated.

A number of factors have been observed as **'triggers'** for the development of PHT, including anorectic drugs (e.g. fenfluramine), cocaine, amphetamines and HIV infection. PHT may also be associated with portal hypertension, possibly due to a failure of the liver to remove vasoactive substances (e.g. serotonin), exposing the pulmonary arterial endothelium to higher concentrations.

Abnormalities of endothelial function are well described in IPHT (impaired production of prostacyclin and nitric oxide, excessive synthesis of endothelin), which could lead to vasoconstriction, subsequent vascular growth and remodelling. However, it is unknown whether these abnormalities cause the disease or are secondary to the progressive vascular damage that occurs as the disease progresses.

Sleep apnoea, due to intermittent nasopharyngeal obstruction, occurs particularly in obese individuals, causing snoring and poor quality sleep; in some, the chronic nocturnal hypoxaemia results in PHT. Extremely rarely, PHT may be due to progressive occlusion of the pulmonary venous rather than arterial vessels (**pulmonary veno-occlusive disease**), the aetiology of which is unknown.

Clinical features

Although the progression of IPHT is very variable, patients usually do not become symptomatic until the condition is well advanced. **Dyspnoea** is common, and central **anginal** chest discomfort and **syncope** may occur on exertion as the severity of PHT worsens. The patient may notice tissue cyanosis. Conversely, patients with secondary PHT usually present earlier with symptoms related to the underlying aetiology of their PHT (e.g. lung disease, congenital heart disease, venous thrombosis and pulmonary embolism (PE)). Whatever the aetiology, signs of PHT include:

• elevated jugular venous pressure (JVP);
• sinus tachycardia or AF;

- normal or low systemic blood pressure;
- poor peripheral circulation (cold extremities);
- central or just peripheral cyanosis;
- RV third heart sound (S3) and/or fourth heart sound (S4);
- loud pulmonary (P2) component of second heart sound (S2);
- tricuspid regurgitation;
- peripheral oedema;
- possibly hepatic enlargement and ascites.

Clubbing may occur in certain chronic lung diseases and in cyanotic congenital heart disease, where additional signs specific to the underlying cardiac abnormality may also be found.

Diagnosis (see Fig. 16.1)

The **electrocardiogram** (Fig. 16.2; see also Chapter 3) may show right axis deviation, right atrial or RV hypertrophy, but will often be unremarkable. The presence of a barrel chest in chronic lung disease diminishes electrical voltages on the ECG and may obscure evidence of hypertrophy.

The **chest radiograph** (Fig. 16.3) may show dilatation of the main pulmonary arteries in any cause of PHT, evidence of underlying lung disease or patchy pulmonary perfusion defects (chronic thromboembolic PHT).

Pulmonary function tests are often slightly abnormal in IPHT, but will usually be more

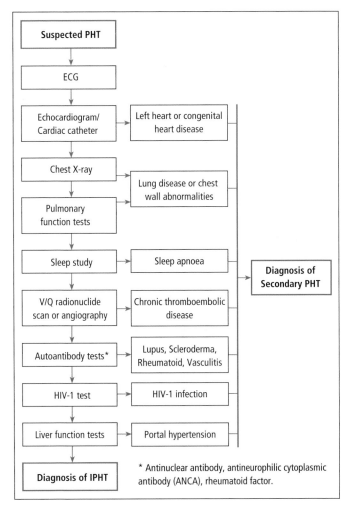

Fig. 16.1 Algorithm for investigation of suspected pulmonary hypertension.

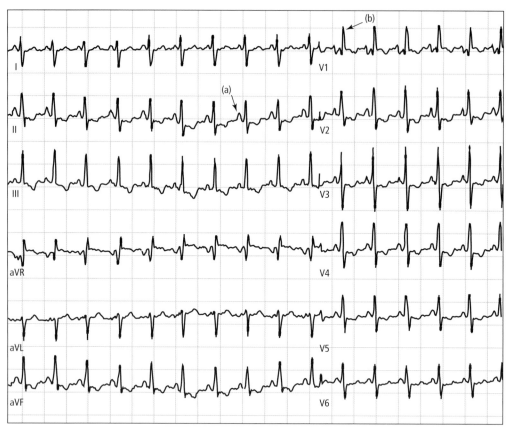

Fig. 16.2 ECG taken from a patient with chronic PHT showing p pulmonale (a), RV hypertrophy (b) with strain pattern and right-axis deviation.

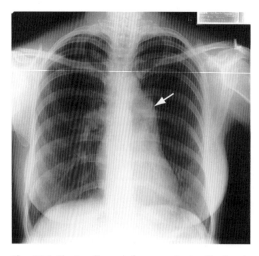

Fig. 16.3 Chest radiograph from a patient with chronic PHT showing enlargement of the main pulmonary artery.

abnormal in patients with underlying lung disease. Carbon monoxide diffusing capacity is particularly low when PHT is present.

Ventilation–perfusion (V/Q) lung scanning (see Fig. 16.4) is undertaken if pulmonary embolism is suspected (patchy perfusion).

Computed tomography (CT) scanning is increasingly used both to image the pulmonary arteries and to look for evidence of underlying lung parenchymal disease. Congenital cardiac abnormalities may also be demonstrable.

Echocardiography may show underlying cardiac disease (congenital or acquired) and allows pulmonary artery pressure to be estimated (see Chapter 4).

Right heart catheterization is undertaken to confirm a diagnosis of PHT, and to assess its severity and the vasodilatory response to drugs or high concentration of inspired oxygen. Pulmonary arteriography may show evidence of thromboembolic disease.

Hypoxaemia associated with IPHT may be at least partially improved by inspiration of 100% oxygen (FiO_2), unlike in conditions of arteriovenous admixture (congenital cardiac shunts) where pulmonary venous blood is already maximally oxygenated. In children, this difference in response to an increase in FiO_2 may be used to help distinguish cardiac from pulmonary causes of hypoxaemia.

Prognosis

The prognosis in IPHT is variable, but depends on its severity, rate of progression and response or otherwise to vasodilator therapy. Average survival from diagnosis may be as low as 1–3 years without treatment, whereas patients treated with, for example, epoprostenol (prostacyclin) often have markedly improved prognosis (55 vs. 28% 5-year survival when compared with untreated).

Treatment

For secondary causes of PHT, treatment should be directed towards the underlying aetiology. Lung diseases may respond to steroids, bronchodilators, domiciliary oxygen and antibiotics, and congenital or acquired cardiac defects may be correctable surgically or ameliorated by a variety of pharmacological agents (see Chapter 18). **Oxygen** is a potent pulmonary vasodilator and, for any cause of PHT, supplementary domiciliary administration of oxygen, using either gas cylinders or an air concentrator, may improve symptoms. There is no evidence that supplementary oxygen alters prognosis.

In IPHT, oral **vasodilator drugs** are often used, but should be started with caution and under medical supervision because the vasodilator may dilate the systemic, but have little effect on the pulmonary, vasculature, causing a marked fall in systemic blood pressure. When PVR is high, a compensatory increase in cardiac output may be impossible because of the fixed PVR and RV impairment. Acute cardiac decompensation and sometimes death may result. A beneficial symptomatic or haemodynamic response to vasodilators may indicate that the pulmonary vessels are still capable of some vasodilatation and may identify patients at an earlier stage in their disease process. The importance of selecting patients for vasodilator therapy, having experience in using the various agents available and the advantages of concentrating experience of this rare condition, strongly argues for the management of IPHT patients to be supervised by a few highly specialist centres.

In most centres, vasoreactivity is quantified by administration of a potent, short-acting vasodilator (IV epoprostenol or adenosine, or inhaled nitric oxide) under haemodynamic monitoring. Inhaled nitric oxide has the advantage of being selective for the pulmonary vascular bed. For those who are found to be responsive, oral **calcium channel blockers** can be used, particularly the dihydropyridines (nifedipine, amlodipine) or diltiazem if tachycardia is present. Verapamil is not advised because of its negative inotropism. For both responders and non-responders, other agents may also be used.

- **Prostacyclin and its analogues**: epoprostenol (prostacyclin) acts via specific receptors linked to adenylate cyclase, producing vasodilatation secondary to increased intracellular cAMP, and potentially beneficial effects on vascular remodelling, reducing ongoing endothelial damage and modulating platelet function. It is given by continuous intravenous infusion (by external pump) or by intermittent inhalation (iloprost, a prostacyclin analogue). Side-effects include jaw pain, diarrhoea and arthralgias.
- **Endothelin receptor antagonists**: endothelin (ET) has long-term effects on vascular smooth muscle cell proliferation. Bosentan is a novel orally administered ET receptor antagonist, which has shown encouraging results (liver function tests require monitoring).
- **Phosphodiesterase inhibitors**: sildenafil (Viagra) is an orally administered cGMP phosphodiesterase (PDE type 5) inhibitor that enhances nitric oxide-mediated vasodilatation and inhibits proliferation of vascular smooth muscle cells.

Doses of all these agents may need to be titrated to high levels over time. ACE inhibitors have not been shown to be beneficial.

Surgical treatment for primary PHT has included a variety of procedures, such as double (preferred) or single lung transplantation, with or without additional heart transplantation (depending on the severity of associated cardiac dysfunction), and for chronic thromboembolic PHT has involved disobliteration of the proximal pulmonary arteries by thromboendarterectomy. The results of all these surgical procedures have been encouraging, but case selection is important. Creation of an intracardiac right-to-left shunt by **balloon atrial septostomy** has been performed in a few patients with syncope or severe right heart failure in an attempt to increase systemic blood flow by bypassing the pulmonary vascular obstruction, despite the consequent arterial desaturation. Procedural mortality can be high (15–20%).

Patients with IPHT are at increased risk of intrapulmonary thrombosis and thromboembolism, due to sluggish blood flow, dilated right heart chambers, venous stasis and a sedentary lifestyle. Even a small thrombus can cause haemodynamic deterioration in a patient with a compromised pulmonary vascular bed. Patients with IPHT should therefore be anticoagulated with **warfarin** to achieve an international normalized ratio (INR) of 2.0–2.5. By inference, patients with secondary PHT (and no contraindication to warfarin) may also benefit from anticoagulation, but evidence for this is unavailable.

Pulmonary embolism

Introduction

The incidence of pulmonary embolism (PE) is difficult to ascertain because cases occur in a wide variety of hospital and community settings, and it has been estimated that at least half of all PEs go unreported. A 20-year study in the USA showed that the age-adjusted rate of deaths reported as being due to PE decreased from 191 per million in 1979 to 94 per million in 1998 overall. During the study period, the age-adjusted mortality rates for blacks were consistently 50% higher than those for whites, and those for whites were 50% higher than those for people of other races (Asian, American Indian, etc.). Within racial strata, mortality rates were consistently 20–30% higher among men than among women. Each year about 1 per 1000 of the UK population will have a PE, mainly during or soon after a period of hospitalization; the incidence rises with age. In an acute general hospital, PE may contribute to 1% of all admissions and to 10–15% of deaths.

Aetiology

The classical clinical triad that predisposes to venous thromboembolism was described by Rudolph Virchow in 1856 as:
1 local trauma to a vessel wall;
2 hypercoagulability; and
3 blood stasis.

Most patients with PE have clinical conditions associated with these predisposing factors such as:
• major trauma;
• recent surgery;
• obesity;
• immobility;
• smoking;
• increasing age;
• malignant disease;
• oral contraceptive pill;
• pregnancy;
• hormone replacement therapy;
• less common conditions (e.g. hyperviscosity syndromes, nephrotic syndrome).

Some patients with PE but without obvious predisposing clinical risk factors have hypercoagulable clotting disorders. Resistance to activated protein C, caused by mutation of the factor V gene (**Leiden mutation**), may be present in up to 5% of the population, increases the risk of thromboses by 8–10 times, and is found in 20–40% of those presenting with thromboses. Other prothrombotic conditions include elevated levels of antiphospholipid antibodies or factor VIII, defective fibrinolysis and deficiencies of antithrombin III, protein C, protein A or plasminogen. In general, primary coagulation abnormalities are uncommon and routine screening is considered not cost-effective, except for patients less than 50 years of age, those with a family history of thromboembolism and those with recurrent episodes of PE in the absence of an obvious cause.

Pathophysiology

The clinical effects of PE depend on:
- the extent of pulmonary vascular obstruction;
- the release of vasoactive and bronchoconstricting humoral agents from activated platelets (e.g. serotonin, thromboxane A2);
- the presence of pre-existing cardiopulmonary disease;
- the age and general health of the patient.

RV afterload increases significantly when >25% of the pulmonary circulation is obstructed, and PHT is exacerbated by associated vasoconstriction due to hypoxaemia and the presence of inflammatory mediators. This results initially in a rise in RV pressure, followed by RV dilatation and tricuspid regurgitation and, as the RV begins to fail, a fall in RV pressure. An otherwise normal RV is incapable of increasing pulmonary artery pressure much above 50–60 mmHg in response to sudden major obstruction of the pulmonary circulation, whereas in chronic thromboembolic or primary PHT RV pressure may rise gradually to suprasystemic (>100 mmHg) levels. A combination of reduced pulmonary blood flow and displacement of the interventricular septum into the left ventricular (LV) cavity by a dilating RV, impairs LV filling. Thus, the dyspnoea of patients with acute severe obstruction of the pulmonary circulation may be eased by manoeuvres that increase systemic venous return and LV preload, such as lying flat, tilting with the head down and infusion of intravenous colloid. This contrasts with the dyspnoea of patients with LV failure, which is eased by manoeuvres that reduce LV preload, such as sitting upright and diuretic therapy.

Clinical features

The clinical differences between the various presentations of PE are given in Table 16.1. The differential diagnosis of PE is broad and covers conditions as benign as minor anxiety states to more life-threatening diseases (Box 16.2). Many patients with PE have concomitant illnesses or are recovering from surgical procedures, which complicate the interpretation of physical findings. For instance, leg veins harvested for coronary bypass surgery result in swelling and tenderness of the operated leg, features compatible with thrombosis, even in the absence of a deep venous throm-

Table 16.1 Clinical differences between the various presentations of PE.

	Acute minor PE	Acute major PE	Chronic PE
Dyspnoea	Mild	Severe	Chronic, progressive
Chest pain	Pleuritic	Acute, dull, central	Exertional, dull, central
Tachycardia	Mild	Usually marked	Variable
Blood pressure	Normal	Low	Normal until late
Cyanosis	No	Common	Common
Oedema	No	Not acutely	Common
JVP	Normal	Raised	Raised
Heart sounds	Normal	S3	S3, S4, P2+
Chest radiograph	Often normal	Often abnormal	Abnormal
ECG	Usually normal	Often abnormal	Abnormal
PA systolic BP	Normal	30–50 mmHg	>70 mmHg

BP, blood pressure; ECG, electrocardiogram; JVP, jugular venous pressure; P2, pulmonary second sound; PA, pulmonary artery; PE, pulmonary embolism; S3, third heart sound; S4, fourth heart sound.

Box 16.2 Differential diagnosis of PE

- Myocardial infarction
- Pneumonia
- Asthma
- Pneumothorax
- Acute pulmonary oedema
- Aortic dissection
- Pleurisy
- Fractured rib
- Musculoskeletal pain
- Right- or left-heart disease
- Cor pulmonale

bosis (DVT). Cardiac surgery patients are often dyspnoeic and have chest pain postoperatively, making the diagnosis of PE more difficult. PE results in varying degrees of haemodynamic disturbance. A clinical classification has been suggested that describes the haemodynamic consequences of the embolus; however, many smaller emboli are not detected clinically.

Acute minor PE is a consequence of obstruction of small distal pulmonary arteries, often resulting in parenchymal lung infarction. When symptoms occur, they include tachypnoea, pleuritic chest pain and haemoptysis. There is usually no haemodynamic disturbance, and physical examination is often normal but may reveal a tachycardia, pleural rub and mild pyrexia.

Acute major PE results from significant obstruction to the proximal pulmonary arteries and usually causes severe dyspnoea, dull central chest pain, tachycardia, gallop rhythm, raised venous pressure and tachypnoea. When the degree of pulmonary arterial obstruction is sudden and severe, syncope or death may occur.

Chronic thromboembolic PHT is rare, occurring in approximately 0.1% of survivors of acute PE. It usually presents with a gradual onset of dyspnoea, with or without a history of previous venous thrombosis or pulmonary emboli. It is a result of chronically increasing pulmonary arterial obstruction, caused by unresolved or recurrent emboli, or thrombosis *in situ*. Exertional chest discomfort may occur, and clinical findings are those of RV pressure overload.

Investigations

Electrocardiography may show a sinus tachycardia or be normal in minor PE, but shows characteristic abnormalities in around 30% of patients with massive PE. These include the S1, Q3, T3 pattern (S wave in lead I, Q wave and inverted T wave in lead III), right bundle branch block, p pulmonale and right axis deviation. Non-specific changes, including sinus tachycardia, AF and T wave inversion in the anteroseptal leads (V_1–V_3), are seen in 80–90% of cases of proven PE.

Echocardiography: right heart dilatation may be noted and an estimation of RV pressure may be possible if tricuspid regurgitation is detected. The presence of RV dysfunction is associated with a worse outcome. Occasionally, thrombus may be seen in the right heart. If a patent foramen ovale or atrial septal defect is seen, special consideration needs to be given to the management of possible paradoxical embolism from the venous to the systemic circulation.

Chest radiography changes are often non-specific. Dilatation of a major proximal pulmonary arteries, and areas of pulmonary oligaemia may suggest major arterial obstruction. Wedge-shaped opacities in the peripheral lung fields due to pulmonary infarction, with or without a small pleural effusion, may occur with minor PE. In chronic thromboembolic PHT, the cardiothoracic ratio may be increased and there may be features suggesting RV dilatation, patchy oligaemia and dilatation of the main PAs. When PE is suspected, a normal chest radiograph in an acutely breathless, hypoxaemic patient increases the likelihood of PE. The chest radiograph is often more helpful when it suggests alternative diagnoses (e.g. lobar pneumonia).

Isotope radionuclide V/Q lung scanning (Fig. 16.4): a normal perfusion scan rules out significant PE. However, abnormal perfusion occurs in conditions other than PE, such as chronic lung disease and pneumonia and, when an assessment of ventilation is made simultaneously, evidence of V/Q mismatch greatly increases the likelihood of PE being the cause of reduced perfusion. Radionuclide scans are usually reported as representing a

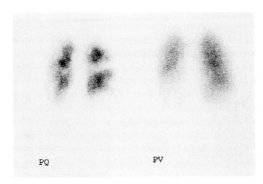

PQ PV

Fig. 16.4 Radionuclide V/Q lung scan showing normal ventilation (PV) but patchy perfusion defects (PQ) due to PE.

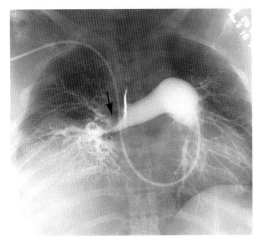

Fig. 16.5 Pulmonary angiogram showing massive PE occupying most of the right main pulmonary artery.

low, moderate or high likelihood of PE. When suggestive of PE, radionuclide scanning tends to underestimate the angiographic severity and haemodynamic disturbance of PE.

Pulmonary angiography (Fig. 16.5): patients with a normal isotope perfusion scan are extremely unlikely to have PE. The diagnosis of PE can be considered confirmed in patients in whom the index of clinical suspicion is high and whose isotope lung scan suggests PE is probable. These two groups of patients require angiography only exceptionally. However, where the index of clinical suspicion is moderate or high and the isotope scan is equivocal, angiography should be considered.

Magnetic resonance imaging (MRI) and **CT scanning**, particularly spiral (helical) contrast-enhanced CT, are increasingly used and may detect clinically unsuspected emboli. CT scanning is the investigation of choice in patients with suspected PE who also have pre-existing pulmonary disease because it allows an assessment of the co-existing lung disease, as well as helping determine whether PE is present.

D-dimer: in conditions where thrombus is formed, plasmin-mediated proteolysis of fibrin releases D-dimeric fragments. Increased levels of D-dimer have been found in 90% of patients with PE proved by V/Q lung scanning. However, although elevated levels are sensitive for the presence of PE, they are not specific. Levels are also elevated for up to 1 week postoperatively, in myocardial infarction, sepsis and other systemic illnesses. Used in conjunction with the clinical assessment, a normal D-dimer may have a negative predictive accuracy of 97% and may therefore be useful in excluding the presence of venous thrombosis.

Management (see Fig. 16.6)

General considerations

Acute PE is often fatal, with a mortality rate of around 30% in those untreated. Most patients who die from PE do so within the first few hours of the event, due to recurrent PE; treatment with anticoagulants decreases the mortality rate to 2–8%. Thus, it is imperative that effective therapy be instituted as quickly as possible. The clinical severity of PE is highly variable, ranging from asymptomatic to severe hypoxaemia and shock. As a result, management varies from patient to patient and requires clinical judgement. A clear history of the patient's symptoms and risk factors should be obtained. With few exceptions, patients suspected of having PE should have a chest radiograph and ECG, and be referred for either V/Q isotope lung scanning or CT scanning. Where the index of clinical suspicion is high, anticoagulation should be started, pending the results of investigations. Apart from supportive therapy (e.g. analgesia and oxygen), the three immediate treatment options for PE are anti-

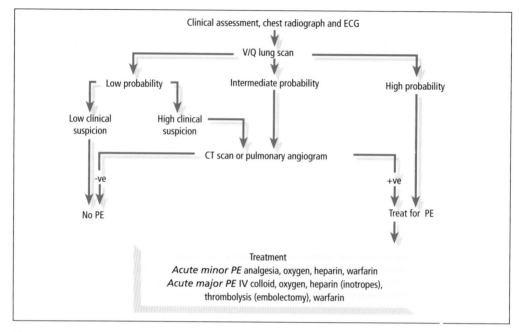

Clinical assessment, chest radiograph and ECG

V/Q lung scan

Low probability   Intermediate probability   High probability

Low clinical suspicion   High clinical suspicion

CT scan or pulmonary angiogram

-ve   +ve

No PE   Treat for PE

Treatment
Acute minor PE analgesia, oxygen, heparin, warfarin
Acute major PE IV colloid, oxygen, heparin (inotropes),
thrombolysis (embolectomy), warfarin

Fig. 16.6 Management algorithm for suspected acute PE.

coagulation with heparin, thrombolytic therapy and occasionally pulmonary embolectomy.

Anticoagulation

Heparin probably reduces mortality by reducing the likelihood of further emboli. It accelerates the action of antithrombin III and prevents further fibrin deposition, allowing the body's fibrinolytic system to lyse an existing clot. There is a tendency to under-anticoagulate patients. Those with DVT and PE may require more unfractionated heparin to achieve adequate anticoagulation than those without active thrombosis, owing to the presence of high plasma concentrations of factor VII and heparin-binding proteins. Intravenous unfractionated heparin (IV UFH) was the preferred initial treatment for acute PE, but low molecular weight heparin (LMWH) decreases mortality, recurrent PE and major bleeding compared with IV UFH, so is now the preferred option in most haemodynamically stable cases of acute PE. LMWHs are less prone to binding than UFH, so resistance is unlikely. Their half-lives are also longer, the dose response is more predictable and they cause fewer bleeding

side-effects. IV UFH may still be preferred in patients with persistent hypotension (i.e. massive PE) and patients with PE and severe renal failure; thrombus size is more often reduced by IV UFH than SC LMWH (more important where the thrombus load is greatest), and severe renal failure can alter the pharmacokinetics of SC LMWH requiring that anti-Xa activity be monitored. Since aPTT testing is more readily available than anti-Xa assays, IV UFH may be more manageable. As many as 10–20% of patients receiving UFH will develop mild and transient thrombocytopenia, and 2–3% of patients exposed to heparin for >4 days may develop the more severe immune-mediated type of heparin-induced thrombocytopenia (HIT) syndrome (see also Chapter 7).

Thrombolysis

Although no trial has been large enough conclusively to prove that lysis of acute PE reduces mortality, most would agree that pulmonary emboli clear more rapidly with thrombolytic therapy. Achieving more rapid resolution of PE seems desirable because prolonged haemodynamic disturbance harms the patient and, if further emboli occur, they will have a smaller haemodynamic effect if previous ones have been partially lysed. A second advantage of thrombolysis is that potentially dangerous iliofemoral venous thrombi may be lysed, though there is the perceived risk of detachment of thrombus from the vessel wall, resulting in further PE.

Thrombolytics obviously increase the risk of bleeding complications, and their use should therefore be carefully considered on an individual patient basis. Potential patients include those with major PE who have, or have had:

- syncope;
- persistent hypotension;
- severe hypoxaemia;
- right ventricular dysfunction;
- free-floating right heart thrombus;
- patent foramen ovale.

In other words, thrombolysis should particularly be considered for those with evidence of large emboli causing haemodynamic disturbance, or where the consequences of further emboli could be particularly serious. Whilst early reperfusion is improved, there is no definite evidence that thrombolytic therapy results in better long-term restoration of pulmonary blood flow than heparin treatment and the action of the patient's endogenous fibrinolytic mechanisms.

Pulmonary embolectomy

Some patients are so severely compromised haemodynamically that they may not survive the 1 or 2 hours required to derive benefit from thrombolysis. Also, thrombolysis is contraindicated in some patients, and others deteriorate despite its administration. For the minority of patients with massive PE who fall into these groups, surgical pulmonary embolectomy may be life-saving. Some have reported using a catheter inserted into the pulmonary artery partially to fragment the clot and improve pulmonary blood flow; smaller fragments may then respond more rapidly to thrombolysis.

Procedures on the inferior vena cava (IVC)

Once a PE has occurred, residual thrombus is almost always present in the deep veins, as has been demonstrated at autopsy in >90% of cases. Percutaneous insertion of devices into the IVC, such as filters and umbrellas, have been used to reduce further emboli from the deep pelvic/femoral veins reaching the pulmonary circulation. These techniques have been less widely used in the UK than in other European countries or the USA. The rate of recurrence of PE using treatment regimens not involving these devices is remarkably low (about 5%), and it is uncommon for treated patients to die from further embolism after hospital discharge or for them to progress to chronic thromboembolic PHT. In the acute phase of massive PE, any procedure on the IVC that reduces venous return may potentially be detrimental. However, for patients at high risk of further emboli, those in whom anticoagulation is contraindicated, those who have recurrent emboli despite adequate anticoagulation or in those with severe bleeding associated with anticoagulation, an IVC filter may be beneficial. IVC filters may decrease recurrent PE but may increase the subsequent risk of DVT. They have not been shown to reduce mortality.

Specific presentations

Acute minor PE

By definition, patients will not have haemodynamic disturbance. They should be given analgesia, oxygen and heparin; usually LMWH (enoxaparin: 1 mg/kg subcutaneously twice daily, or 1.5 mg/kg once daily — see above). When warfarin is started during active thrombosis, the levels of protein C and protein S fall, creating a thrombogenic potential. Oral loading with warfarin should therefore be covered by simultaneous heparin IV for a minimum of 5 days. Oral anticoagulation is given to achieve an INR of 2.0–3.0 and is usually continued for 3–6 months. If PE occurs in the absence of obvious risk factors, patients should be treated for at least 6–12 months, and indefinite anticoagulation should be considered. In patients with known protein C deficiency, it is important to initiate oral anticoagulation gradually while heparin therapy is ongoing because of the risk of warfarin-induced skin necrosis. LMWH may be continued long-term, rather than warfarin, in certain circumstances such as pregnancy and malignancy.

Acute major PE

Where necessary, **resuscitation** should be undertaken before investigation. Patients should be given oxygen and moved to an Intensive Care Unit (ICU) or High Dependency Unit (HDU) where haemodynamic and respiratory monitoring can be performed. A central venous line should be inserted to measure venous pressure and allow the judicious administration of intravenous colloid and inotropes, and thrombolytic agents. If thrombolytic therapy is planned, a jugular rather than infraclavicular approach should be used. If central venous monitoring is not available, transcutaneous arterial oximetry may provide an assessment of resolution. If possible, the insertion of arterial lines should be avoided when thrombolysis has been given.

Massive PE carries a high early mortality, and vigorous therapy should be pursued. **Intravenous heparin** (see above) is preferred (bolus dose of 5000 IU followed by infusion of 30000–40000 IU per 24 h, with dose adjusted to achieve an aPTT of 2.0–2.5 or adequate anti-Xa (level depends on local assay). Streptokinase, recombinant tissue-type plasminogen activator (t-PA) and recombinant human urokinase are the **thrombolytic agents** that have been most commonly used and best studied (others include lanetoplase, tenecteplase, and reteplase — see also Chapter 6). There is no evidence that intrapulmonary arterial infusion confers greater benefit than peripheral venous infusion. For streptokinase, administer 250000 units intravenously over the initial 30 min, then 100000 units/h for 24–72h; if t-PA is used, give 100 mg IV over 2 h. Heparin should be resumed when the thrombolytic dosing is completed and the aPTT is less than twice the upper limit of normal; a loading dose is not given.

Chronic thromboembolic PHT

Owing to its insidious nature, chronic thromboembolic PHT commonly presents late, at a stage when there is little alternative to surgical pulmonary thromboendarterectomy or lung or heart–lung transplantation. Although vasodilators have been used to treat chronic PHT, they are ineffective if the primary abnormality is pulmonary arterial occlusion by fixed organized thrombus, although they may help recruit remaining pulmonary vessels. Rigorous attention to oral anticoagulation control (INR 2.5–3.0) is vital. Domiciliary oxygen may help symptomatically.

Deep venous thrombosis

If a diagnosis of PE has been established, there is little to be gained by investigating the deep veins, because almost all these patients have DVT, although many are asymptomatic. In an autopsy study of patients who died of PE, 83% had a leg DVT but only 19% had shown symptoms. Similarly, PE may be asymptomatic in patients with DVT. In a treatment trial of proximal leg DVT, 40% of patients had asymptomatic PE, the diagnosis of PE being based on abnormal V/Q scans.

Investigations

If the diagnosis of PE is less clear, or radionuclide lung scanning or pulmonary angiography is not available, investigations of the deep veins may be helpful. If the clinical suspicion of PE and radionuclide lung scanning are equivocal, investigations suggesting the presence of DVT, especially proximal to the calf, indicate the need for anticoagulation. About 75% of patients who present with clinically suspected DVT do not have the condition. Only 50% of patients with DVT show the classical symptoms of a tender, swollen calf with positive Homans' sign, and these symptoms may be present in those without DVT. Thus, if DVT is suspected, further investigations are needed.

Contrast venography has been the gold standard investigation against which the newer techniques of impedance plethysmography, radiofibrinogen leg scanning and Duplex imaging (Doppler flow assessment combined with ultrasound scanning) have been assessed. Their accuracy in detecting DVT depends on operator experience.

Ultrasonography is less invasive than venography and more accurate than impedance plethysmography. In experienced hands, and with the use of colour duplex Doppler, ultrasonography of the femoral, popliteal and calf trifurcation veins is highly sensitive (>90%) for detecting proximal vein thrombosis but less sensitive (80% in symptomatic and 40–50% in asymptomatic patients) in detecting calf vein thrombosis. If the findings are normal but the clinical suspicion of venous thrombosis is high, the test should be repeated after 3–5 days. A normal investigation and normal plasma D-dimer value almost excludes thrombosis. Diagnosing recurrent venous thrombosis is often difficult because investigations may be abnormal as a result of previous episodes. In the absence of an obvious cause of DVT, occult malignancy should be sought, especially if the DVT is recurrent. Surgical procedures carrying the greatest risk of DVT include pelvic, hip and knee operations; without prophylaxis, 60–80% of these patients develop DVT. Patients suffering major trauma, myocardial infarction, stroke and thrombophilic disorders are also at risk. In these patients, low-dose subcutaneous heparin (5000 IU twice or three times a day), anti-embolism stockings and intermittent pneumatic leg compression are beneficial. The perioperative use of subcutaneous heparin can prevent about 66% of DVT, with significant reduction in fatal PE. LMWH is of particular benefit as prophylaxis in orthopaedic patients.

Treatment

Anticoagulation: treatment for an established proximal DVT is intravenous heparin, given initially as a bolus of 5000 IU and followed by a continuous infusion of at least 30 000 IU/day for 4–7 days. The dose should be adjusted on the basis of laboratory tests. Patients receiving heparin who have subtherapeutic anticoagulation in the first 24 h may have 15 times the rate of thrombotic recurrence of those who are adequately anticoagulated. Intermittent subcutaneous administration of heparin, 17 500 IU twice a day, especially with the LMWH varieties, is also effective and may allow patients to be discharged earlier. Three meta-analyses of data from trials comparing LMWH with conventional UFH suggested that LMWHs are more

effective at preventing recurrence and cause fewer bleeding side-effects. Small falls in platelet levels are common in the early stages of UFH treatment, but only 3% of patients have an immune, immunoglobulin G- (IgG)-mediated, thrombocytopenia which can be profound and should be suspected when the platelet count falls below 100 000/mm^3 or less than 50% of baseline levels. The use of LMWH considerably reduces the occurrence of this complication. Oral anticoagulation with warfarin should be started immediately, aiming for an INR of 2.5–3.0. The optimal duration of oral anticoagulant therapy is uncertain. The results of three randomized trials suggest that treatment should be for at least 3 months and possibly 6 months. Those with recurrent episodes should take warfarin in the long term. Pregnant women requiring anticoagulation should be treated with UFH or LMWH, which do not cross the placenta and are safe for the fetus; warfarin can cause fetal bleeding and is potentially teratogenic. Heparin taken for more than 4 weeks may cause osteoporosis.

Thrombolytic agents may be associated with more rapid and complete lysis of DVT and less post-phlebitic syndrome, but despite this are seldom used in patients with DVT; the clinical relevance of achieving earlier relief of venous obstruction is uncertain, thrombolytics increase the risk of major bleeding and the risk of death and early recurrence in patients with DVT is low if anticoagulants are started promptly. Most patients are unwilling to accept the increased risk of death or disability due to bleeding to prevent the post-phlebitic syndrome. The post-phlebitic syndrome, caused by venous hypertension due to venous valvular incompetence and residual venous obstruction, is a chronic complication of DVT consisting of pain, swelling and occasionally ulceration of the lower legs. It occurs in >50% of patients with proximal DVT and in about 33% of those with calf vein thrombosis. Massive proximal lower extremity or iliofemoral thrombosis, associated with severe symptomatic swelling, or limb-threatening ischaemia, are the usual indications for considering thrombolysis (see massive PE above). If thrombolytic therapy is to be administered, it should be administered within 2 weeks of onset of the DVT. The angiographic response to thrombolysis is greatest when there is a short interval between the onset of symptoms and the initiation of therapy.

Treatment of calf DVT is controversial. Diagnostic studies suggest that only 20% of calf vein thrombi extend into proximal veins within 2 weeks of presentation. The remainder are probably small and resolve without consequence. One trial suggested that the morbidity rate is lower in those who are anticoagulated for a calf DVT compared with those who are not, but the number of patients studied was small. If anticoagulants are not given, the extension of the thrombus proximal to the calf can be assessed by ultrasonography.

Further reading

British Thoracic Society guidelines for the management of suspected acute pulmonary embolism. *Thorax* 2003; 58: 470–84. http://www.brit-thoracic.org.uk/bts_guildelines_pe_html

European Society of Cardiology Task Force Report: Guidelines on diagnosis and management of acute pulmonary embolism. *European Heart Journal* 2000; 21: 1301–36. http://www.escardio.org/knowledge/guidelines/Diagnosis_and_Management_Acute_Pulmonary_Embolism.htm

Guidelines for diagnosis and treatment of primary pulmonary hypertension. *European Heart Journal* 2004; 25: 2243–78. http://www.escardio.org/knowledge/guidelines/Diagnosis_Treatment_Pulmonary_Arterial_Hypertension.htm

Chapter 17

Pregnancy and the heart

Normal pregnancy

Pregnancy and the peripartum period are associated with many cardiovascular changes. **Blood volume** increases by an average of 50% and is greater than the increase in red cell mass, leading to some dilution of haemoglobin. Haematocrit may fall by up to 35% and haemoglobin levels to around 110–120 g/L. Stroke volume and **cardiac output** increase by 30–50% but are usually lowest in the supine position due to caval compression by the gravid uterus causing reduced venous return. Systemic **blood pressure** falls to a nadir in the middle trimester due to vasodilatation, but later increases towards term and especially with the pain and anxiety of labour. Diastolic pressure falls more than systolic, causing an increase in pulse pressure. The **heart rate** normally increases by 10–20 bpm in the last trimester. Vaginal delivery causes as much haemodynamic stress as a Caesarean section and should not be regarded necessarily as a safer option for the pregnant woman with pre-existing heart disease.

During normal pregnancy, **symptoms** include:

- tiredness;
- reduced exercise tolerance;
- dyspnoea;
- orthopnoea;
- lightheadedness;
- syncope occasionally.

On examination, **signs** include:

- tachycardia;
- wide pulse pressure;
- peripheral oedema;
- elevated jugular venous pressure (JVP);
- palpable right ventricular impulse;
- loud first heart sound (S1);
- increased splitting of the second heart sound (S2);
- mid-systolic flow murmurs.

The **electrocardiogram** (ECG) may show QRS axis deviation and T-wave changes, and **echocardiography** reveals increased left and right ventricular dimensions, mild increases in atrial size, mild functional mitral and tricuspid regurgitation, and small pericardial effusion.

Congenital heart disease

Most patients with non-cyanotic heart disease can be managed through a successful pregnancy, although the associated haemodynamic changes usually result in worsening of symptoms. An unfavourable outcome can be anticipated in cyanotic heart disease, those with severe pulmonary hypertension and in patients with severe symptoms before pregnancy. Elective induction once the fetus is mature, with haemodynamic monitoring and specialized medical care, can improve outcome. Caesarean section is considered in most women with anything other than simple congenital heart disease (e.g. atrial septal defect (ASD)). The need for antibiotic prophylaxis is disputed, but many feel that the risk of giving antibiotics is so small and the potential consequences of endocarditis so potentially catastrophic that, with the exception of a secundum ASD, all patients with congenital heart disease should be given prophylaxis.

Primary pulmonary hypertension

This carries a high maternal mortality during pregnancy (40%), which should ideally be avoided or termination considered. Because oral contraceptives have been suggested as possible aetiological factors in this condition, sterilization by tubal ligation is the preferred form of birth control. If a pregnancy is continued for any reason, treatment is the same as for the underlying condition, with spontaneous vaginal delivery being preferable to induction. If Caesarean section is considered, great care is required with anaesthetic agents which may cause profound hypotension (negative inotropism, systemic vasodilatation).

Rheumatic heart disease

Progress through pregnancy depends on the nature and severity of the valvular disease. The most common lesion is mitral stenosis (MS), the haemodynamic effects of which can be expected to be much worse with the associated increase in blood volume. Unless the MS is severe (valve area <1 cm²), patients can normally be managed through a vaginal delivery. Epidural anaesthesia is the preferred route, because this induces vasodilatation and a consequent beneficial fall in left atrial and pulmonary artery pressures. In severe MS with deteriorating haemodynamics, successful closed surgical mitral valvotomy or percutaneous balloon mitral valvuloplasty have been reported. Care must be taken to minimize any radiation exposure to the pregnant mother and, if procedures involving radiation are necessary, these should be delayed until as late in pregnancy as possible. Open mitral valve operations (valvotomy or replacement) carry a higher risk to mother and fetus.

Patients with mitral or aortic regurgitation and those with anything other than severe aortic stenosis tolerate pregnancy fairly well. Most would recommend prophylactic antibiotics for vaginal or Caesarean delivery for all patients with valvular disease. Oral anticoagulants are potentially teratogenic, and management in pregnant patients requiring anticoagulation for native or prosthetic valve reasons requires specialist cardiological and haematological involvement.

Cardiomyopathies

The majority of patients with **hypertrophic cardiomyopathy** (HCM) can be managed successfully through pregnancy, although worsening of symptoms is common and the risk of ventricular arrhythmias increases. Treatment is similar to that of the non-pregnant female with the condition, taking care to avoid drugs that may be teratogenic or worsen fetal haemodynamics. The risk of endocarditis is increased in HCM, especially of the obstructive type, and most would recommend antibiotic prophylaxis for delivery. **Peripartum cardiomyopathy** is a rare but well-recognized condition of unknown aetiology, which occurs in approximately 1:10000 pregnancies but with higher occurrence in Africa (up to 1%). The incidence is greater in women with twins, those over 30 years of age and in multiparas. It results in a dilated cardiomyopathy, which can be severe and life-threatening, with symptoms often starting in the last trimester but sometimes dismissed as being due to the later stages of normal pregnancy. Hence, the diagnosis may only be revealed after delivery. Treatment is similar to that of any patient with heart failure, hydralazine being a useful vasodilator which is safe in pregnancy. Most will improve to a varying and unpredictable degree on delivery of the fetus. The condition can recur in further pregnancies.

Hypertension

See Chapter 5.

Arrhythmias (see also Chapter 13)

Pregnancy is associated with an increased incidence of arrhythmias both in those with and in those without known pre-existing cardiac disease. In healthy women, frequent atrial and ventricular ectopics may occur. Palpitations, dizziness and even syncope can occur in normal pregnancy and they are only occasionally associated with a documented arrhythmia. Atrial flutter and fibrillation are rare, but re-entry tachycardias are commonly exacerbated in pregnancy. Anti-arrhythmic drugs should be avoided if at all possible, although **digoxin, quinidine, lidocaine (lignocaine) and adenosine** are thought to be safe. Direct current (DC) cardioversion can be performed if an arrhythmia is prolonged or haemodynamically compromising.

Antibiotic prophylaxis in pregnancy

- Ampicillin IV or IM 2.0g with gentamicin IM 1.5mg/kg (not >80mg) 30min before procedure/delivery, with amoxycillin 1.5g orally 6h later or IV 8h later.
- In those allergic to penicillin use vancomycin IV 1.0g over 1h with gentamicin IM 1.5mg/kg (not >80mg) 1h before the procedure and again 8h after.
- For the low-risk patients 3.0g of amoxycillin orally 1h before the procedure, and 1.5g 6h after, is sufficient.

Chapter 18

Congenital heart disease

Introduction

The incidence of congenital heart disease is around 0.8% of live births, making it the most common congenital abnormality. Most of these lesions are simple and require only surveillance, with a small proportion requiring intervention in later life. However, some are severe and complex, and approximately 4 per 1000 children will require intervention in infancy.

Twenty years ago surgery was categorized as palliative or 'corrective'. Nowadays we recognize that most interventions are in fact palliative, and lifelong surveillance is necessary as new complications can develop. These are commonly in the form of progressive valvular and muscle dysfunction, and arrhythmias. The superimposition of acquired cardiac disease, such as systemic hypertension and coronary artery disease, will further increase the complexity of the long-term clinical management of these patients.

This chapter will deal with the common structural abnormalities, and the relationship between pathophysiology, clinical presentation and treatment is highlighted. The long-term clinical problems and their treatment are discussed in the context of the initial structural problems and the early treatment.

The fetal circulation and its adaptation to postnatal life

The fetal circulation (Fig. 18.1)

Knowledge of the fetal circulation is vital to understanding congenital heart disease presenting in the newborn. The placenta oxygenates fetal blood (fetal lungs contain amniotic fluid), which returns to the fetus via the umbilical vein. From there, some flows directly to the liver, but most passes through the ductus venosus to the inferior vena cava and then onwards to the right atrium (RA). Streaming preferentially directs this RA blood across the patent foramen ovale (PFO) to the left atrium (LA); it then flows via the left ventricle (LV) to the ascending aorta. The carotid arteries arise from the aortic arch and thus ensure the developing brain is well oxygenated. Deoxygenated blood from the head and neck returns via the jugular veins and superior vena cava (SVC) to the RA, and then streams preferentially to the right ventricle (RV), then the main pulmonary artery (MPA). Fetal pulmonary vascular resistance (PVR) is high, so blood does not flow to the lung circulation but shunts through the patent ductus arteriosus (PDA) into the descending aorta (DA). It mixes with oxygenated blood from the aortic arch, and flows to

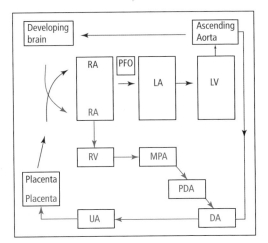

Fig. 18.1 Fetal circulation.

the lower body and, via the umbilical artery (UA), to the placenta again.

Normal adaptation to postnatal life

With the onset of breathing, gas transfer occurs in the alveoli, there is a fall in PVR, and an increase in pulmonary blood flow and pulmonary venous return to the LA. The LA pressure increases and then exceeds that in the RA, causing the flap of tissue overlying the PFO to close the defect. The PDA gradually closes and the circulation rapidly adopts the 'adult', in-series pattern. The PVR reaches its nadir at about 6 weeks when it reaches about 20% of the systemic vascular resistance (SVR), and normally remains at this level for life.

Failure of postnatal adaptation

There are three clinical scenarios that can be attributed to failure of complete adaptation of the circulation from fetal to postnatal life (Box 18.1).

1. Patent foramen ovale (Fig. 18.2)

Complete closure of the PFO occurs in 75% of humans, eliminating any potential RA–LA communication. However, in 25% the flap is to varying degrees non-adherent, resulting in small to very large (up to 2.5 cm) communications at times when

Box 18.1

Failure of post natal adaptation to adult circulation:
- Patent foramen ovale (PFO)
- Patent ductus arteriosus
- Pulmonary hypertension

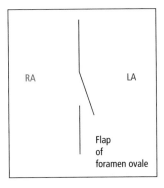

Fig. 18.2 Patent foramen ovale.

RA pressure exceeds that in the LA. Usually PFOs have no clinical consequences, but a few otherwise healthy individuals appear to raise their RA pressure above that of the LA at times, with four potentially adverse sequelae (paradoxical emboli, decompression sickness, migraine and systemic hypoxaemia — see below). Closure of the PFO may be recommended, and increasingly this can be performed using catheter techniques. Investigation is usually by contrast echocardiography; 10 mL of agitated saline is injected into an antecubital vein with simultaneous transthoracic echocardiography, whilst the patient undertakes the valsalva manoeuvre (see page 16). Contrast will be seen entering the right heart then rapidly filling the LA and LV in susceptible patients.

Paradoxical embolism

Thrombus derived from the systemic venous system, most commonly the pelvic veins, normally embolizes to the lungs (pulmonary emboli — see Chapter 16), and when small are filtered from the circulation without clinical sequelae. Larger clots embolizing to the lungs will cause symptoms depending on their size as a result of haemodynamic compromise. **Paradoxical embolism** is a result of venous-derived clot gaining access to the systemic arterial circulation through a connection between the right and left heart, the most common being a PFO. Clots can therefore gain access to any part of the systemic circulation, resulting in a range of conditions including cerebral transient ischaemic attacks (TIAs), stroke, mesenteric embolism, limb ischaemia, etc. Young patients who do not have risk factors for arterial disease may need to be investigated to exclude paradoxical embolism when presenting with one of these conditions.

Decompression sickness
While surfacing, any nitrogen coming out of solution in the venous system is normally exhaled from the lungs. With a PFO and tendency to right-to-left shunting (RA pressure is elevated by immersion), the diver may suffer catastrophic complications from arterial nitrogen embolism (the 'bends').

Migraine
Certain types of migraine have recently been noted to occur more frequently in patients with PFO, and closure may substantially improve symptoms in highly selected patients. The mechanism for this is unclear but seems likely to be related to the passage of vasoactive amines from the hepatic portal venous system to the cerebral circulation without some filtering effect normally provided by the lungs.

Systemic hypoxaemia
A few patients will develop symptomatic hypoxaemia, particularly on exertion, because of right-to-left shunting of a large amount of deoxygenated blood into the systemic circulation across a PFO.

2. Patent ductus arteriosus

Failure of closure of the ductus arteriosus is common in premature infants and occurs less commonly in term babies. As the PVR falls, there is increasing flow from the aorta to the pulmonary arteries, the amount depending on the anatomical size of the ductus. This 'additional' pulmonary blood then flows via the pulmonary veins to the LA and LV, which dilate, and in more severe examples

will elevate LA and pulmonary venous pressure to a level where pulmonary oedema develops. The baby will present with breathlessness and poor weight gain. Where surgery is required, the duct is ligated through a left thoracotomy. Transcatheter closure of the PDA can be undertaken in older infants, children and adults.

3. Persistent pulmonary hypertension (PHT) of the newborn

A very small percentage of newborn babies do not develop the normal progressive fall in PVR, and the pulmonary vascular bed remains vasoconstricted. PHT occurs as a result of progressive vasoconstriction, medial hypertrophy and intimal proliferation. The RV eventually develops suprasystemic pressures and RV failure, and increased RA pressure develops. Where a PFO is present, 'right-to-left' shunting occurs when RA pressure exceeds that of the LA, causing increased cyanosis. Similar shunting and cyanosis will also occur if a PDA is present and pulmonary arterial pressure exceeds aortic. Pulmonary arterial vasodilators have been used in the hope of reducing right-sided pressures and allowing some remodelling of the pulmonary vascular bed, but prognosis remains poor in this condition and heart–lung transplantation may be required.

Conditions causing arteriovenous shunts

This group of abnormalities includes PDA, and atrial and ventricular septal defects. To understand the haemodynamic effects and clinical features associated with each of these, it is important to analyse principles of preload, afterload and myocardial function (see Chapter 8). Left-to-right shunts through these defects are measured as a ratio between pulmonary (Qp) and systemic (Qs) blood flow. A common shunt would be 2:1, i.e. the Qp is twice the volume of Qs. Young infants can have very large shunts where >2:1 would normally be symptomatic and need surgery. The descriptions below assume a normal PVR; this is not always the case and the onset of PHT is discussed in the section on Eisenmenger syndrome (p. 249).

Atrial septal defects (ASDs)

Pathophysiology

After birth, LA pressure exceeds RA pressure and a left-to-right shunt develops through the defect. The RA and RV therefore receive, in addition to the normal systemic venous return, the volume of blood that has crossed the septum (the 'shunt'). The size of the shunt depends on the defect's size and the pressure gradient between the LA and RA. The RA enlarges and increases RV preload (diastolic filling) leading to RV dilatation. RV stroke volume and pulmonary blood flow increase (see Fig. 18.3 and Box 18.2). In a normal circulation, the negative intra-thoracic pressure associated with inspiration promotes systemic venous return and RA

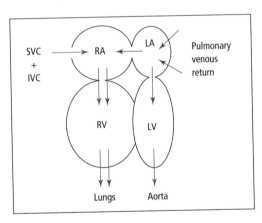

Fig. 18.3 Atrial septal defects.

Box 18.2

In a patient with a large ASD:
- RA preload is increased. **The RA is dilated**
- RV preload is increased. **The RV is dilated**
- RV afterload is normal (if pulmonary vascular disease has not supervened). **The RV is not hypertrophied**
- LA preload is increased (increased pulmonary blood flow) but there is continuous off-loading to the RA. **The LA is not dilated**
- LV preload is normal or reduced. **The LV is not dilated**

---

filling increases; LA filling is reduced. In a large ASD, this differential is lost and respiration has the same effect on filling of both atria. This leads to important auscultatory findings.

Symptoms

Presentation can be at any age but is uncommon in infants. Most ASDs are picked up because of abnormal auscultatory findings, but exercise intolerance and recurrent respiratory symptoms are common. Symptoms increase with age as the degree of left-to-right shunting tends to increase with time. Rarely a patient can present with a cerebral abscess.

Signs (see also Chapter 2)

Signs include an RV heave (RV dilatation), wide and fixed splitting of the second sound (wide because the pulmonary component of the second sound is delayed, and fixed because respiration does not alter the degree of splitting of the second sound in an ASD for reasons stated above), and because of increased pulmonary blood flow, a pulmonary ejection murmur. If there is a very large shunt at atrial level, there may be a tricuspid diastolic flow murmur (maximal at the lower left sternal edge).

Investigations

The chest X-ray may show cardiomegaly with a prominent right atrial border, large central pulmonary arteries and pulmonary plethora (increased pulmonary blood flow). Transthoracic echocardiography will usually show the ASD, and RA, RV and pulmonary artery dilatation. Transoesophageal echocardiography (TOE) is useful in patients with poor precordial windows.

Anatomical subtypes of atrial septal defects

Secundum ASDs

These are the most common type of defect and are in the region of the fossa ovalis, so the defect is usually in the central atrial septum. The atrioventricular (AV) valves are not normally affected but mitral valve prolapse may occur. The ECG would normally show sinus rhythm with incomplete right bundle branch block (iRBBB) and **right** axis deviation. RV hypertrophy will be present only if there is associated PHT (see Eisenmenger syndrome, p. 249 below). Closure of these defects is commonly achieved with a catheter-delivered device.

Partial atrioventricular septal defects (primum ASD)

These occur in the lower part of the atrial septum, adjacent to the AV valves which are usually abnormal; the left is commonly regurgitant. This is the defect most common seen in patients with Down syndrome. Presentation is usually earlier than with the secundum type. Surgery is usually necessary to correct the abnormality because of the usual AV valve involvement. The ECG usually demonstrates sinus rhythm with iRBBB and **left** axis deviation.

Sinus venosus defects

These are usually large and in the part of the septum just underneath the superior vena cava (SVC). The SVC tends to override the septum and the right-sided pulmonary veins may drain anomalously to the RA. Surgery is necessary to close the defect and correct any abnormality of pulmonary venous drainage. ECG shows sinus rhythm with iRBBB and right or left axis deviation.

Anomalous pulmonary venous drainage

When drainage of some of the pulmonary veins is to some part of the right heart, instead of the LA, it is described as partial anomalous pulmonary venous drainage (PAPVD) and when **all** veins drain to the right heart the term total anomalous pulmonary venous drainage (TAPVD) is used. Drainage of the veins can be directly to the RA, the coronary sinus or to any other systemic venous drainage channel (left innominate vein, SVC or IVC). These abnormalities can occur in isolation or in association with an ASD. As the haemodynamic effects (left-to-right shunt) are identical to those of an ASD, their presentation and clinical features are very similar. TOE is the investigation of choice.

When sufficient to cause right heart dilatation, or where associated with a significant ASD, the abnormal vein or veins can be redirected into the LA surgically.

Ventricular septal defects (VSDs)

Defects in the ventricular septum are common; up to 10% of newborns have a small communication when studied with colour Doppler echocardiography. The vast majority close spontaneously and, if they do not, become haemodynamically insignificant as the child grows. A number of adults with smaller defects may develop symptoms with dyspnoea and exercise intolerance, having been asymptomatic for many years.

Pathophysiology

After birth, as the PVR falls, a large defect will present with the signs of a large shunt. As pulmonary artery and RV pressures fall, there is increasing (systolic) flow from the LV, through the VSD and RV to the pulmonary vascular bed. Increased pulmonary venous return to the LA and LV results in their dilatation. In diastole, RV filling (preload) is normal (normal systemic venous return) and so the RV is not usually dilated. LV stroke volume is increased, although a significant proportion is directed back via the VSD to the pulmonary vascular bed. If the shunt is very large, the LV end-diastolic and LA pressures, and pulmonary venous pressures, may rise enough for pulmonary oedema to develop (see Fig. 18.4 and Box 18.3).

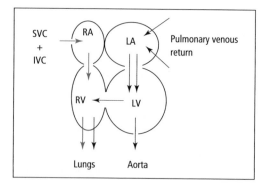

Fig. 18.4 Ventricular septal defects.

> **Box 18.3**
>
> In a patient with a large VSD:
> - RA preload is normal. **The RA is not dilated**
> - RV preload is normal. **The RV is not dilated**
> - RV afterload is normal (if pulmonary vascular disease has not supervened): **The RV is not hypertrophied**
> - LA preload is increased (increased pulmonary blood flow). **The LA is dilated**
> - LV preload is increased. **The LV is dilated in diastole**

Symptoms

Babies with large VSDs will present with poor feeding and low weight gain. They will be sweaty and have hepatomegaly. Some older patients who have been asymptomatic for some years can become symptomatic in later life and this may reflect progressive changes in LV diastolic function. As part of ageing, and particularly with the development of ischaemic heart disease and/or hypertension, LV diastolic pressures rise. Patients with a VSD are very sensitive to this as even the small increase in preload resulting from the VSD may lead to greater than expected increases in LV diastolic pressure, LA and pulmonary venous pressures. Late closure of a VSD may be indicated for symptoms in some of these patients.

Clinical signs (see Chapter 2)

These include a precordial thrill, displaced LV impulse (LV dilatation) and loud pansystolic murmur at the left lower sternal edge. In moderate or large shunts, a mitral diastolic flow murmur at the apex may be present.

Investigations

With small defects, ECG and chest X-ray may be normal. In larger defects, the ECG may show LV hypertrophy and LA enlargement on voltage criteria. Signs of biventricular hypertrophy may be present. Chest X-ray may show cardiomegaly, LV dilatation, prominent pulmonary arteries and plethora. Infants may show pulmonary oedema.

Echocardiography usually shows the defects and any associated abnormalities, with Doppler allowing an assessment of right heart pressure.

Anatomical subtypes of VSD

Perimembranous

These lie in the perimembranous septum behind the septal leaflet of the tricuspid valve (TV) and immediately beneath the aortic valve. Spontaneous partial or complete closure can occur, often by adherence of the TV septal leaflet to the margins of the VSD (so-called 'aneurysmal closure'). Aortic regurgitation (AR) can develop as prolapse of one of its coronary cusps (most commonly the right) into the VSD can occur. Mid-cavity RV obstruction can occur.

Doubly committed VSD

These occur immediately below the pulmonary and aortic valves (also called subpulmonary defect) and can be associated with AR. They are generally large, show less tendency to close than other types of VSD and often require surgical closure.

Muscular VSD

This is found anywhere in the muscular septum, commonly apical (particularly in neonates), and the majority undergo spontaneous closure.

Treatment

Most VSDs requiring intervention in infancy require surgery. In older children and adults, some defects are being closed by transcatheter techniques.

Eisenmenger syndrome

Eisenmenger syndrome is a term used to define a specific sequence of events in patients with long-term left-to-right shunts. These patients begin life with an ASD, VSD or PDA. After the early fall in PVR that occurs in the first few weeks of life, pulmonary blood flow increases and in some the pulmonary vascular bed develops aggressive vasoconstriction. Medial hypertrophy (similar to that noted in fetal and early neonatal life) redevelops and PVR increases. Right heart pressures rise and pulmonary blood flow decreases. Eventually PVR exceeds SVR and the direction of shunting reverses to right to left. The patient becomes increasingly cyanosed, and symptoms of hypoxaemia dominate (fatigue, breathlessness, worsening exercise capacity). Pulmonary vasodilators (oxygen, calcium antagonists, prostacyclin, bosentan, sildenafil) can improve symptoms, but heart–lung transplantation may be required. Other complications include sudden death, polycythaemia, thrombosis, cerebral abscess, right heart failure and severe haemoptysis.

Obstructive lesions

Lesions of the semilunar valves (aortic and pulmonary stenosis), aorta (coarctation) and Fallot's tetralogy are associated with obstruction to flow to either the systemic or pulmonary circulation.

Aortic stenosis (AS)

Congenital abnormalities of the aortic valve are common (4% of the population), the most common being described as the **bicuspid** aortic valve, although the majority of these valves are anatomi-cally tricuspid but have one hypoplastic cusp and commissural fusion leading to functionally bicuspid AS. In adults, normal aortic valves, or those with a minor congenital abnormality, can become progressively stenotic as thickening and calcification develops (see Chapter 10). In this section we will focus on critical AS of the newborn and severe AS in the older infant and child (Fig. 18.5).

Critical AS of the newborn

These valves are severely deformed, and usually functionally bicuspid or even monocuspid. The degree of AS may be so severe that the systemic circulation is dependent on right-to-left shunting through a persistent ductus arteriosus ('duct dependent') after birth, and severe cardiac failure may occur. The LV is frequently hypoplastic, but may be dilated and poorly contractile. Emergency aortic valvotomy is indicated and can be undertaken surgically or percutaneously by balloon dilatation. Not uncommonly, long-term residual LV dysfunction occurs. Valvotomy is only palliative, as restenosis or progressive regurgitation is inevitable and a surgical 'Ross procedure' or mechanical valve replacement will be required, but is delayed where possible to allow growth of the child.

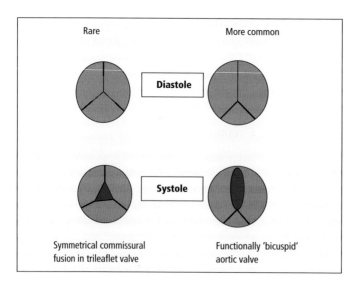

Fig. 18.5 Aortic stenosis.

Severe AS in an older infant or child

Patients presenting after the neonatal period tend to have less deformed valves, less severe stenosis and better LV function than those with newborn AS. Balloon or surgical valvotomy may be indicated for those children with pressure gradients >60–70 mmHg on catheter withdrawal across the valve, or a mean >40 mmHg on Doppler assessment. Intervention with lower gradients may be indicated for the symptomatic or where LV dysfunction develops.

Coarctation of the aorta

Narrowing (coarctation) of the aorta is usually in the distal aortic arch, immediately after the origin of the left subclavian artery and just proximal to the site of the ductus arteriosus, but varying degrees of aortic hypoplasia can occur elsewhere. Ductal tissue can be present circumferentially around the aorta at the site of the PDA and, as ductal closure occurs, constriction of the aorta leads to clinical coarctation. Broadly, two clinical presentations occur: critical neonatal coarctation and less severe coarctation presenting later in infancy or onwards ('adult type').

Neonatal coarctation (see Fig. 18.6)

Neonatal coarction presents with severe congestive cardiac failure and acidosis due to poor lower body and renal perfusion. The infant is often well at birth because aspects of the fetal circulation persist for longer than in the normal neonate; the PDA may be patent for a few days and PVR may remain high so some right-to-left shunting (PDA to the descending aorta) may provide adequate lower body and renal perfusion. Femoral pulses may be palpable at this time, so delaying diagnosis. However, when PVR does fall and/or the PDA closes (usually a few days), the child will become critically ill. Emergency medical treatment aims to increase PVR (hypoventilation to raise the CO_2 and normoxaemia) and reopen the ductus arteriosus (IV prostaglandin), but urgent surgery to resect the coarctation through a left thoracotomy will be required. Balloon dilatation can be effective in a minority.

'Adult' coarctation

These children and adults present after ductal closure but are able to perfuse the lower body adequately, but sub-optimally, through the coarct segment. However, upper body hypertension and LV hypertrophy results. Signs include weak femoral pulses, radiofemoral delay and a systolic murmur at the upper left sternal edge, radiating to the back. In the longer term increased flow through existing arteries (e.g. internal mammaries, which arise from subclavian arteries, and intercostals) collateralizing with the descending aorta develops and flow through these can also be heard over the posterior chest. Enlargement of the intercostals creates the 'rib notching' that may be seen in older patients on chest X-ray. Surgery or balloon dilatation (with or without stent placement) should be undertaken to avoid the long-term complications of hypertension. Hypertension may persist even after correction of the coarct and should be treated conventionally (see Chapter 5).

Pulmonary valvar stenosis (PS)

Unlike AS, PS is almost always congenital in origin and may be part of a more generalized syndrome (e.g. Noonan syndrome). Occasionally, carcinoid

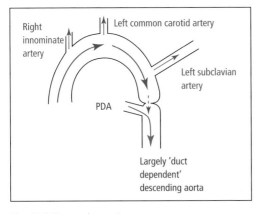

Fig. 18.6 Neonatal coarction.

Right innominate artery

Left common carotid artery

Left subclavian artery

PDA

Largely 'duct dependent' descending aorta

syndrome can affect the pulmonary valve, but rheumatic involvement is very rare.

Critical PS in the newborn and infant

Severe PS presents differently in the newborn from the older infant, children and adults. There is such poor forward flow through the pulmonary valve (PV) that the patient is 'duct dependent' (aorta to pulmonary artery) and RV pressure can be supra-systemic. Tricuspid regurgitation and impaired diastolic function result in right-to-left shunting through the PFO, causing cyanosis. Emergency treatment aims to maintain patency of the PDA (IV prostaglandins) before urgent percutaneous balloon valvuloplasty or surgery is undertaken. Longer term, progressive pulmonary regurgitation (PR) and RV dysfunction may occur, and some will require a PV replacement in later life.

PS in the older infant and adult

Pathophysiology

The greater the PS, the greater the degree of RV hypertrophy, and over time the RV may fail, becoming dilated and poorly contractile.

Clinical features (see also Chapter 2)

Patients presenting out of infancy are usually asymptomatic unless PS is severe. Occasionally, exertional dyspnoea, dizziness or even syncope can occur. A prominent ejection systolic murmur at the upper left sternal edge will be heard, often associated with a systolic ejection click. The pulmonary component of S2 may be soft or absent. A palpable RV heave may be present in moderate or severe cases, and JVP may be raised with a dominant 'a' wave.

Investigations

The ECG may show RV and RA hypertrophy. The chest radiograph may show post-stenotic dilatation of the main pulmonary artery even in mild cases, but pulmonary oligaemia will be seen only in the more severe. RA and RV enlargement are late findings. Echocardiographic findings include

thickening and restricted opening of the PV leaflets, RV hypertrophy, RA dilatation and post-stenotic pulmonary artery dilatation. Doppler ultrasound velocity measurements can estimate the gradient across the PV. Occasionally, TOE is required to distinguish PV stenosis from muscular infundibular narrowing of the RV outflow tract, a distinction which is important as it affects management.

Treatment

In moderate and severe cases, percutaneous balloon dilatation of the PV is often successful. In very dysplastic valves, particularly those associated with Noonan syndrome, or where there is significant infundibular stenosis, surgical intervention may be required. Long-term follow-up of patients with previous surgical valvotomy or balloon valvuloplasty is mandatory; progressive PR, RV dilatation and dysfunction, or restenosis may develop, and PV replacement may be required.

Tetralogy of Fallot

This is the most common **cyanotic** congenital cardiac lesion, although not the most common to present in the neonatal period (see transposition, p. 254 below).

Pathophysiology

There is a large subaortic VSD and the aorta arises partly from the LV and partly from the RV ('overriding aorta'; see Fig. 18.7). Embryologically the aorta is more anteriorly placed. Hypoplasia of the RV outflow tract (RVOT) occurs, resulting in a combination of valvar and subvalvar (infundibular) PS. The greater the degree of RVOT obstruction the less antegrade flow of deoxygenated blood from the RV to the pulmonary arteries and the greater the degree of right-to-left shunting through the VSD and into the aorta. A baby with a critically narrow RVOT will be 'duct dependent' and require prostaglandin therapy. The degree of RVOT obstruction and cyanosis tends to progress as the baby grows.

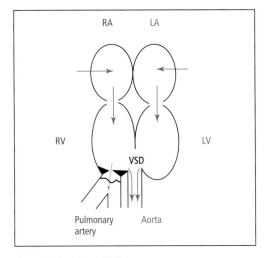

Fig. 18.7 Tetralogy of Fallot.

of cases. Diagnosis is made on transthoracic echocardiography where the large overriding aorta and VSD will be seen, and there will be a narrow RVOT and turbulence across it on Doppler interrogation.

Management

Surgical 'correction' is possible in most cases presenting outside the neonatal period, and comprises patch closure of the VSD and surgery to the RVOT. If the PV annulus is a good size, then a pulmonary valvotomy and resection of the infundibular obstruction may be possible. More commonly (in approximately 70% of cases) the annulus and infundibular region will be hypoplastic and a 'transannular' patch will be required. PR is common postoperatively, but is usually well tolerated in the long term.

Follow-up

Long-term follow-up is mandatory. Redevelopment of the subpulmonary obstruction can occur in a small number of cases, but progressive PR with associated RV dilatation and dysfunction is more common and may necessitate PV replacement. Arrhythmias, both atrial and ventricular, are common and are treated conventionally (see Chapter 13).

Abnormal atrioventricular and ventriculoarterial connections

In the normal heart, there is atrioventricular (AV) concordance, i.e. the morphological RA drains via a tricuspid valve into a morphological RV, and the morphological LA drains via a mitral valve into the morphological LV. Similarly, there is ventriculoarterial (VA) concordance, i.e. the morphological RV gives rise to the pulmonary arteries and morphological LV gives rise to the aorta. There are a number of congenital cardiac abnormalities that result in AV and/or VA connection abnormalities, and two of the more common of these these will now be discussed.

Clinical features

These depend almost exclusively on the degree of RVOT obstruction; if severe, there is little forward pulmonary blood flow and the right-to-left shunt through the VSD will be large, the patient very cyanosed and early treatment will be required. The neonate may be 'duct dependent' and require prostaglandin and even early surgery to create a systemic-to-pulmonary artery shunt (e.g. Blalock–Taussig shunt). Most cases are less critical and present with cyanosis over a period of months as the degree of infundibular PS progresses. Rarely, patients can present with cyanosis in later childhood. An ejection systolic murmur associated with infundibular/valvar pulmonary stenosis dominates (the VSD is large, ventricular pressures are equal and so there is no VSD murmur), and is loudest at the mid- and upper left sternal edge and radiates through to the back. Later presentation with cyanosis may be associated with clubbing.

Investigations

ECG will show RV hypertrophy and right axis deviation. Chest X-ray will demonstrate cardiomegaly with an upturned apex, typical of RV hypertrophy, and pulmonary vasculature will probably be reduced. A right aortic arch is present in about 20%

Transposition of the great arteries (VA discordance)

This is the most common congenital heart lesion causing cyanosis in the newborn period.

Pathophysiology (see Fig. 18.8)

The great vessels are transposed, with the aorta arising from the RV and the pulmonary artery from the LV. If the foramen ovale is functionally closed and the PDA closes early, then the infant will die of severe hypoxaemia (because the systemic and pulmonary circulations are disconnected, and work in parallel). In fact, most newborns are well because initially they have both a PFO and PDA. The PFO allows a left-to-right shunt at the atrial level, enabling oxygenated blood returning from the lungs to the LA to gain access to the systemic circulation via the RA and RV. The PDA shunts in the normal way, from the aorta to the pulmonary artery (because of the usual fall in PVR after birth), enhancing pulmonary blood flow and pulmonary venous return to the LA.

Clinical features

There is usually moderate or severe cyanosis with no signs of respiratory distress. The second sound is accentuated (the aorta is anteriorly placed and A2 therefore easily heard). There are usually no murmurs, although a ductal murmur may be present. There may be an RV heave. ECG will show the normal neonatal RV dominant pattern. **Chest radiograph** may show the upturned apex of RV hypertrophy, and normal or increased pulmonary vascularity. The mediastinum may be narrow as the aorta sits directly in front of the pulmonary artery (in the normal infant the mediastinum is wider because the pulmonary artery crosses over in front of the aorta and then to its left). If atrial mixing is poor (usually as a result of ductal closure or because the atrial communication is restrictive), the infant may become acidotic and extremely unwell.

Treatment

Urgent balloon catheter dilatation of the atrial septum (septostomy) is undertaken to promote atrial

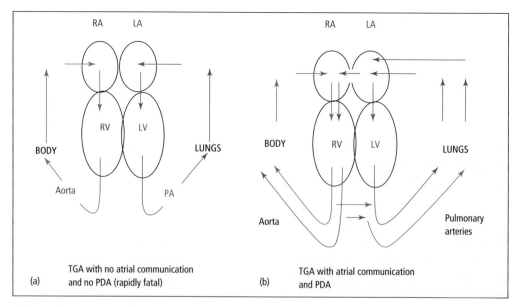

(a) TGA with no atrial communication and no PDA (rapidly fatal)

(b) TGA with atrial communication and PDA

Fig. 18.8 (a) Transposition of the great arteries with no atrial communication and no patent ductus arteriosus (rapidly fatal). (b) Transposition of the great arteries with atrial communication and patent ductus arteriosus.

shunting and this stabilizes the majority of babies until more definitive surgery is undertaken. Historically there are two surgical procedures that have been undertaken.

• **Prior to the early 1980s, the Senning or Mustard procedure**: otherwise known as 'atrial switch' or 'physiological correction' procedures. The atrial septum is removed and the SVC and IVC blood flow is redirected with a patch of pericardium ('baffle') through the mitral inflow and into the LV. This enables deoxygenated blood to reach the pulmonary circuit. Oxygenated venous return from the lungs returns to the LA and flows freely over the baffle, across to the RA, into the RV and to the aorta. The child is pink but has an RV as the systemic ventricle and the tricuspid as the systemic AV valve. Many patients have reached adult life having undergone a Mustard or Senning operation, but follow-up is mandatory to monitor RV dysfunction, tricuspid regurgitation and arrhythmias. Transplantation may be required in later life.

• **After the early 1980s, the arterial switch procedure**: otherwise known as the 'anatomical correction' procedure because it restores VA concordance. The aorta and pulmonary arteries are transected above their respective valves and 'switched' and resutured to the appropriate ventricle. The most critical part of the procedure is related to relocation of the coronary arteries; they arise below the transection line above the original aortic valve and have to be translocated to the new or 'neo' aorta with a cuff of arterial wall and without causing a 'kink'. Unlike the atrial correction, both anatomy and physiology are restored to normal. Complications following this operation appear to be less than those after the atrial repair but longer follow-up is required. Aortic regurgitation occurs in up to 10%, and supravalve PS and branch PS can occur as a result of distortion/fibrosis in the region of the pulmonary artery anastomosis. Coronary abnormalities occur in around 3% of patients due to their relocation. It remains to be seen whether LV dysfunction or acquired coronary disease is going to be more prevalent than in normal individuals. Arrhythmias appears to be much less common.

Congenitally corrected transposition (AV and VA discordance or 'double discordance')

Pathophysiology (see Fig. 18.9)

There is discordance of the AV connection and discordance of the VA connection. The anatomical RV and tricuspid valve are on the left, draining the LA and ejecting into the aorta (the RV is the systemic ventricle). The LV and mitral valve are on the right, connecting to the RA and pulmonary artery. Progressive RV dysfunction and tricuspid valve regurgitation can occur, and various degrees of electrical AV block are common. Other congenital cardiac abnormalities are often associated, including VSD and pulmonary stenosis.

Clinical findings

In the absence of any other associated congenital abnormalities, this can go undiagnosed until adult life. However, in the second to fourth decade of life progressive RV failure occurs. Management is directed at treating the RV failure/systemic AV valve regurgitation with diuretics, ACE inhibitors and β-blockers, although if the predominant problem is

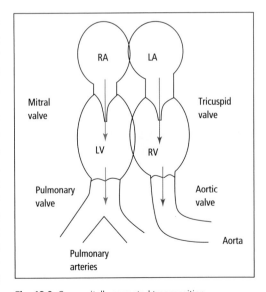

Fig. 18.9 Congenitally corrected transposition.

valve regurgitation, surgical repair or valve replacement may be indicated.

The 'single ventricle' circulation and the Fontan procedure

True single ventricles are exceptionally rare, but a number of complex congenital cardiac problems are associated with what is effectively a single ventricle because one of them is so hypoplastic as to be of no functional value. In these circumstances the main ventricle has to be used to deliver blood to the body and so another arrangement is necessary to deliver deoxygenated blood to the lungs. This is the basis of the Fontan procedure. This area is one of the most complex encountered in the management of congenital heart disease. In this section only one type of 'single ventricle' condition will be discussed, together with the role of the Fontan procedure in its management.

Tricuspid atresia and the Fontan circulation

Tricuspid atresia with normal VA connections is the most common form of single ventricle (Fig. 18.10). There is no right AV connection and so systemic venous return crosses the atrial communication and joins the pulmonary venous return in the LA. This admixture enters the LV which delivers blood to the lungs via a VSD and to the body from the aorta (when there is VA concordance). The RV is usually very hypoplastic and has no use in the future Fontan circulation. Presentation in infancy will depend on how much restriction to pulmonary blood flow exists after birth (the size of the VSD and the presence or otherwise of pulmonary valvar or subvalvar stenosis).

The child may require a number of procedures before the Fontan circulation can be completed. For example, there may be very poor pulmonary blood flow because of a severely restrictive VSD, and a systemic-to-pulmonary artery shunt may be required in the neonatal period. Conversely, there may be excessive flow through a large VSD and the pulmonary vascular bed may require protection, for example with a pulmonary artery band. Fig. 18.11

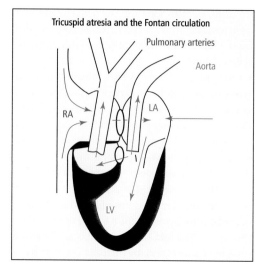

Fig 18.10 Tricuspid atresia with normal VA connections.

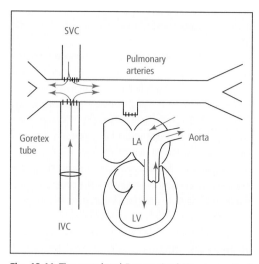

Fig. 18.11 The completed Fontan circulation in a patient with the most common type of tricuspid atresia.

therefore represents the circulation in a patient with tricuspid atresia who has completed the Fontan pathway. In the Fontan circulation, pulmonary blood flow is 'driven' by the venous circulation: via a 'cavopulmonary' shunt (SVC to pulmonary artery), and via a Goretex tube which connects the IVC to the pulmonary artery. Flow occurs through this circuit without the aid of a pumping chamber using a combination of factors, including venous pressure, negative intrathoracic pressure and energy derived from the arterial circulation (from the LV). It clearly depends on a normal pulmonary vascular resistance, good LV and mitral valve function, and normal respiratory physiology. The Fontan procedure can be applied to other types of single ventricle physiology including those with a dominant RV, but are beyond the scope of this chapter.

Follow-up

Patients can have extremely good functional status after the Fontan procedure, but long-term follow-up is essential as complications are common (arrhythmias, LV dysfunction, mitral valve regurgitation and a low cardiac output state). Anticoagulation is important in the adult because of the propensity to venous thromboembolic disease, liver disease and protein-losing enteropathy secondary to high venous pressures. Cardiac transplantation will be necessary in some.

Other congenital cardiac abnormalities

Ebstein's anomaly

One or more leaflets of the tricuspid valve are displaced into the RV with varying degrees of dysplasia and there is a functionally small right ventricular cavity and frequently severe tricuspid regurgitation. The portion of the right ventricle above the valve is 'atrialized' and acts functionally as the right atrium. Ebstein's anomaly is often associated with an ASD and so cyanosis may develop due to right-to-left shunting. Wolff–Parkinson–White syndrome is a recognized association. Mild forms may be asymptomatic, but atrial arrhythmias, tricuspid regurgitation and RV failure are common in adults. Mild forms may not require any treatment, but improved surgical techniques for atrial reduction and tricuspid valve reconstruction allow increasingly successful intervention in severe cases.

Marfan syndrome

See Chapter 15.

Sinus of Valsalva aneurysm

Aneurysm of the sinus of Valsalva in the aortic root may go unrecognized unless detected coincidentally by echocardiography. Problems arise only where distortion of the aortic valve annulus causes aortic regurgitation or the aneurysm ruptures, usually into the RA or RV. Rupture of a sinus of Valsalva aneurysm can occur at any age, but usually occurs in young men before the age of 30 years. Large ruptures can cause dramatic, immediate haemodynamic upset, but small perforations may be asymptomatic and recognized only by the presence of a continuous murmur at the left sternal edge. Surgery is recommended even for relatively small perforations because of the risk of deterioration and infective endocarditis.

Coronary artery fistulae

Fistulae from the coronary circulation usually drain directly into the RA, coronary sinus or pulmonary artery. The coronary artery involved is usually grossly dilated and tortuous, due to high blood flow. Although rare, these can present as a continuous murmur or with symptoms of myocardial ischaemia, as a result of a coronary steal phenomena, where perfusion to parts of the myocardium is reduced because of preferential run-off into the low resistance fistulous circulation. Surgery is generally required if symptoms are limiting.

Chapter 19

Heart disease in the elderly

Demographic changes

Although there has been an increase in the UK population of 8% over the past 30 years from 55.9 million to 60.2 million, the increase in the elderly as a percentage of the total has been disproportionately high. The percentage of people aged 65 years or more increased by 13%, whereas the percentage aged less than 16 years fell by 6%. Those aged 85 years or over increased by 12% during the same period. Furthermore, life expectancy at the age of 65 years has reached its highest ever level. Based on 2003–2005 figures, 65-year-old men can, on average, expect to live a further 16.8 years, and women a further 19.6 years (Fig. 19.1).

Thus, the proportion of elderly patients is increasing and this, coupled with the increase in life expectancy, will lead to a major and increasing burden on health care resources. Effectively targeting these patients is made more difficult by the relative lack of trial data relating to the elderly, together with the difficulty in demonstrating benefit in terms of improved life expectancy, event-free survival, etc. It is quality of life, rather than longevity, that is important to elderly patients.

Ageing trends in the UK, Europe and North America are not necessarily reflected in other populations where life expectancy may be poor. Furthermore, in countries where birth rates are particularly low (e.g. Japan), the proportion of elderly patients may be even more dramatic.

In understanding the diseases of old age, it is important to differentiate conditions which occur naturally as part of the ageing process and diseases that are commonly acquired in later life. Degenerative disease of the conducting tissue and calcification of a structurally normal tricuspid aortic valve are normal accompaniments of the ageing process; cardiac amyloid and mitral annulus calcification are further examples, whereas coronary heart disease (CHD) is not. Heart failure as a consequence of a dilated cardiomyopathy is recognized as more common in the elderly, increasing in prevalence from 1% in the fifth decade to 10% in those aged over 80 years.

Normal cardiac ageing (see Box 19.1)

The mechanism of ageing is poorly understood; no unifying hypothesis satisfactorily explains all the observed changes. Important contributors include:
- genetic influences;
- external factors (e.g. exposure to ionizing radiation, toxins, diet);
- mutations;
- hormones;
- autoimmune factors;
- programmed cell death (apoptosis).

There are a number of structural changes that can be regarded not as pathology but as part of the natural ageing process. An increase in cardiac mass

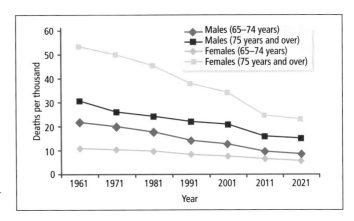

Fig. 19.1 UK death rates by gender and age (Office of National Statistics).

Box 19.1 Normal cardiovascular ageing

- Arteries (dilation, tortuosity)
- Cardiac chambers (reduced ventricular cavity size, changes in left atrium shape and compliance, atrial dilation)
- Conducting tissue (fibrosis of fibres and nodes, loss of SA pacemaker cells)
- Myocardium (hypertrophy, fibrosis, collagen accumulation)
- Valves (calcification, chordal elongation and rupture)

---

due to a degree of ventricular hypertrophy is associated with a reduction in ventricular cavity volume. These changes result in an increase in ventricular stiffness, leading to reduced compliance. On microscopy there is evidence of myocyte hypertrophy, myocyte fall-out and an increase in fibrosis and collagen deposition. Calcium is deposited in valve leaflets and elsewhere (e.g. mitral annulus), and conduction tissue fibrosis may be associated with a loss of pacemaker cells in the sinoatrial (SA) node.

Pathophysiological changes include:
- a loss of aortic elasticity;
- an increase in systolic blood pressure;
- mild degrees of valvular regurgitation;
- abnormalities of intracardiac conduction.

Pattern of cardiac disease in the elderly

Although government targets focus on the need for revascularization, the increasing age of the population has resulted in valve replacement accounting for a significant and increasing proportion of surgical procedures (Fig. 19.2). 'Senile' degeneration of an anatomically normal (tricuspid) aortic valve is becoming numerically more important in an ageing population, such that severe calcific aortic stenosis is now seen in 2–6% of the elderly. Aortic regurgitation as a consequence of a degenerative aortopathy is now one of the most common causes of aortic regurgitation seen in the ageing population. Similarly, mitral regurgitation as a consequence of a 'floppy' valve is far more common than rheumatic mitral valve disease in the elderly UK population.

Systemic hypertension (see Chapter 5)

Blood pressure increases with age. However, it is clear that a significant number of elderly patients have a pathological elevation in blood pressure, which is associated with significant cardiovascular mortality, and in whom successful treatment has been shown to be beneficial. In reported series, 30–70% of persons aged 65 years or more have a significant elevation in blood pressure (systolic >160 mmHg, diastolic >90 mmHg). In treating the

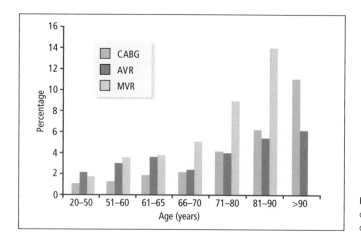

Fig. 19.2 Age and the early mortality of CABG and valve replacement operations.

elderly hypertensive, a simple, well-tolerated and cost-effective drug regimen should be the goal. Once-daily medication without postural side-effects might include an angiotensin-converting enzyme (ACE) inhibitor, an angiotensin II receptor blocker, a long-acting calcium antagonist or a thiazide diuretic. Even the treatment of isolated systolic hypertension has been shown to reduce cardiovascular (myocardial infarction) and cerebrovascular (stroke) mortality. Associated left ventricular hypertrophy on echocardiography is an additional risk factor and may indicate the need to intervene.

Hypertrophic cardiomyopathy
(see Chapter 8)

A subgroup of patients with hypertrophic cardiomyopathy present in the elderly age group. Symptoms and signs are similar to those of younger patients, although ventricular hypertrophy is less marked, sudden death is less frequent and the prognosis is more favourable. Females predominate and many are hypertensive. Treatment options are similar to those of younger patients.

Heart failure (see Chapter 9)

Congestive cardiac failure is one of the most common reasons for acute hospital admission in the elderly patient. The typical symptoms of breathlessness, orthopnoea, nocturnal dyspnoea and fluid retention may not be present; rather, complaints of fatigue, anorexia and weight loss may make diagnosis difficult. The prevalence of heart failure increases from 1% in younger patients to 10% in those aged 80 years or more. Ventricular dysfunction (either diastolic or systolic) is frequently missed in the elderly, leading to undertreatment; this is inexcusable with the widespread availability of echocardiography. Most elderly patients with heart failure have a dilated cardiomyopathy or occult CHD. Unrecognized aortic stenosis with few clinical signs is a well-recognized diagnostic trap. A restrictive cardiomyopathy as a consequence of amyloid (Fig. 19.3) infiltration is usually identifiable with confidence on an echocardiogram. Symptoms of heart failure are characteristically associated with abnormalities of conduction. Cardiac amyloidosis is untreatable and 50% of patients are dead within 6 months.

Elderly patients with heart failure may improve dramatically with treatment, although improvement in prognosis is more difficult to define. Cautious use of diuretics (including spironolactone), ACE inhibitors, angiotensin II inhibitors and low-dose β-blockade is the mainstay of treatment. Digoxin is best avoided unless the patient is in atrial fibrillation.

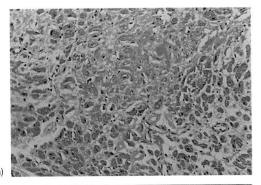

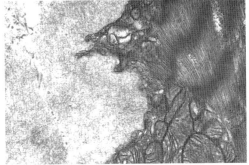

Fig. 19.3 Cardiac amyloid: (a) Congo red stain; (b) electron microscopy.

Box 19.2 Drugs underused in the elderly following myocardial infarction

- Aspirin
- ACE inhibitors
- β-Blockers
- Heparin
- Thrombolysis

Coronary heart disease (see Chapter 6)

CHD accounts for at least one-third of deaths in the elderly. The atypical presentation in this age group, coupled with an apparent reticence to offer proven effective treatment, leads to CHD being the cause of major mortality in these patients. This observation is all the more disappointing as many therapies (including aspirin, β-blockade, ACE inhibition, thrombolysis and primary percutaneous intervention) have been shown to be more effective in the elderly compared with their younger counterparts (see Box 19.2).

Angina presenting in the elderly is frequently atypical, with less striking chest pain and more frequent breathlessness, and non-specific symptoms including fatigue and somnolence. Morbidity and mortality are similar in patients presenting with typical and atypical symptoms. Similarly, the electrocardiogram (ECG) may only show 'non-specific' repolarization changes or left bundle branch block (LBBB). It is important to be aware of the changing prevalence of CHD in older women, who are affected as commonly as men. Co-morbidity, including diabetes, hyperthyroidism, anaemia, systemic hypertension and unrecognized aortic stenosis, may all contribute to myocardial ischaemia. Routine investigation such as treadmill exercise testing may not be feasible because of immobility; in this age group, radionuclide myocardial perfusion scanning, dobutamine stress echocardiography or stress MRI may be more helpful. Cardiac catheterization may be associated with technical difficulties relating to arterial access, arterial tortuosity and aortic ectasia, combined with potential nephrotoxity of contrast agents due to impaired renal function. Standard treatment with anti-anginal agents should be adjusted to reflect the changes that occur in drug metabolism in the elderly.

These include:
- impaired absorption;
- reduced lean body mass;
- impaired hepatic or renal metabolism;
- altered protein binding;
- reduced receptor density.

Percutaneous coronary intervention and coronary artery bypass grafting (CABG) are effective strategies in selected patients (see below). There are very real difficulties in making a definitive diagnosis of acute myocardial infarction in the elderly. Up to 40% of patients experience no chest pain at all, and in a further minority pain is atypical and may be mistaken for pain arising from the gastrointestinal tract or pulmonary embolism. Breathlessness is the primary complaint of many patients as a consequence of left ventricular dysfunction, or episodes of altered consciousness from undetected arrhythmia following occult myocardial infarction. Subtle changes in mood, confusion or other constitutional symptoms are also well recognized. In the

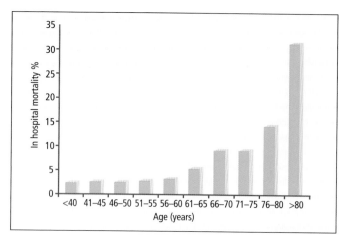

Fig. 19.4 Age-related mortality following myocardial infarction.

elderly, the electrocardiographic changes resulting from myocardial infarction are often ST segment depression rather than elevation; furthermore, cardiac enzyme levels may be disproportionately low, or falsely positive (particularly in the case of troponin). Increasing age is a major determinant of mortality, confirmed in both the GISSI and the GUSTO studies (Fig. 19.4).

Arrhythmias and conduction disease
(see Chapter 13)

Atrial fibrillation is the most common arrhythmia seen in the elderly, with a prevalence of 10% in patients aged 70 years, increasing to 15% by the age of 80 years. Although drug treatment is typically aimed at controlling ventricular rate, at least one attempt at direct current (DC) or chemical cardioversion is usually worthwhile. Trial data clearly indicate that there is a significant thromboembolic risk in the elderly patient which can be reduced with low-dose anticoagulation using warfarin (target international normalized ratio (INR) 2.0–2.5). In patients with a contraindication to anticoagulants, aspirin is a reasonable, although less efficacious, alternative. The role of alternative more powerful antiplatelet agents (e.g. clopidogrel) is as yet unclear. Permanent pacing is one of the most cost-effective procedures available, and should be offered to all patients with complete 3° atrioventricular block, or symptomatic SA disease. The latter group may require additional anti-arrhythmic medication to treat concomitant atrial arrhythmias.

Valvular heart disease (see Chapter 10)

Systolic murmurs are common in the elderly and do not usually indicate significant pathology. Ejection systolic murmurs arise from a thickened or sclerotic aortic valve, and late systolic murmurs relate to mild mitral regurgitation secondary to chordal elongation, rupture or abnormal papillary muscle geometry. As the age of the population increases, calcification of a structurally normal aortic valve predominates as the cause of haemodynamically significant aortic stenosis. Calcification of a congenitally bicuspid valve typically presents in patients in their 60s, whereas calcification of a structurally normal valve typically presents in patients aged 70 years or more. Medical treatment has little to offer. Valve replacement, usually using a biological valve, should be reserved for patients with symptoms (breathlessness, chest pain or syncope). Perioperative mortality in selected patients is in the range of 3–8% in this population. Stroke is the major and feared complication, which may occur in 5–10% of patients.

Mitral annulus calcification is usually asymptomatic but easily identified on a lateral chest radiograph (Fig. 19.5) or, with echocardiography, mitral annulus calcification may be associated with mild mitral regurgitation and it may rarely be a source of thromboembolism.

Intervention in the elderly patient

Heart disease in the elderly remains underinvestigated and undertreated. The increasing financial burden of treating the elderly population will inevitably lead to some form of health care targeting (rationing) as the mean age of the population increases. Biological rather than chronological age is the main determinant of a successful outcome following intervention, together with presence of pre-procedural co-morbidity. In selected patients, results of commonly performed procedures, including CABG, percutanous coronary intervention and valve replacement, are little different from those of a younger population. There is a slight increase in peri-procedural stroke rate and renal dysfunction, but this should not preclude intervention in the otherwise fit patient. Many forms of medical intervention, including thrombolysis, and the use of aspirin, β-blockers and ACE inhibitors in patients following myocardial infarction, may be particularly effective in the elderly. Similarly, the presence of significant systemic hypertension (often isolated systolic hypertension) should be treated as there is clear evidence that late morbidity and mortality are reduced as a result of a reduction in myocardial infarction, heart failure and stroke.

The appreciation of the thromboembolic stroke risk in the patient in atrial fibrillation has led to the more frequent use of anticoagulants, even in an elderly population (see Chapter 10). Permanent pacing is most commonly performed in the elderly (Fig. 19.6).

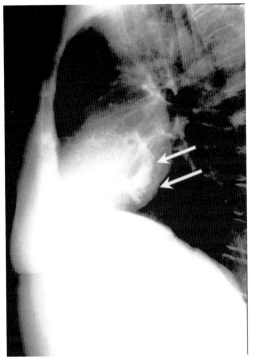

Fig. 19.5 Mitral annulus calcification (lateral chest radiograph).

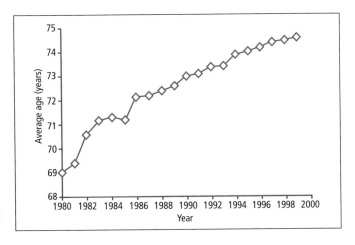

Fig. 19.6 Permanent pacing: age at time of first pacemaker implant.

Chapter 20

Cardiac tumours

Myxoma

Myxomas are tumours which usually appear as pedunculated intracardiac masses, the stem often arising from the atrial septum (atrial myxomas). They are:

- the most common form of cardiac tumour but are rarely malignant;
- found most commonly in the left atrium (approximately 90% of cases), then right atrium and then ventricles, but infrequently are present in more than one chamber;
- neoplastic in origin but the precise cell of origin remains undefined;
- histologically a mucoid stroma with stellate-shaped cells and pleomorphic nuclei;
- more common in near relatives of affected individuals.

Myxomas may directly interfere with the blood flow through the cardiac chambers and give rise to symptoms from the haemodynamic consequences (which depend on the chamber involved). When the tumour mass is in the left atrium, it may give rise to clinical signs which mimic mitral stenosis. On clinical examination, auscultatory features are:

- a 'tumour plop', analogous to the opening snap of a stenosed mitral valve;
- splitting of the first heart sound (S1);
- accentuation of the pulmonary component of the second heart sound (S2);

- accompanying mitral flow murmurs (commonly a diastolic murmur but also a regurgitant systolic murmur);
- elevation of the JVP with a prominent 'a' wave and steep 'y' descent may occur.

Right atrial tumours may mimic tricuspid valve stenosis while ventricular myxomas may block outflow of blood from the ventricles. Very rarely they can grow so large as to occupy an entire cardiac chamber. The consequences of tumour embolization are generally obvious (cerebrovascular accident, occlusion of arterial flow to a limb). Noteworthy is the possibility of pulmonary hypertension, complicating obstruction of the pulmonary arterial bed. Systemic features include arthralgia, anaemia, fever, constitutional malaise and weight loss. These symptoms are probably related to tumour secretion of the inflammatory cytokine interleukin-6. A raised erythrocyte sedimentation rate (ESR) is common, but a normal ESR does not exclude the diagnosis. Coupled with the cardiac murmurs, these clinical features may suggest a differential diagnosis of bacterial endocarditis.

Echocardiography is the investigation of choice. Myxomas are usually visible on transthoracic views, but better images are obtained by trans-oesophageal echocardiography. Urgent surgical intervention is mandatory. Surgical excision requires removal of the tumour pedicle and a surrounding lip of tissue. It is usually curative, but long-term follow-up is advisable as late recurrences are possible.

Sarcoma

These are:
- rare in the heart;
- arise most commonly in the right atrium;
- commonly present with symptoms related to obstruction to venous flow;
- arise before the third decade of life.

Definition of the tumour type depends on the primary cellular component and includes angio-sarcoma, fibrosarcoma or rhabdomyosarcoma. Treatment is palliative. Surgical excision can be attempted, but is usually limited by the extent of surgical damage that would be involved.

Rhabdomyoma

These are:
- the most common cardiac tumours of infants and children;
- derived from cardiac embryonic tissue;
- found equally frequently in both ventricles, and nearly all are multiple;
- found in both atria (about 30%);
- strongly associated with tuberous sclerosis (a familial syndrome characterized by hamartomas of various organs, epilepsy, mental deficiency and adenoma sebaceum).

Although benign, surgical management may require extensive resection.

Metastatic disease

Metastasis of cancer tissue to the heart is a rare presentation of malignant disease but does occur occasionally in established neoplasms, most commonly:
- bronchial carcinoma;
- breast carcinoma;
- malignant melanoma;
- leukaemia;
- lymphoma.

The most common cardiac consequences of metastatic disease are:
- arrhythmias (usually atrial fibrillation or heart block);
- malignant pericardial effusion (forms slowly and may reach large volumes before presentation with haemodynamic effects).

Further reading

Goldhaber SZ, Braunwald E, eds. *Cardiopulmonary Diseases and Cardiac Tumors: Atlas of Heart Diseases*. Vol. 3, Philadelphia: Current Medicine, 1995.

Chapter 21

Surgery and anaesthesia

Introduction

Surgery is associated with stress to the cardiovascular system, and not surprisingly patients with underlying cardiovascular disease are potentially at risk during and after the procedure. Understanding the broad principles of risk assessment and modification are important not only for those directly involved in the management of such patients but for anyone likely to refer a patient for a surgical procedure. As the surgical population ages and the prevalence of co-existent cardiac disease rises, greater numbers of patients will present for surgery with coronary artery disease (CAD) or poor cardiac function. Outcome will only be improved with careful preoperative evaluation, and appropriate preoperative optimization and postoperative circulatory control.

The main principles can be considered with respect to patients undergoing anaesthesia for non-cardiac surgery. A later section covers aspects of cardiac surgery and anaesthesia.

Anaesthesia for non-cardiac surgery

The major perioperative cardiovascular complications are:
- myocardial infarction;
- pulmonary oedema;
- ventricular dysrhythmias;
- cardiac death.

In general, these complications arise from myocardial ischaemia or poor cardiac function.

Preoperative assessment (Table 21.1)

The aims of assessment are to answer the following questions:
- Does the patient have, or is at risk of having, CAD (see Chapter 6)?
- Does the patient have valvular disease (see Chapter 10)? Antibiotic endocarditis prophylaxis will be needed.
- Is cardiac function adequate to maintain oxygen delivery during surgery (see Chapters 4 and 9)?
- Does the patient have a history of cardiac arrhythmia (see Chapter 13)?

The cardiovascular risks of the surgery proposed need to be weighed against the risks to the patient from the condition for which it is indicated. For example, a patient with a non-life-threatening condition, such as varicose veins, and a history of significant angina should be considered for coronary revascularization prior to varicose vein surgery, whereas a patient with recent myocardial infarction presenting with a perforated peptic ulcer should have life-saving abdominal surgery despite the cardiac risks.

The following are worth noting:
- 60% of vascular, and 10% of non-vascular surgical patients have coronary artery disease.

Table 21.1 Clinical Predictors of Increased Perioperative Cardiovascular Risk

Major risk predictors	Intermediate risk predictors	Minor risk predictors
Unstable coronary syndromes	Mild angina pectoris	Advanced age
acute or recent MI with	Previous MI based on the	Abnormal electrocardiogram
evidence of important	history or the presence of	left ventricular hypertrophy
ischemic risk by	pathologic Q waves	left bundle branch block
clinical symptoms or	Compensated or previous CHF	ST-T-wave abnormalities
noninvasive study	Diabetes mellitus, particularly	Rhythm other than sinus
unstable or severe angina	insulin-dependent diabetes	rhythm (e.g., AF)
Decompensated CHF	Renal insufficiency	Low functional capacity:
Significant arrhythmias		(e.g., inability to climb
high-grade		one flight of stairs holding a
atrioventricular block		bag of groceries)
symptomatic ventricular		History of stroke
arrhythmia in the		Uncontrolled systemic
presence of underlying		hypertension
heart disease		
supraventricular		
arrhythmias with		
uncontrolled ventricular rate		
Severe valvular disease		

- 5% of unselected patients undergoing non-cardiac surgery suffer a cardiovascular complication.
- 20–60% of those at risk, or who have coronary disease, suffer perioperative myocardial ischaemia.
- Myocardial ischaemia occurs three times more frequently **postoperatively** than preoperatively, and five times more frequently than during surgery. Whilst there may be various explanations for this, it highlights the importance of postoperative cardiac observation.
- Postoperative myocardial ischaemia or infarction is a predictor of longer-term cardiac morbidity.
- The majority of postoperative myocardial infarcts occur in the first two postoperative days.
- The stress associated with surgery can cause the following:
– repeated episodes of myocardial ischaemia, resulting in diffuse subendocardial necrosis (non-Q-wave myocardial infarction)
– coronary plaque rupture, vessel occlusion or full thickness myocardial infarction (Q-wave).

Patients should therefore be assessed preoperatively (ideally well in advance of their surgery, if elective) and formal cardiac assessment or investigations arranged as appropriate. Predictors of postoperative myocardial ischaemia (ECG changes or troponin rise) include:
- preoperative diabetes or left ventricular hypertrophy;
- postoperative anaemia or hypothermia;
- increased sympathetic tone;
- increased pro-coagulant activity;
- an increase in inflammatory cytokines.

Improving cardiac outcome

1 **β-Blockers** started preoperatively and continued for at least 7 days postoperatively reduce the likelihood of myocardial infarction and cardiac death, particularly in high-risk populations undergoing vascular surgery. Proposed mechanisms of action include:
- blunting the increase in heart rate, blood pressure and contractility associated with surgery;

- anti-arrhythmic effect;
- reduced endothelial injury;
- increased prostacyclin;
- inhibition of platelet accumulation;
- inducing a switch from free fatty acid metabolism to glucose oxidation.

In practical terms, patients already taking β-blockers preoperatively should have these continued. Patients undergoing vascular surgery who have, or are at risk of having, coronary disease should be started on a β-blocker, unless contraindicated.

2 α₂ agonists (mivazerol, clonidine and dexmetatomidine) reduce perioperative mortality and myocardial infarction after non-cardiac and vascular surgery. Proposed mechanisms of action include:

- reduced haemodynamic instability;
- less central sympathetic discharge;
- less peripheral noradrenaline release;
- dilatation of post-stenotic coronary vessels.

3 Aspirin reduces acute coronary events, inflammation and platelet aggregation.

4 Statins reduce perioperative mortality after major vascular surgery by 20% due to:

- atheromatous plaque stabilization;
- reduced endothelial dysfunction;
- reduced inflammation.

Perioperative factors

A patient under general anaesthesia should be unconscious, pain-free and relaxed. Homeostatic control and the anaesthetist's management of the cardiovascular and respiratory systems ensure the continual delivery of oxygenated red cells (DO_2) to the tissues to maintain cellular respiration and adequate CO_2 removal. Anaesthesia is generally associated with a reduction in heart rate and BP, and control of pain. Research has shown that deliberately induced myocardial ischaemia, followed by a period of reperfusion, temporarily induces an increased ability to withstand subsequent ischaemic episodes. This is known as ischaemic preconditioning (IP). IP is modulated by the actions of adenosine, bradykinin, opioids, $α_1$-adrenoceptor agonists and nitric oxide synthase. Most inhala-

tional anaesthetic agents (especially isoflurane and sevoflurane) and high doses of opioids (e.g. fentanyl) appear to have actions analogous to IP.

Cardiac dysfunction and delivery of oxygenated red cells (DO_2)

Deterioration in cardiac performance after surgery will reduce the delivery of tissue oxygen and organ dysfunction may follow.

$$DO_2 = (\text{cardiac output}) \times (\text{arterial oxygen content})$$
$$= (HR \times SV) \times (Hb \times 1.34 \times \text{saturation})$$

For the average male with:

Heart rate (HR)	75/min
Stroke volume (SV)	70 mL/beat
Haemoglobin (Hb)	150 g/L
Arterial oxygen saturation	98%
Body surface area	1.8 m²

DO_2 is 1034 mL/min or 574 mL/m²/min.

Surgery promotes an inflammatory reaction, an increased oxygen consumption, which in turn requires an increased DO_2. The greater the degree of 'oxygen debt', the higher the risk of postoperative organ dysfunction and mortality. The splanchnic circulation is the most sensitive system to a reduction in DO_2. Intestinal microvillus anatomy is denuded, the mucosal barrier deteriorates and bacteraemia and endotoxinaemia follow, worsening the pro-inflammatory state.

A combination of fluids to increase and optimize preload, and inotropes to optimize cardiac contractility, will tend to optimize DO_2. There is some evidence that the drug dopexamine also has a preferential effect on improving gut blood flow and hence preserving the intestinal barrier.

Cardiac surgery and anaesthesia

Similar considerations apply to patients undergoing cardiac surgery as to those having non-cardiac operations. However, the patient requiring a cardiac operation is obviously known already to have cardiac disease and is likely to have been investigated fully to assess their cardiovascular risk, and for this risk to have been reduced as far as possible by appropriate management.

The main indications for cardiac surgery include:

- congenital heart disease;
- coronary artery disease;
- valvular heart disease;
- penetrating and blunt cardiac trauma;
- aneurysms, dissections and transections of the thoracic aorta.

Preoperative evaluation

The history and examination of patients with cardiac disease follows standard guidelines and are described in Chapters 1 and 2. In addition, the range and extent of investigations will be specific to individual patients, and include both quantitative and qualitative assessment of cardiac performance. Typical preoperative evaluation of these patients will have included:

- resting ECG (±exercise ECG)
- chest X-ray
- cardiac catheterization
- echocardiogram
- haematology
  - full blood count (including platelets)
  - coagulation screen (INR and activated partial thromboplastin ratio (APTR))
- biochemistry
  - U&E, creatinine
  - glucose
- additional relevant investigations such as:
  - pulmonary function tests
  - carotid Doppler studies
  - sickle cell screen.

Risk stratification

Following assessment and investigation, it is possible to stratify the risk of postoperative death. This is expressed as a percentage, which may range from 1–2% for some procedures to >25% for more serious emergencies. The significant factors influencing risk are:

- type of cardiac operation proposed;
- age of the patient (risk rises with age);
- urgency of surgery (planned elective operations carry less risk than emergency surgery);

- LV function (risk rises with severity of LV dysfunction);
- female gender;
- whether the surgery is first-time or redo cardiac surgery (greater risk)
- the presence of other co-morbidities such as:
  - preoperative creatinine >200 mmol/L
  - vascular disease
  - poor pulmonary function
  - neurological disease.

These factors have been incorporated into simple additive systems, such as the EuroSCORE, or complex statistical algorithms, which permit comparison of outcome data among different surgical centres and different surgeons. It is important to recognize that even for those at highest risk, the majority of patients survive.

Preoperative medication

The choice of which drugs to stop and which to continue immediately prior to surgery lies with the anaesthetist, and is obviously influenced by patient-specific factors, but the following rules apply in general.

- Anti-anginal drugs are best continued up to surgery to offer control of the circulation at a time when anxiety or operative stimuli may provoke myocardial ischaemia.
- Digoxin has a half-life of 5 days and its concentration is unlikely to be influenced whether continued or not.
- On the day of surgery stop:
  - diuretics to reduce preoperative hypovolaemia;
  - ACE inhibitors as the systematic vascular resistance may be unacceptably low during cardiopulmonary bypass (CPB);
  - oral hypoglycaemics (all may induce symptomatic hypoglycaemia, metformin increases lactate concentrations during surgery, sulphonylureas close K_{ATP} channels and block ischaemic and anaesthetic pre-conditioning). Insulin may be needed to control blood glucose concentrations;
- Anticoagulants:
  - warfarin should be discontinued for 4 days in order to normalize the INR, but heparin may

need to be substituted to reduce the risk of thrombosis or embolism;
  • low molecular weight heparins should be stopped for 24 h.
• Aspirin and clopidogrel (antiplatelets) should ideally be stopped for 5 days, but this needs to be weighed against the resultant increased thrombotic tendency.
• Sedative premedication may include, alone or in combination:
  • morphine;
  • benzodiazepines;
  • hyoscine.

Induction of anaesthesia

Titration of anaesthetic induction minimizes their potentially adverse haemodynamic consequences.
• Midazolam or propofol induce unconsciousness.
• Fentanyl provides analgesia.
• Longer-acting neuromuscular blocking drugs provide relaxation and permit tracheal intubation.

Maintenance of anaesthesia

• Inhalational agents such as isoflurane or sevoflurane in an oxygen/air mix maintain unconsciousness.
• Propofol by IV infusion may be used to maintain unconsciousness when the inhalational route is not appropriate, for example during CPB.
• Certain centres use thoracic epidural analgesia to supplement IV analgesia.
• Many use aprotinin to reduce postoperative blood loss.
• Broad-spectrum antibiotic prophylaxis is mandatory.

Lines and monitoring

All patients require close respiratory and cardiovascular and monitoring.
• Endotracheal intubation permits intermittent positive pressure ventilation (IPPV), mandatory once the chest is opened.

• Airway gas monitoring allows control of anaesthesia and ventilation.
• A large IV (14 G) cannula permits infusion to maintain preload.
• Peripheral arterial line allows instantaneous BP measurement and arterial gas sampling.
• Central venous access for central venous pressure measurement and drug administration.
• Urinary catheter to monitor urine output.
• Temperature is monitored centrally (nasopharynx or oesophageal) and peripherally (axilla).
• Pulmonary artery catheterization may be used to measure the cardiac output, and intraoperative transoesophageal echocardiography provides anatomical and functional assessment of cardiac performance.

Tissue oxygen delivery (DO$_2$)

The process of cardiac surgery is complex but can be considered in three phases with reference to DO$_2$.
1 **Pre-cardiopulmonary bypass (CPB)**: the preparations are made for the corrective part of surgery. The lungs, diseased heart and circulation provide DO$_2$.
2 **Cardiopulmonary bypass (see below)**: corrective surgery can begin, blood bypasses the lungs and the oxygenator and pump in the CPB circuit ensure continued DO$_2$.
3 **Following CPB**: the wound is repaired, the lungs and heart (in the setting of the pathophysiological consequences of CPB and surgery) provide DO$_2$.
  The adequacy of DO$_2$, CO$_2$ removal, coagulation and metabolic and electrolyte status is repeatedly monitored during cardiac surgery:
  • arterial blood gas analysis;
  • activated clotting time (ACT) for monitoring heparin effect;
  • thromboelastogram (TEG) provides quantitative and qualitative information on the coagulation status;
  • haemoglobin or haematocrit;
  • lactate and glucose.

Surgical strategies

Since the heart moves, usually it has to be stopped or stabilized to ensure a suitable surgical target. There are generally two alternatives:

1 Local (off pump) immobilization of the target vessel for coronary artery bypass grafting (OPCAB). The heart continues to eject.

2 Global immobilization of the entire heart, essential for valve surgery, and requiring CPB and cardioplegia (see below).

Cardiopulmonary bypass

A schematic view of the CPB circuit is shown in Fig. 21.1. As the circulation bypasses the lungs there is no need to continue IPPV. Maintenance of anaesthesia can be continued with propofol or an inhalational agent with the oxygen/air into the oxygenator. Extra-corporeal circulation requires the systemic administration of 300 IU/kg of heparin as anticoagulation. The extra-corporeal circuit is run by a perfusionist, who controls the circulation and DO_2 during the period of CPB. Specifically changes can be made, to the following:

• Constituent contents of the circuit, which may include crystalloid solutions, colloid or blood components.

• Venous line resistance, which, if low will allow free venous drainage to the reservoir, or, if high, venous return will fill the right ventricle.

• The speed of pump rotation will affect the rate of return of oxygenated blood to the patient.

• The fractions of oxygen and air; generally 60% oxygen is delivered to the oxygenator.

• The flow of gas to the reservoir; the greater the flow, the lower the $PaCO_2$, and vice versa.

• Suction of blood from the operative field. Shed blood can be scavenged with suckers and re-transfused.

• Systemic vascular resistance (SVR). Standing orders may permit the perfusionist to administer drugs to the circuit including phenylephrine.

• The delivery of cardioplegia.

Cardioplegia

Once CPB is established, the coronary arteries are perfused with cardioplegia, which causes diastolic cardiac arrest. If the heart is electrically silent, it does not move and requires minimal energy, and it can survive without a blood supply. Doses of cardioplegia are repeated every 20–25 min. Traditionally a cold electrolyte solution, cardioplegia is now often in an oxygenated blood base at 4 °C. Important components are potassium (20 mmol/L), magnesium, calcium and procaine.

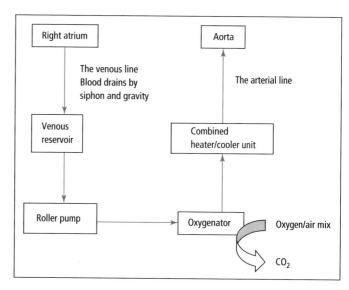

Fig. 21.1 A schematic view of the CPB circuit incorporating a membrane oxygenator.

As surgery progresses, immobilization is no longer needed, the coronary blood supply can be re-established and the cardioplegia eluted. As cardiac electrolytes return to normal, spontaneous cardiac activity begins.

Separation from CPB

This process re-establishes the lungs and heart to provide DO_2; IPPV is restarted, the haematocrit is optimized and the temperature is raised to 35–37 °C. The stroke volume is optimized by adjusting preload (venous filling) and using inotrope infusions. High afterload rarely occurs. Low SVR is more common and may reduce coronary perfusion; vasoconstrictors may be needed. The heart rate may need to be increased with temporary epicardial pacing.

Following separation from CPB

The effect of heparin is reversed with protamine, haemostasis is secured, pleural drains are inserted, and the surgically split sternum is sutured with wire.

There are complex pathophysiological consequences of CPB that affect management:

• Temperature control (excessive warming causes neurological injury, hypothermia impairs haemostasis).
• Anaemia is common. Intraoperative cell salvage or diuresis raises the haemoglobin to an acceptable 80–90 g/L.
• Coagulopathy (thrombocytopenia, dilution of clotting factors, residual heparin effect) is multifactorial and may require blood component therapy.
• Cardiac dysfunction is not unusual. The strategies for management include monitoring of cardiac output (with use of inotropes and vasodilators) and intra-aortic balloon counter-pulsation (see Chapter 9).

• Pulmonary dysfunction, particularly pre-existing pulmonary dysfunction.
• Neurological dysfunction. Subtle neuropsychological consequences of CPB are common and have been found in 50% of patients. Cerebral infarcts are found in 2–5% of patients postoperatively.
• Renal dysfunction. CPB worsens renal function, proportionately more so with impaired preoperative renal function.

Postoperative care

Postoperative care is aimed at achieving patient analgesia, haemodynamic stability, control of cardiac dysrhythmias, maintenance of systolic pressure (110–140 mmHg), optimizing gas exchange, monitoring of chest drainage, control of bleeding and maintenance of urine output and fluid balance.

Complications of cardiac surgery

• Atrial fibrillation occurs in 25% of patients.
• Bleeding requiring return to theatre (5%).
• Cardiac tamponade may require the reopening of the chest in the postoperative care area.
• Renal failure requiring haemofiltration (2%).
• Wound infections.
• Gastrointestinal complications:
  • transient ileus;
  • peptic ulceration/perforation;
  • transient abnormalities of hepatic enzymes.

Further reading

Mackay JH, Arrowsmith JE, eds. *Core Topics in Cardiac Anaesthesia*. London: Greenwich Medical Media, 2004.

Chapter 22

Cardiology, the law and occupation

Cardiology and driving

The effects of illness in relation to the legal requirements for driving a motor vehicle in the UK are outlined in the handbook *Medical Aspects of Fitness to Drive: A Guide for Medical Practitioners* (published by The Medical Commission on Accident Prevention). The latest edition (4th, 1998) has been influenced by the arrival of the European Union driving licence. The *At a Glance Guide to the Current Medical Standards of Fitness to Drive* was recently updated (August 2006), and copies are obtainable from the Driver and Vehicle Licensing Agency (DVLA) (The Medical Advisor, Drivers Medical Unit, DVLA, Longview Road, Morriston, Swansea SA99 1TU, UK), or on-line at http://www.dvla.gov.uk/medical/ataglance.aspx. Medical aspects of licensing are now also available in the Motoring section of the Directgov website (http://www.direct.gov.uk/Motoring/DriverLicensing/MedicalRulesForDrivers/fs/en)

Road traffic accidents

Medical conditions are an uncommon cause of motor vehicle accidents, accounting for approximately 1 hospital admission per 250 serious accidents. Of these, the most common events (39%) occur in association with grand mal epilepsy, whereas heart conditions account for only 10% of accidents that involve collapse at the wheel.

There has been a dramatic increase in the numbers of older drivers in recent years: the number of male drivers over 65 years increased by 200% between 1965 and 1985, and the number of female drivers in the same age group over a similar time period increased by 600%. Females over the age of 74 years are the most likely group to be involved in an accident.

Legislation relating to driving in the UK

The Secretary of State for Transport has the legal responsibility for granting a driving licence, which is administered by the DVLA in Swansea. It is the responsibility of the applicant to declare any medical condition that may affect their ability to drive safely. Should the holder of a licence develop a condition that is detrimental to safe driving, it is their responsibility to notify the licensing authorities. This is a major issue in the UK where a single full driving licence may be held without renewal from the age of 17 to 70 years. The Secretary of State can request medical reports from a doctor or insist that the patient undergoes a medical examination if there is doubt relating to their fitness to drive. Patients with a progressive medical condition may be issued with time-restricted licences lasting 1, 2 or 3 years. After the age of 70 years, licences are usually renewable on a 3-year basis. Individual cases are considered by a team of medical advisors at the DVLA, and there is a right of appeal through a court if a licence is refused or revoked.

In terms of cardiovascular disease, the main prescribed disabilities that may be a bar to driving relate to sudden attacks of giddiness or fainting as a result of underlying heart disease.

Medico-legal aspects: the doctors' responsibility

The DVLA, not the doctor, determines an individual's fitness to drive. Although the doctor may be asked to provide a report to the DVLA, this will not include the request for an opinion as to the fitness to drive. Doctors providing a report for a motor vehicle insurance company should be aware that there is a potential liability if they certify a patient fit to drive and there is a subsequent accident, if it is found that the doctor's advice fell outside the national guidelines. A doctor owes the patient a duty of confidentiality, but occasionally the doctor may feel it necessary to notify the DVLA if a patient continues to drive when medically unfit or having had a licence revoked. In these circumstances, the doctor should first warn the patient, prior to notifying the DVLA.

Classes of driving licence

In the UK, there is a medical distinction between Group I drivers (motorcyclists, cars, minibuses and light goods vehicles), and Group II drivers (goods vehicles >3.5 t laden weight, bus and coach drivers). The criteria for Group II entitlement are more stringent than for those holding the normal (Group I) licence.

Cardiovascular disease

Since the first edition of the *Medical Aspects of Fitness to Drive: A Guide for Medical Practitioners*, there has been a relaxation in the guidelines relating to driving and heart disease, particularly in the areas of valve replacement, revascularization (cardiac artery bypass graft (CABG)), percutaneous coronary intervention, permanent pacemakers

---

> **Box 22.1**
>
> Car drivers who have suffered the following cannot drive for 1 month:
> - Acute myocardial infarction
> - Cardiac surgery (CABG, valve replacement)

---

and 'automatic' implantable cardioverter defibrillators (AICDs).

In general, Group I drivers should stop driving for 1 month after a cardiac event (e.g. acute myocardial infarction, CABG — see Box 22.1), and can then resume driving without notifying the DVLA as long as there is no ongoing disability. Group II drivers must notify the DVLA immediately after the event and the licence may be revoked pending the report of a cardiologist. Investigation in these circumstances will usually include a maximum symptom-limited treadmill exercise test using the Bruce protocol whilst the patient is off cardioactive medication. A satisfactory result is deemed to be the completion of stage III of the full Bruce protocol (9 min exercise) without cardiac symptoms, an appropriate haemodynamic response, no significant ST segment shift, and no exercise-induced arrhythmias. Cardiac catheterization (coronary arteriography) is no longer required for reinstatement of the Group II licence except in exceptional circumstances.

The guidelines for driving licence holders with cardiovascular disease are shown in Table 22.1.

Cardiology and occupation

Pilots and flying

In the UK, the responsibility for pilot and air traffic controller certification rests with the Civil Aviation Authority (CAA) (Safety Regulation Group, Medical Department, Aviation House, Gatwick Airport South, West Sussex, RH6 0YR. Also at caa.aeromed-sect@srg.caa.co.uk). Cardiac problems in pilots tend to be treated on an individual basis. Initial examinations for commercial (Class I and II) pilots are usually conducted by the CAA medical department, whereas the evaluation of private (Class III) pilots is the responsibility of recognized general

Table 22.1 Guidelines for Group I and II licence holders with cardiovascular disease.

Cardiovascular disorder	Group I entitlement	Group II entitlement
Angina	Cease driving when symptoms occur at rest Recommence driving when symptoms controlled DVLA need not be notified	Refusal or revocation with continuing symptoms (treated/untreated) Re-licensing may be permitted when symptom-free for 6/52 with a negative exercise/functional test
Angioplasty/stent	Cease driving for 1/52 DVLA need not be notified	Disqualifies from driving for 6/52 Re-licensing may be permitted when symptom-free for 6/52 with a negative exercise/functional test
CABG	Cease driving for 4/52 DVLA need not be notified	Disqualifies from driving for 3/12 Re-licensing may be permitted when symptom-free for 3/12 with a negative exercise/functional test and an LVEF ≥40%
ACS (including AMI)	Cease driving for 4/52 Driving can recommence 1/52 after NSTEMI treated by PCI DVLA need not be notified	Disqualifies from driving for 6/52 Re-licensing may be permitted when symptom-free for 6/52 with a negative exercise/functional test
Pacemaker	Cease driving for 1/52 NB: includes box change DVLA need not be notified	Disqualifies from driving for 6/52 Re-licensing may be permitted thereafter
AICD	Driving may occur when the device has been implanted for 6/12, if: **1.** The device has not delivered a shock within 6/12 (except during testing) **2.** Any previous therapy has not been accompanied by incapacity in the preceding 2 years **3.** A period of 1/12 off driving must occur following revision of the device (or electrode) **4.** A period of 1/52 off driving must occur following a box change DVLA need not be notified (see full guidance)	Permanently bars
Successful catheter ablation	Cease driving for 1/52 DVLA need not be notified	Disqualifies from driving for 6/52 Re-licensing may be permitted thereafter
Arrhythmia (SA disease, AV block, AF/flutter, SVT, VT)	Driving must cease if the arrhythmia has caused or is likely to cause incapacity Resume driving when controlled for 4/52 DVLA need not be notified	Disqualifies from driving if the arrhythmia has caused or is likely to cause incapacity Resume driving when controlled for 3/12

ACS, acute coronary syndrome; AF, atrial fibrillation; AICD, 'automatic' implantable cardioverter defibrillator; AMI, acute myocardial infarction; AV, atrioventricular; CABG, coronary artery bypass graft; DVLA, Driver and Vehicle Licensing Agency; NSTEMI, non ST-elevation myocardial infarct; PCI, percutaneous coronary intervention; SA, sinoatrial; SVT, supraventricular tachycardia, VT, ventricular tachycardia.

Extracted from: *At a Glance Guide to the Current Medical Standards of Fitness to Drive*. DVLA August 2006 (http://www.dvla.gov.uk/medical/ataglance.aspx)

practitioners with a flying interest (Authorized Medical Examiners (AME)). A Medical Advisory Panel is the final arbiter of the decision-making process as to whether a licence is granted, revoked, refused or, in some cases, issued with restrictions applied. Detailed guidelines are issued by the CAA for most of the more common cardiac conditions.

Other occupations

A number of other occupations are subject to fulfilling medical standards in relation to cardiovascular disease. These include the police, firefighters, taxi drivers, seafarers, train drivers, workers on offshore platforms and divers. There is usually a medical officer affiliated to the specific group who is aware of the requirements necessary to continue in an occupation or to hold a particular licence.

Appendix

Useful websites

Organizations (UK)		
British Cardiovascular Society	www.bcs.com	UK national society principally representing professionals working in cardiovascular disease
		For links to subspecialties follow 'Affiliate List'
		See also 'Links Directory'
British Heart Foundation	http://www.bhf.org.uk	Main UK charity investing in research, and support and care for heart patients
Department of Health (England)	http://www.dh.gov.uk/en/index.htm	Government department providing health and social care guidance and publications
National Institute for Health and Clinical Excellence	http://www.nice.org.uk	National Health Service (England) organization publishing guidance on wide-ranging topics related to patient care
National Library for Health (cardiovascular disease section)	http://www.library.nhs.uk/cardiovascular	Information and systematic reviews on evidence-based medicine (UK)
British Medical Journal Clinical Evidence	http://www.clinicalevidence.com	Summaries of current evidence-based management guidelines
The Healthcare Commission	http://www.healthcarecommission.org.uk	Independent inspection body for both the National Health Service and independent health care organizations in England
Heart	http://heart.bmj.com/	International, but UK-based, journal publishing research on cardiovascular disease
The Lancet	http://www.thelancet.com	Prestigious UK general medical journal, often attracting major cardiovascular research
Resuscitation Council (UK)	http://www.resus.org.uk	Guidelines on resuscitation and practice
Drugs and Therapeutics Bulletin	http://dtb.bmj.com	UK publication covering reviews on all aspects of prescribing
British National Formulary	http://bnf.org/bnf	Comprehensive and widely used prescribing guidance

Organizations (non-UK)		
American College of Cardiology	http://www.acc.org	US society principally representing professionals working in cardiovascular disease
American Heart Association	http://www.americanheart.org	US organization with strong public-focused content on cardiovascular disease
European Society of Cardiology	http://www.escardio.org/	European society representing national societies and subspecialty professional groups (follow tab 'ESC Constituent Bodies')
TheHeart.org	http://www.theheart.org/index.do	Covers latest international research and publications relating to cardiovascular disease
New England Journal of Medicine	http://content.nejm.org	Prestigious US general medical journal, often attracting major cardiovascular research
Laboratory tests	http://www.labtestsonline.org	Comprehensive guide to lab tests and their use for patients

Index

Skärm

superior vena cava (SVC) 5, 10, 12, 14, 42, 179
  congenital heart disease 248, 255
  fetal circulation 244
  heart failure 143
  transposition of the great arteries 255
  tricuspid atresia 256–7
supraventricular arrhythmia 147
supraventricular tachycardia (SVT) 33–5, 192, 193–4, 198, 202, 215
  driving regulations 275
  see also atrial fibrillation; atrial flutter
surgery 151, 266–72
  anaesthesia 266–8
  anticoagulation 125
  aortic aneurysms 224–5
  aortic dissection 222, 224
  aortic trauma 226
  atrial flutter 196
  cardiac carcinoid 171
  constrictive pericarditis 134, 135
  contraindication for thrombolysis 112
  coronary artery fistulae 257
  DVT risk 239
  dilated cardiomyopathy 132
  heart failure 145, 151, 153
  hypertrophic cardiomyopathy 134
  infective endocarditis prophylaxis 177
  pacemakers 190
  postoperative care 267, 272
  pulmonary embolism 232, 233–4, 237
  pulmonary hypertension 232
  pulmonary stenosis 252
  syphilitic aortitis 226
  TOE 49
  transposition of the great arteries 255
  see also cardiac surgery
Swan–Ganz catheter 153
S waves 37, 234
sympathetic hyperactivity 68
sympathetic nervous system 139–40, 146
syncope 2, 4–5, 184, 262
  aortic dissection 222
  aortic stenosis 157
  bradycardia 188, 190
  CHD 86
  driving 274
  heart failure 150
  hypertropic cardiomyopathy 133–4
  MI 105

pregnancy 241, 243
pulmonary embolism 234, 237
pulmonary hypertension 228, 232
pulmonary stenosis 252
see also vasovagal syndrome
Syndrome X 85
syphilis 9, 155, 224
  aortic regurgitation 161
  aortitis 225–6
systemic lupus erythematosus (SLE) 74, 86, 131, 136
  acute pericarditis 179
  bradycardia 187
  infective endocarditis 172
  hydralazine 148
  pulmonary hypertension 229
systemic sclerosis 131, 136, 179, 181
systemic vascular resistance (SVR) 221, 245, 271, 272

tachycardia 4, 5, 16, 33–5, 184, 186, 191–4
  adrenaline 215
  antidromic 198
  aortic blood pressure 221
  aortic regurgitation 162
  atrioventricular nodal re-entry 199–200
  atrioventricular re-entry 196–9
  automatic 191
  bundle branch 205
  catheter ablation techniques 193–4
  CHD 86–7, 90
  counterclockwise macro re-entrant atrial (CCMAT) 195–6
  CPR 215
  ECG 30
  ectopic atrial 193–4
  fascicular 205
  heart failure 138, 139, 142
  incisional 196
  infective endocarditis 173
  intra-atrial re-entry 193, 194
  MI 105
  orthodromic 198
  pacemaker–mediated 191, 193–4
  pregnancy 241
  pulmonary embolism 233, 234
  pulmonary hypertension 228, 231
  reflex 74
  sinus 5, 9, 191–3
  sinus node (SN) re-entry 193–4
  treatments 193
  see also atrial tachycardia; supraventricular tachycardia; ventricular tachycardia

Takayasu's aortitis 225
tamponade, cardiac see cardiac tamponade
TAXUS stent 102
technetium-99m 64
technetium pyrophosphate 109
teicoplanin 176
temperature control 218–19, 270, 271
tenectaplase 111, 123, 238
terazosin 74
tetany 2
tetralogy of Fallot 252–3
thallium–201 64, 91
thermodilution technique 55–6
thiamine 138
thiazide diuretics 260
  heart failure 146
  hypertension 74, 76, 77
  mitral stenosis 165
thienopyridine 122
thiocyanate 78
third heart sound (S3) 18–23
  angina 86–7
  dilated cardiomyopathy 131
  heart failure 142
  MI 105, 116, 117, 118
  pericarditis 181
  pulmonary embolism 109, 233
  pulmonary hypertension 229
  restrictive cardiomyopathy 134
thoracic aortic dissection 4
thoracic pump 209–10
thrill 10, 158, 166, 249
thrombin 120
  inhibitors 123
thrombocytopenia 174, 272
  heparin–induced 122, 236, 239
thromboelastogram (TEG) 270
thromboembolism 115, 214
  aetiology 219–20
  atrial fibrillation 194, 262
  Fontan procedure 257
  heart failure 149, 153
  infective endocarditis 173
  MI 116
  mitral annulus calcification 168, 262
  mitral regurgitation 167
  mitral stenosis 164, 165
  pulmonary embolism 233
  pulmonary hypertension 228, 231, 232
  see also thrombosis
thromboendarterectomy 232, 238
thrombolysis 51, 123–4, 208
  contraindications 112
  CPR 217–18
  MI 104, 110, 111–12, 115, 117, 118, 261
  pulmonary embolism 236–7, 238

300

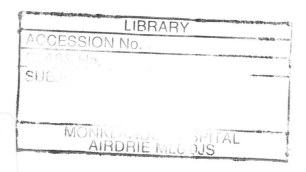